ECG Interpretation of Wide QRS Complex Tachycardia

Lucian Muresan
Editor

ECG Interpretation of Wide QRS Complex Tachycardia

A collection of 50 ECGs

Springer

Editor
Lucian Muresan
Department of Cardiology
Emile Muller Hospital
Mulhouse, France

ISBN 978-3-031-97029-0 ISBN 978-3-031-97030-6 (eBook)
https://doi.org/10.1007/978-3-031-97030-6

This Springer imprint is published by the registered company Springer Nature Switzerland AG
The registered company address is: Gewerbestrasse 11, 6330 Cham, Switzerland

Preface

Despite recent advances in the field of cardiology, with an increasing focus on imaging techniques such as magnetic resonance imaging and positron emission tomography, the standard 12-lead electrocardiogram continues to be an extremely valuable and commonly used tool in the evaluation of patients with a wide range of cardiac conditions.

Since the first attempts at recording the electrical activity of the heart by Augustus Waller in May 1887 in London, to the first published reports by Einthoven in 1901 on 3-lead ECG recordings using a string galvanometer and then the standard use of the modern 12-lead ECG recordings starting 1954, millions of ECGs are routinely recorded each year, still being a part of the standard of care of patients with heart disease.

Presently, ECG recording still has an important place among the first diagnostic tests to be used in several areas of clinical medicine, such as Emergency Medicine, Cardiology, Intensive Care, Geriatrics, Internal Medicine, Neurology, Nephrology, and Pneumology, to name a few. It can directly establish the diagnosis of, or contribute (along with diagnostic tests such as transthoracic and transesophageal echocardiography, blood cardiac marker analysis and cardiac computed tomography) to establishing the diagnosis of most major emergencies in the field of cardiology, such as acute myocardial infarction, life-threatening arrhythmias, cardiac tamponade and acute cor pulmonale. It still represents the most useful diagnostic test in identifying the whole spectrum of cardiac arrhythmias, from benign supraventricular arrhythmias, such as isolated premature atrial contractions, to life-threatening arrhythmias, such as ventricular tachycardia and ventricular fibrillation. It can play a major role in correctly differentiating malignant ventricular arrhythmias from non-severe arrhythmias that mimic the former group, such as supraventricular tachycardias with bundle branch block, antidromic atrioventricular reentrant tachycardias, and rapid ventricular paced rhythms.

It is extremely important in clinical practice that practitioners working in direct patient care, especially the ones from Emergency Departments, Cardiology Units, and Intensive Care Units, are well trained in recognizing life-threatening arrhythmias and are able to make the correct diagnosis in a short time, in order to provide appropriate treatment.

The purpose of this ECG book is to help the readers consolidate their knowledge in the field of cardiac arrhythmias. It focuses on wide QRS complex tachycardias, more specifically on correctly identifying their nature and their underlying mechanism (ventricular tachycardia, supraventricular tachycardia with pre-existing or functional bundle branch block, and pre-excited tachycardias) by examining and interpreting several clues and characteristic features. The target audience the authors had in mind while writing this book includes medical students, medical residents / interns, medical specialists (especially cardiologists, physicians working in intensive care departments, emergency medicine, internal medicine, geriatrics, nephrology, neurology, and pneumology), as well as fellows in cardiac electrophysiology and electrophysiologists.

We hope that each reader will find among the pages of this book at least a few valuable pieces of information that will help them advance on their unique professional journey.

We would like to express our very warm and special thanks to our dear nurse team for the recording of the ECG presented in this book: Céline Arnold, Mathilde Aybar, Perle Barbieri, Saliha Birouk-mokhbi, Marie Bosshertz, Anaïs Bonnet, Myriam Boubout, Nadia Chebel, Marie D'amore, Roukia Fakhour, Melanie Farley, Clémence Godart, Myriam Guise, Fatos Guzel, Asma Hamadi, Valerie Hoff, Guillaume Hoireau, Elisa Kury, Philippe Monteillet, Aurélie Munch, Maria Mundeke Katende, Julie Murer, Laurence Petitjean, Césarine Pommier, Beyza Sahin Havanur, Leonie Stauder-Utard, Trommenschlager Adeline, and Justine Wuillemin. Their effort and constant dedication to patient care made this book possible. Thank you!

Mulhouse, France
November 2024

Lucian Muresan

Contents

Introduction

Lucian Muresan

The present book focuses on dealing with one of the most difficult areas in ECG interpretation, that of cardiac arrhythmias. It was designed to serve as a practical guide on how to approach ECG interpretation of wide QRS complex tachycardia. It contains a unique collection of 50 ECGs on the topic of cardiac arrhythmias, more exactly on the topic of wide QRS complex tachycardias.

Several valuable books on the topic of ECG interpretation exist, mostly focused on teaching the basis of ECG interpretation. There are also several books containing a collection of ECGs (usually from 50 to 100), describing and teaching ECG interpretation for a wide range of cardiac diseases. Their strong point is that they cover a large area of cardiology; therefore, the reader becomes familiarized with the domain. Their weak point is that several important diseases are not fully covered, and there is only a brief explanation of some very important notions that cardiologists should have in this domain (ECG interpretation).

This book contains a collection of 50 ECGs, recorded from patients presenting to the hospital with different cardiac arrhythmias, all of them having a wide QRS complex tachycardia recorded. All of the 50 ECGs presented are analyzed and explained in detail, guiding the reader in a step-by-step manner towards the correct diagnosis: ventricular tachycardia, supraventricular tachycardia with pre-existing or functional bundle branch block, pre-excited tachycardias, or rapid ventricular paced rhythms.

The format of the book was specifically designed with a strong teaching purpose in mind. Each of the 50 chapters starts with a brief description of the clinical characteristics of the patient, providing the most important elements from history taking (past medical history, family history, medication use), and clinical examination. Subsequently, an ECG showing a wide-QRS complex tachycardia is then provided, followed by a question about the nature of the arrhythmia presented on the ECG, with a list of five possible answers. A helping ECG is then provided, usually recorded during sinus rhythm after the termination of the tachycardia, offering hints about the nature of the wide-QRS complex tachycardia. Finally, the correct answer is provided, followed by a detailed analysis and description of the ECG, based on the best currently existing ECG algorithms for the differential diagnosis of wide QRS complex tachycardia. The most used algorithms/criteria in this book are the Brugada algorithm, the Vereckei algorithm, the modified Vereckei algorithm, the Basel algorithm, and the R wave to peak-time criterion. References from the medical literature are provided at the end of each chapter for further reading.

L. Muresan (✉)
Department of Cardiology, Emile Muller Hospital, Mulhouse, France

L. Muresan (ed.), *ECG Interpretation of Wide QRS Complex Tachycardia*,
https://doi.org/10.1007/978-3-031-97030-6_1

The key concepts that are to be kept in mind when analyzing an ECG showing a wide-QRS complex tachycardia are:

1. In the presence of a history of remote myocardial infarction, the probability that the wide QRS complex tachycardia is ventricular in nature is >90%.
2. When atrio-ventricular dissociation can be identified during a wide QRS complex tachycardia, the nature of the tachycardia is highly likely to be ventricular.
3. For Left Bundle Branch BLock morphology wide QRS complex tachycardias, a QRS duration of >160 ms is in favor of a ventricular origin.
4. For Right Bundle Branch Block morphology wide QRS complex tachycardias, a QRS duration of >140 ms is in favor of a ventricular origin.
5. The presence of ventricular pre-excitation on an ECG recorded during sinus rhythm before or after the recording of the ECG showing a wide QRS complex tachycardia is in favor of pre-excited tachycardia.
6. The presence of a bundle branch block on an ECG recorded during sinus rhythm before or after the recording of the ECG showing a wide QRS complex tachycardia that is identical to the morphology of the QRS during tachycardia is strongly in favor of a supraventricular tachycardia with bundle branch block.
7. The presence of capture/fusion beats recorded during the wide QRS complex tachycardia is in favor of a ventricular nature of the tachycardia.
8. A morphology typical of (either left or right) bundle branch block is likely in favor of a supraventricular tachycardia with pre-existing/functional bundle branch block.
9. Extreme (north-west) axis deviation is an argument in favor of ventricular tachycardia.
10. "FBI-tachycardia" (fast, broad, and irregular) is likely to be pre-excited atrial fibrillation.
11. The presence of a ventricular paced rhythm on a previously recorded ECG, that has an identical QRS morphology to the one recorded during a wide QRS complex tachycardia is strongly in favor of a supraventricular tachycardiawith ventricular pacing/endless loop tachycardia.

It is important to keep in mind that these elements are not absolute and that exceptions to these rules exist in specific contexts.

We wish you a pleasant reading!

ECG 1

Ronan Le Bouar

1 Case Presentation

An 81-year-old male patient with a history of ischemic heart disease (severe stenosis of the proximal LAD coronary artery, RCA, and CX artery), with mild-to-moderate LV systolic dysfunction (LVEF of 45%), ischemic stroke, COPD, diabetes mellitus, and chronic lower limb ischemia is admitted to the Cardiology Department due to an episode of palpitations with sudden onset and regular rhythm, accompanied by chest pain, dyspnea, and anxiety, that had started 30 min before arriving to the Emergency Department. His ECG recorded at admittance to the Cardiology Department is presented in Fig. 1.

Question: What is the nature of the rhythm presented in Fig. 1?

(a) Ventricular tachycardia originating from the inferior lateral and apical LV wall
(b) Ventricular tachycardia originating from the left ventricular outflow tract
(c) Ventricular tachycardia originating from the inferior septal and apical LV wall
(d) Antidromic tachycardia using a right-sided bypass tract
(e) Atrial tachycardia with 1:1 atrioventricular conduction and left bundle branch block

Hint: A second ECG recorded several minutes later is presented in Fig. 2.

Correct answer: b. Ventricular tachycardia originating from the left ventricular outflow tract

Explanation: The ECG in Fig. 1 shows a regular wide QRS complex tachycardia with a heart rate of 193 bpm and LBBB morphology. The width of the QRS complex is 138 ms (not 188 ms, as automatically measured by the electrocardiograph). The QRS axis is at +90°. The differential diagnosis of this regular wide QRS complex tachycardia with LBBB morphology includes: ventricular tachycardia (myocardial-related VT), supraventricular tachycardia (atrial flutter, atrial tachycardia, AVNRT, and AVRT) with functional or pre-existing bundle branch block and antidromic tachycardia (in pre-excitation syndromes).

The morphology of the left bundle branch block of the QRS complex during tachycardia from Fig. 1 is not that of a typical one [1]: the QRS duration is indeed of >120 ms, and the QRS has a "QS'" morphology in lead V1 and a unique notched R wave in lead I. However, the QRS complex has a "QS" pattern in lead aVL, and the QRS transition takes place in V2—V3, elements

R. Le Bouar (✉)
Department of Cardiology, Emile Muller Hospital, Mulhouse, France
e-mail: Lebouarr@ghrmsa.fr

L. Muresan (ed.), *ECG Interpretation of Wide QRS Complex Tachycardia*,
https://doi.org/10.1007/978-3-031-97030-6_2

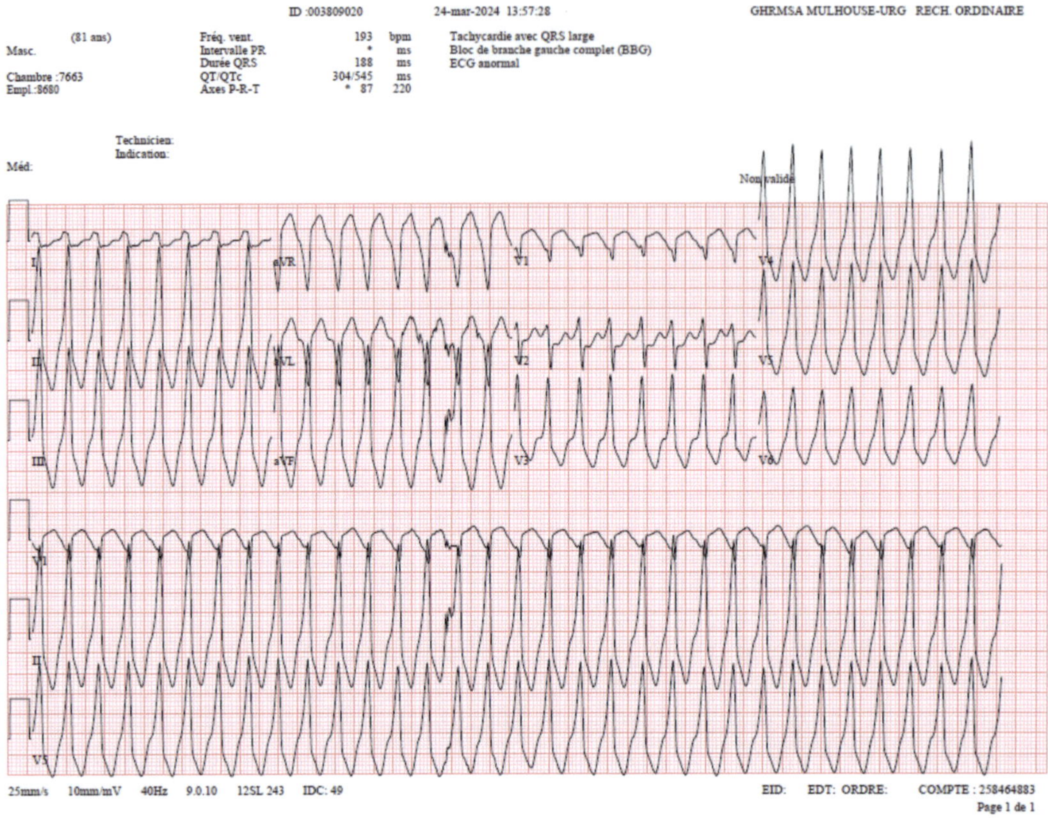

Fig. 1 Twelve-lead ECG recorded at admittance to the Cardiology Department

that are not in favor of a typical left bundle branch block. This makes SVT with LBBB unlikely.

The ECG from Fig. 2 shows a sinus rhythm with a ventricular rate of 90 bpm, QRS axis at −35°, absence of LV hypertrophy, ST segment elevation in lead aVR, and ST segment depression in II, III, aVF, and V2–V6, compatible with ongoing myocardial ischemia (triple-vessel disease or proximal left main disease); there are no signs of ventricular pre-excitation (no short PR interval and no delta waves). This makes antidromic tachycardia unlikely as the correct diagnosis for the tachycardia from Fig. 1.

Applying the Brugada algorithm [2] to the tachycardia from Fig. 1, it can be seen that: (1) There is no absence of an RS complex in the precordial leads (otherwise said, there are rS complexes in lead V2); we therefore move to the second step of the algorithm: (2) This step analyzes the absence of an R to S interval > 100 ms in any precordial lead. This is actually the case, as can be seen in lead V2, where the RS interval is of 105 ms (Fig. 3).

Other arguments in favor of ventricular tachycardia from the Brugada algorithm are: (1) An r wave of >0.04 s in lead V1 or V2 (Fig. 4); (2) A notched S downstroke in V1 or V2, which is present in lead V1 (Fig. 5), and a duration of >60 ms from the onset of the QRS to the nadir of the S wave in lead V1 (Fig. 6) [3].

The Vereckei algorithm [4] for the differential diagnosis of wide QRS complex tachycardias also suggests VT as the correct answer. The first step of the algorithm looks for A–V dissociation, which is not seen on the present ECG. The second step of the algorithm looks for an initial predominant R wave in lead aVR, which is also not the case (Fig. 7).

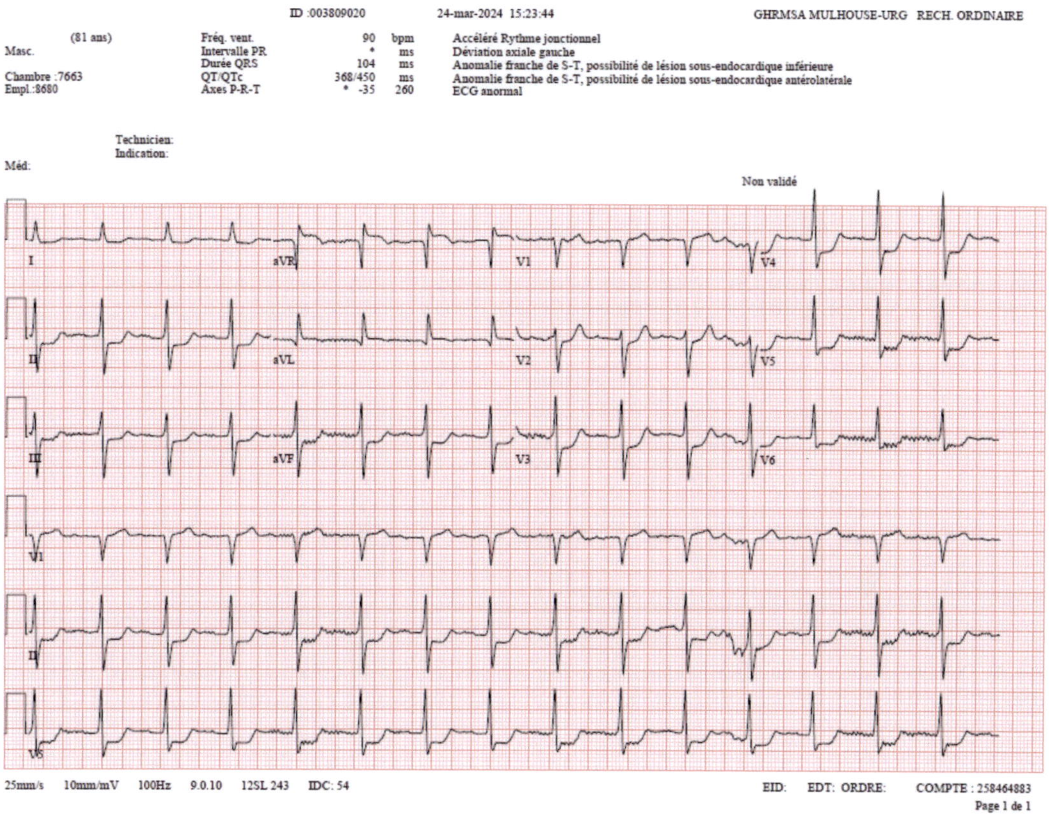

Fig. 2 Twelve-lead ECG recorded after the end of the episode of palpitations

Fig. 3 Detailed analysis of the QRS morphology in lead V2 during the wide QRS complex tachycardia. The RS interval measures 105 ms. This is a criterion diagnostic of ventricular tachycardia

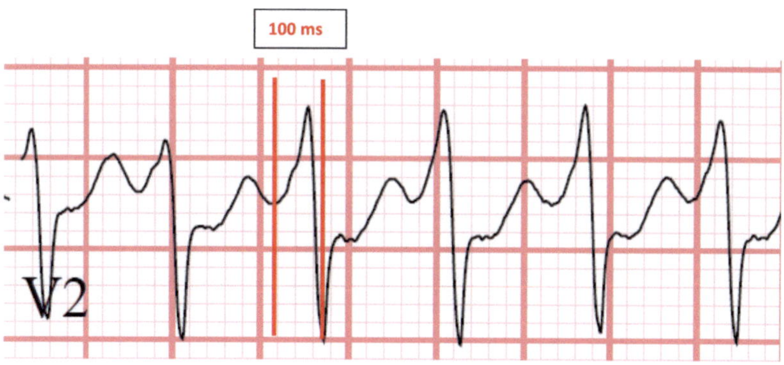

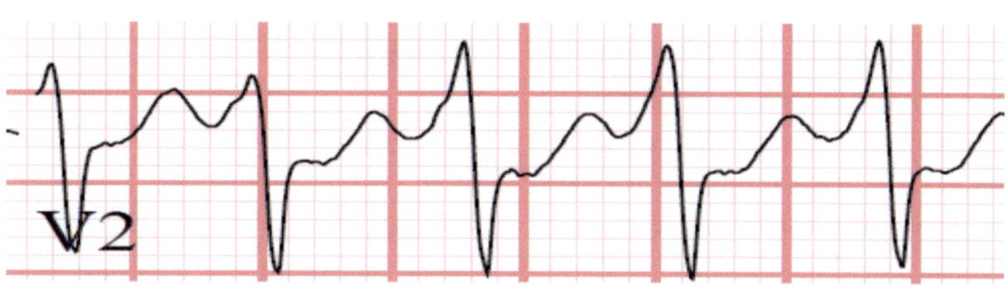

Fig. 4 Detailed analysis of the QRS morphology in lead V2 during the wide QRS complex tachycardia, showing an r wave of >0.04 s, the criterion in favor of ventricular tachycardia

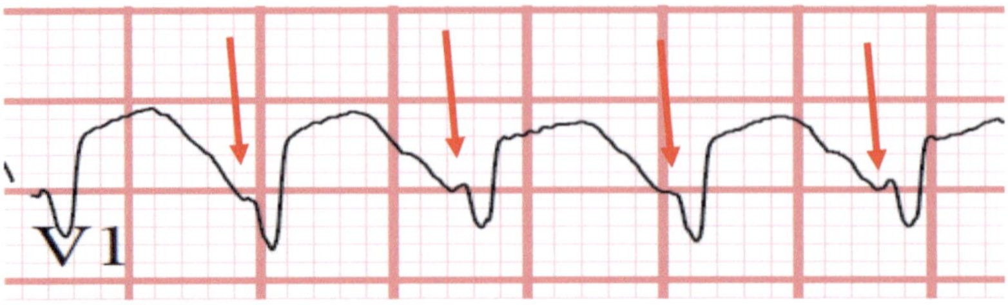

Fig. 5 Detailed analysis of the QRS morphology in lead V1 during the wide QRS complex tachycardia. A notch is present on the downstroke of the S wave, the argument in favor of ventricular tachycardia

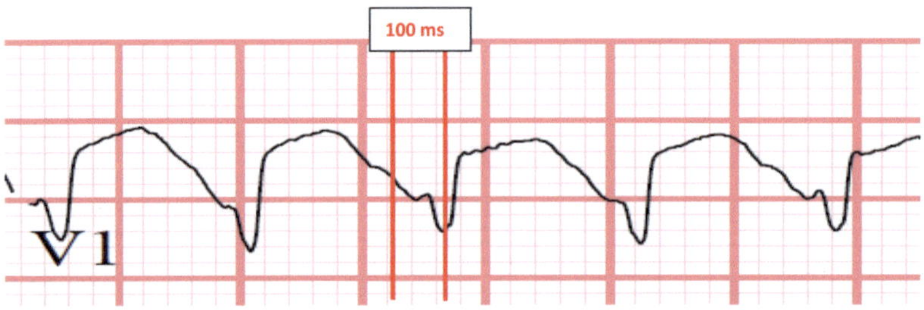

Fig. 6 Detailed analysis of the QRS morphology in lead V1 during the wide QRS complex tachycardia, showing a duration of >60 ms from the onset of the QRS to the nadir of the S wave in lead V1, the argument in favor of VT

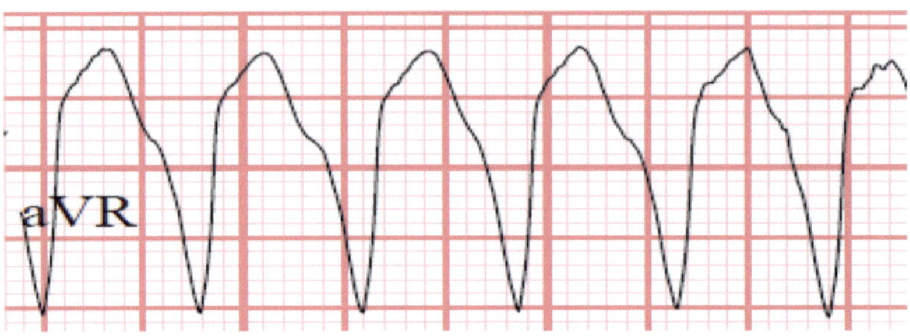

Fig. 7 Detailed analysis of the QRS morphology in lead aVR during the wide QRS complex tachycardia showing the absence of an initial tall R wave, the criterion not in favor of ventricular tachycardia (but not excluding it either)

The third step of the algorithm "QRS morphology unlike BBB or fascicular block" does not suggest SVT with RBBB, based on the arguments exposed above. Therefore, the diagnosis is that of ventricular tachycardia.

Another argument in favor of ventricular tachycardia for a wide QRS complex tachycardia with LBBB QRS morphology is a QRS duration of over 160 ms, which is also the case [5].

The correct diasgnosis is therefore ventricular tachycardia. Its morphology is typical for an origin that is at the level of the left ventricular outflow tract [6–10].

The patient underwent electrical cardioversion.

Coronary angiography was urgently performed which showed severe left main disease and critical stenosis of the proximal RCA. The patient underwent emergent triple CABG.

References

1. Surawicz B, Childers R, Deal BJ, Gettes LS, Bailey JJ, Gorgels A, et al. AHA/ACCF/HRS recommendations for the standardization and interpretation of the electrocardiogram: part III: intraventricular conduction disturbances: a scientific statement from the

American Heart Association Electrocardiography and Arrhythmias Committee, Council on Clinical Cardiology; the American College of Cardiology Foundation; and the Heart Rhythm Society. Endorsed by the International Society for Computerized Electrocardiology. J Am Coll Cardiol. 2009;53(11):976–81.
2. Brugada P, Brugada J, Mont L, Smeets J, Andries EW. A new approach to the differential diagnosis of a regular tachycardia with a wide QRS complex. Circulation. 1991;83(5):1649–59.
3. Kindwall KE, Brown J, Josephson ME. Electrocardiographic criteria for ventricular tachycardia in wide complex left bundle branch block morphology tachycardias. Am J Cardiol. 1988;61(15):1279–83.
4. Vereckei A, Duray G, Szenasi G, Altemose GT, Miller JM. Application of a new algorithm in the differential diagnosis of wide QRS complex tachycardia. Eur Heart J. 2007;28(5):589–600.
5. Eckardt L, Breithardt G, Kirchhof P. Approach to wide complex tachycardias in patients without structural heart disease. Heart. 2006;92(5):704–11.
6. Hachiya H, Aonuma K, Yamauchi Y, Harada T, Igawa M, Nogami A, et al. Electrocardiographic characteristics of left ventricular outflow tract tachycardia. PACE. 2000;23(11 Pt 2):1930–4.
7. Kumagai K, Fukuda K, Wakayama Y, Sugai Y, Hirose M, Yamaguchi N, et al. Electrocardiographic characteristics of the variants of idiopathic left ventricular outflow tract ventricular tachyarrhythmias. J Cardiovasc Electrophysiol. 2008;19(5):495–501.
8. Ouyang F, Mathew S, Wu S, Kamioka M, Metzner A, Xue Y, et al. Ventricular arrhythmias arising from the left ventricular outflow tract below the aortic sinus cusps: mapping and catheter ablation via transseptal approach and electrocardiographic characteristics. Circ Arrhythm Electrophysiol. 2014;7(3):445–55.
9. Anderson RD, Kumar S, Parameswaran R, Wong G, Voskoboinik A, Sugumar H, et al. Differentiating right- and left-sided outflow tract ventricular arrhythmias: classical ECG signatures and prediction algorithms. Circ Arrhythm Electrophysiol. 2019;12(6):e007392.
10. Mariani MV, Piro A, Della Rocca DG, Forleo GB, Pothineni NV, Romero J, et al. Electrocardiographic criteria for differentiating left from right idiopathic outflow tract ventricular arrhythmias. Arrhythmia Electrophysiol Rev. 2021;10(1):10–6.

ECG 2

Crina Muresan

1 Case Presentation

This is the same patient from case 1. An 81-year-old male patient with a history of ischemic heart disease (severe stenosis of the proximal LAD coronary artery, RCA, and CX artery), with mild-to-moderate LV systolic dysfunction (LVEF of 45%), ischemic stroke, COPD, diabetes mellitus, and chronic lower limb ischemia is admitted to the Cardiology Department due to an episode of sustained monomorphic ventricular tachycardia in the context of an NSTEMI. Coronary angiography demonstrated severe triple vessel disease, and the patient underwent triple CABG. Four days after the surgical intervention, the patient presented a new episode of palpitations. This is presented in Fig. 1.

Question: What is the nature of the rhythm presented in Fig. 1?

(a) Ventricular tachycardia originating from the inferior lateral and apical LV wall.
(b) Ventricular tachycardia originating from the anterior septal basal LV wall.
(c) Ventricular tachycardia originating from the inferior septal and apical LV wall.
(d) Antidromic tachycardia using a right-sided bypass tract.
(e) Atrial tachycardia with 1:1 atrioventricular conduction and left bundle branch block.

Hint: A second ECG recorded several minutes later is presented in Fig. 2.

Correct answer: b. Ventricular tachycardia originating from the anterior septal basal LV wall

Explanation The ECG in Fig. 1 shows a regular wide QRS complex tachycardia with a heart rate of 193 bpm and LBBB morphology. The width of the QRS complex is 130 ms (not 118 ms as automatically measured by the electrocardiograph). The QRS axis is at +90°. The differential diagnosis of this regular wide QRS complex tachycardia with LBBB morphology includes: ventricular tachycardia (myocardial-related VT), supraventricular tachycardia (atrial flutter, atrial tachycardia, and AVNRT, aAVRT) with functional or pre-existing bundle branch block, and antidromic tachycardia (in pre-excitation syndromes).

The morphology of the left bundle branch block of the QRS complex during tachycardia from Fig. 1 is not that of a typical one [1]: the QRS duration is indeed >120 ms, and the QRS has a "QS'" morphology in lead V1 and a unique notched R wave in lead I. However, the QRS

C. Muresan (✉)
Department of Cardiology, Emile Muller Hospital, Mulhouse, France
e-mail: crina.muresan@ghrmsa.fr

L. Muresan (ed.), *ECG Interpretation of Wide QRS Complex Tachycardia*,
https://doi.org/10.1007/978-3-031-97030-6_3

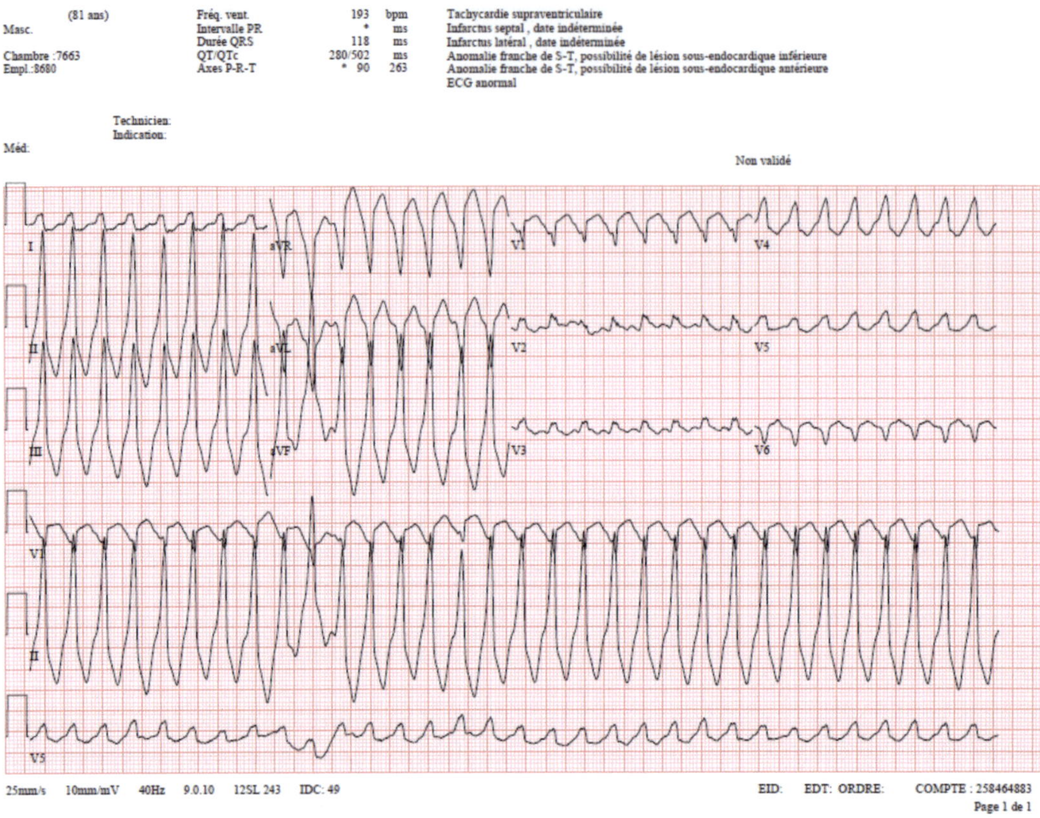

Fig. 1 Twelve-lead ECG recorded at admittance to the Cardiology Department

complex has a "QS" pattern in lead aVL, and the QRS transition takes place in V2, elements that are not in favor of a typical left bundle branch block. This makes SVT with LBBB unlikely.

The ECG from Fig. 2 shows a sinus rhythm with a ventricular rate of 59 bpm, QRS axis at −10°, absence of LV hypertrophy, and flattened T waves in lead II, III, and aVF; there are no signs of ventricular pre-excitation (no short PR interval and no delta waves). This makes antidromic tachycardia unlikely as the correct diagnosis for the tachycardia from Fig. 1.

Applying the Brugada algorithm [2] to the tachycardia from Fig. 1, it can be seen that: (1) There is an absence of an RS complex in the precordial leads (otherwise said, there are no RS complexes present). This is a strong argument in favor of ventricular tachycardia.

Other arguments in favor of ventricular tachycardia from the Brugada algorithm are: (1) An r wave of >0.04 s in lead V1 or V2 (Fig. 3); (2) A notched S downstroke in V1 or V2, which is present in lead V1 (Fig. 4); and a duration of >60 ms from the onset of the QRS to the nadir of the S wave in lead V1 (Fig. 5) [3].

The Vereckei algorithm [4] for the differential diagnosis of wide QRS complex tachycardias also suggests VT as the correct answer. The first step of the algorithm looks for A–V dissociation, which is not seen on the present ECG. The second step of the algorithm looks for an initial predominant R wave in lead aVR, which is also not the case (Fig. 6).

The third step of the algorithm "QRS morphology unlike BBB or fascicular block" does not suggest SVT with RBBB, based on the argu-

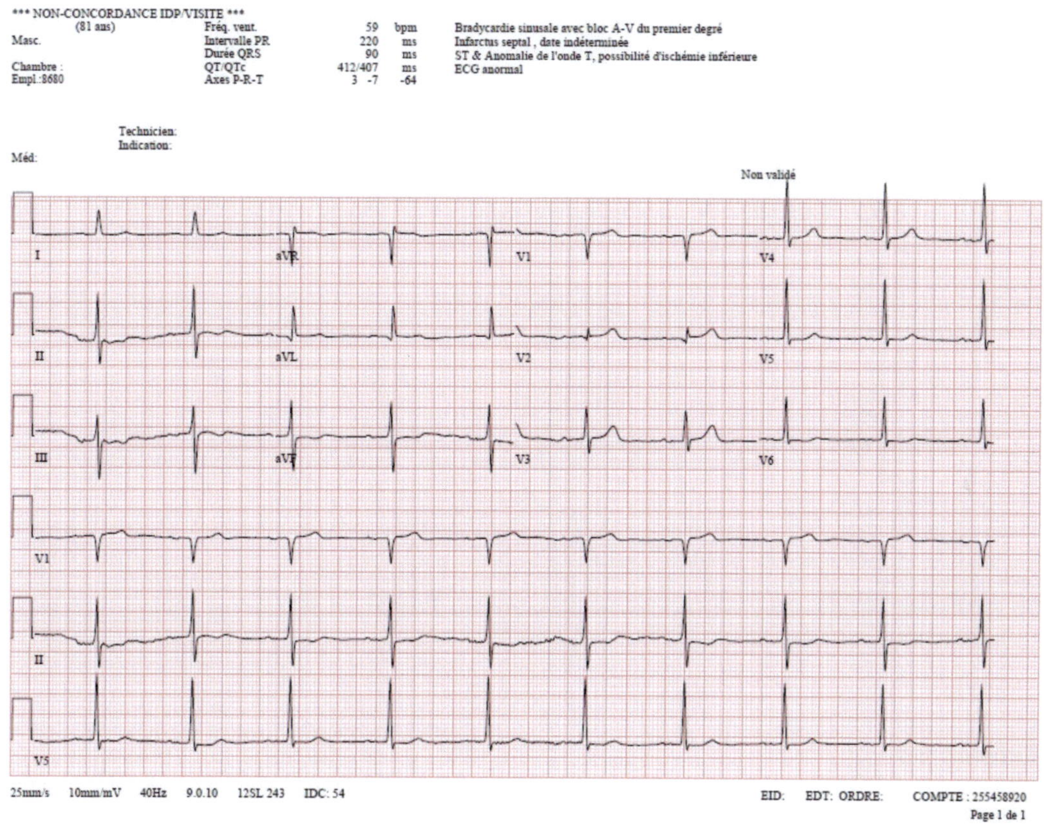

Fig. 2 Twelve-lead ECG recorded after the end of the episode of palpitations

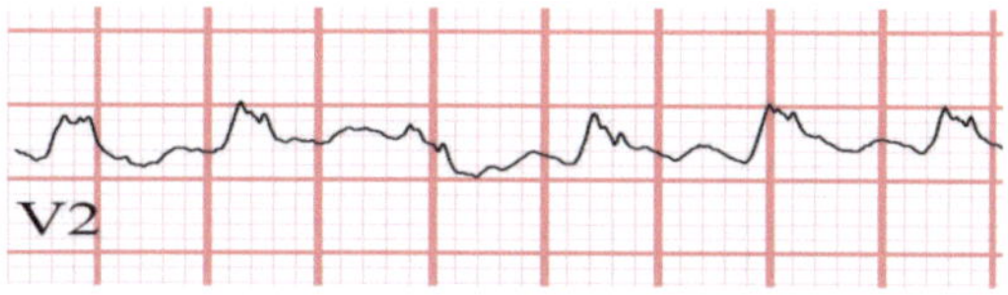

Fig. 3 Detailed analysis of the QRS morphology in lead V2 during the wide QRS complex tachycardia, showing an R wave duration of > 0.04 s.

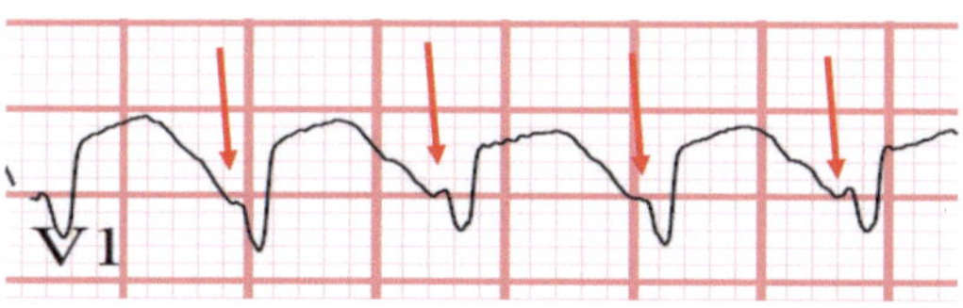

Fig. 4 Detailed analysis of the QRS morphology in lead V1 during the wide QRS complex tachycardia. A notch is present on the downstroke of the S wave, argument in favor of ventricular tachycardia

ments exposed above. Therefore, the diagnosis is that of ventricular tachycardia.

The correct diasgnosis is therefore ventricular tachycardia.

The origin of tachcyardia is at the level of the left ventricle (despite the LBBB-like pattern in lead V1), at the level of the septum (relatively narrow QRS, with an early QRS transition in lead V2 and positive QRS complex in lead I), anterior LV (positive QRS complexes in lead II, III, and aVF), and basal wall (positive QRS complexes starting from lead V2).

The patient underwent electrical cardioversion and a catheter ablation procedure.

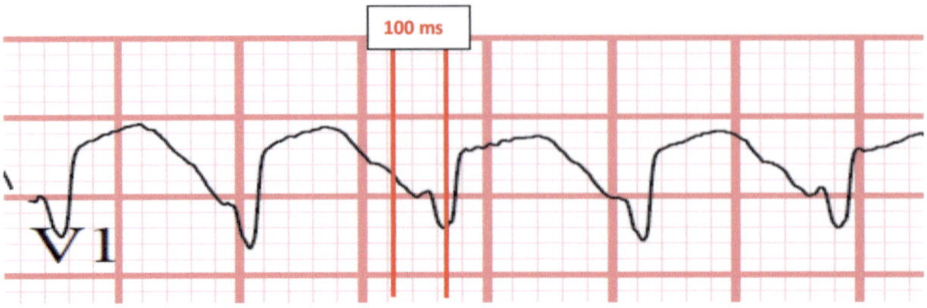

Fig. 5 Detailed analysis of the QRS morphology in lead V1 during the wide QRS complex tachycardia, showing a duration of >60 ms from the onset of the QRS to the nadir of the S wave in lead V1, argument in favor of VT

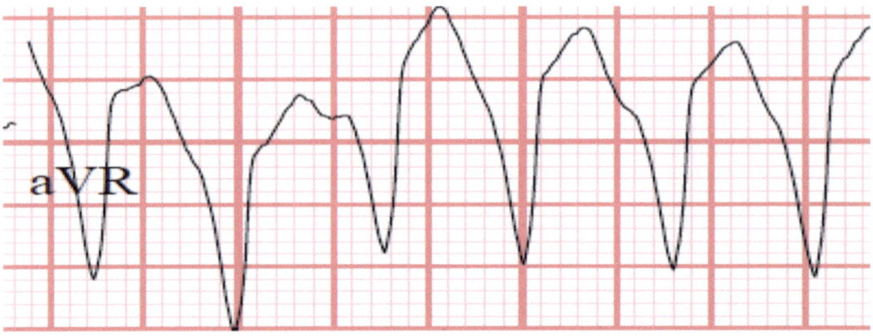

Fig. 6 Detailed analysis of the QRS morphology in lead aVR during the wide QRS complex tachycardia showing the absence of an initial tall R wave, criterion not in favor of ventricular tachycardia (but not excluding it either)

References

1. Surawicz B, Childers R, Deal BJ, Gettes LS, Bailey JJ, Gorgels A, et al. AHA/ACCF/HRS recommendations for the standardization and interpretation of the electrocardiogram: part III: intraventricular conduction disturbances: a scientific statement from the American Heart Association Electrocardiography and Arrhythmias Committee, Council on Clinical Cardiology; the American College of Cardiology Foundation; and the Heart Rhythm Society. Endorsed by the International Society for Computerized Electrocardiology. J Am Coll Cardiol. 2009;53(11):976–81.
2. Brugada P, Brugada J, Mont L, Smeets J, Andries EW. A new approach to the differential diagnosis of a regular tachycardia with a wide QRS complex. Circulation. 1991;83(5):1649–59.
3. Kindwall KE, Brown J, Josephson ME. Electrocardiographic criteria for ventricular tachycardia in wide complex left bundle branch block morphology tachycardias. Am J Cardiol. 1988;61(15):1279–83.
4. Vereckei A, Duray G, Szenasi G, Altemose GT, Miller JM. Application of a new algorithm in the differential diagnosis of wide QRS complex tachycardia. Eur Heart J. 2007;28(5):589–600.

ECG 3

Jacques Levy

1 Case Presentation

A 71-year-old male patient with a history of ischemic cardiomyopathy with severe LV systolic dysfunction (LVEF of 22%), remote inferior myocardial infarction, triple CABG for severe coronary artery disease (occlusion of the proximal LAD, significant stenosis of the right coronary artery and of the circumflex artery), implanted with a Boston Scientific Resonate CRT-D for the primary prevention of sudden cardiac death (programmed in DDD 50–130 bpm mode), and chronic ischemia of the lower limbs is admitted to the Cardiology Department for an episode of palpitations accompanied by chest pain, dyspnea, anxiety, and lightheadedness that had occurred 20 min prior to his presentation to the hospital. His ECG recorded at admittance to the Cardiology Department is presented in Fig. 1.

Question: What is the nature of the tachycardia presented in the ECG?

(a) Pacemaker-mediated tachycardia
(b) Ventricular tachycardia originating from the inferior lateral LV wall
(c) Ventricular tachycardia originating from the inferior septal LV wall
(d) Antidromic tachycardia using a left-sided bypass tract
(e) Atrial tachycardia with a right bundle branch block

Hint: A second ECG recorded after electrical cardioversion is presented in Fig. 2.

Correct answer: c. Ventricular tachycardia originating from the inferior septal LV wall

Explanation The ECG in Fig. 1 shows a regular wide QRS complex tachycardia with a heart rate of 130 bpm and RBBB morphology. The width of the QRS complex is 178 ms. The QRS axis is at −90°. The differential diagnosis of this regular wide QRS complex tachycardia with RBBB morphology includes: ventricular tachycardia (myocardial-related VT and bundle branch reentry VT), supraventricular tachycardia (atrial flutter with 1:1 AV conduction, atrial tachycardia with 1:1 AV conduction, AVNRT, and AVRT) with functional or pre-existing bundle branch block, antidromic tachycardia (in pre-excitation syndromes), and pacemaker-mediated tachycardia.

The morphology of the right bundle branch block of the QRS complex during tachycardia from Fig. 1 is not that of a typical one [1]: the QRS duration is indeed >120 ms; there is a monomorphic notched R wave in lead V1, and the QRS complex has a “RS” morphology in lead

J. Levy (✉)
Department of Cardiology, Emile Muller Hospital, Mulhouse, France
e-mail: Levyj@ghrmsa.fr

L. Muresan (ed.), *ECG Interpretation of Wide QRS Complex Tachycardia*,
https://doi.org/10.1007/978-3-031-97030-6_4

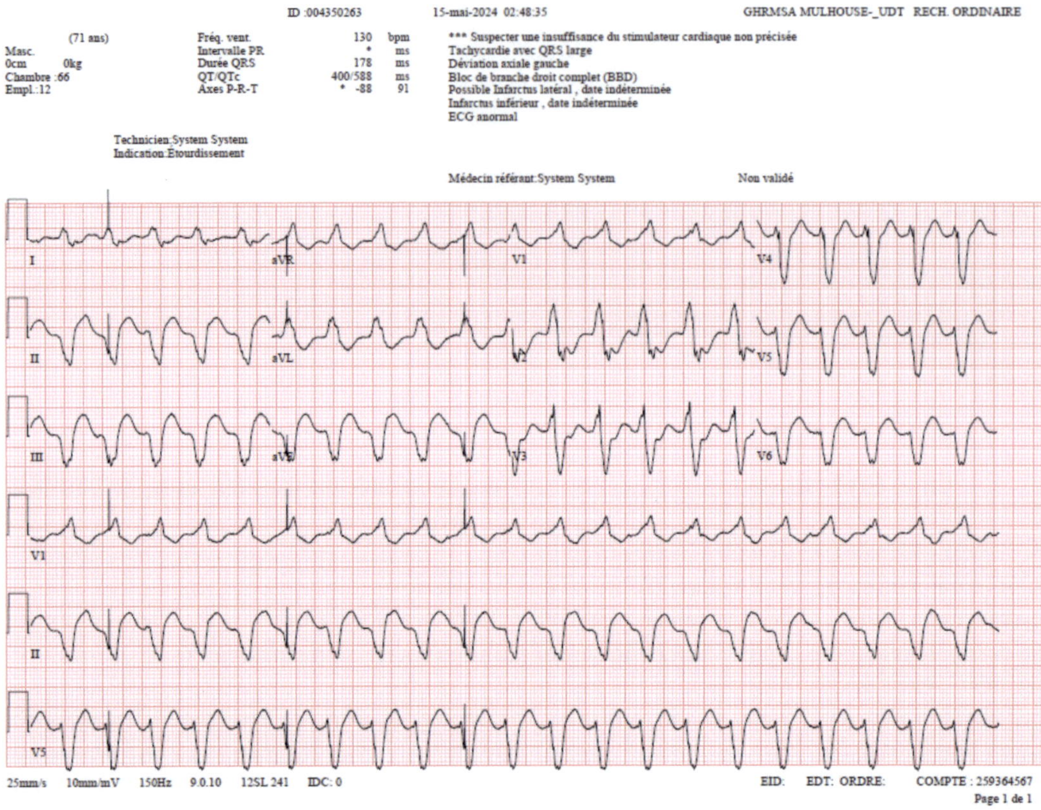

Fig. 1 Twelve-lead ECG recorded at admittance to the Cardiology Department

V6 and DI; however, the R/S ratio is <1 in lead V6, and there is a "unique R" pattern in lead aVL, which is not characteristic for a typical RBBB. This makes SVT with RBBB unlikely.

The ECG from Fig. 2 shows a sinus rhythm with ventricular-paced complexes. The morphology of the QRS complex is not the same as the one recorded by the ECG from Fig. 1. Despite a heart rate of 130 bpm (which also represents the upper pacing rate of the CRT-D), this observation, together with the fact that the QRS complexes from Fig. 1 are not preceded by pacing spikes, excludes answer a—"Pacemaker-mediated tachycardia"—as the correct answer. There are no signs in favor of ventricular pre-excitation on the ECG from Fig. 2 (delta waves, short PR interval), which makes answer d—"Antidromic tachycardia using a left-sided bypass tract"—highly improbable.

Applying the Brugada algorithm [2] to the tachycardia from Fig. 1, it can be seen that: (1) There is no absence of an RS complex in the precordial leads (otherwise said, there are "RS" or "rS" complexes in leads V2–V6); we therefore move to the second step of the algorithm: (2) This step analyzes the absence of an R to S interval > 100 ms in any precordial lead. This is actually the case (Fig. 3).

Other arguments from the Brugada algorithm in favor of the diagnosis of ventricular tachycardia are: the presence of atrioventricular dissociation (Fig. 4) and, for an RBBB morphology wide QRS complex tachycardia, the presence of an "rS" complex, in lead V6. This can also be expressed as a ratio of R/S < 1 in lead V6 (Fig. 5).

The Vereckei algorithm [3] for the differential diagnosis of wide QRS complex tachycardia also suggests VT as the correct answer. The first step of the algorithm looks for A–V dissociation, which is seen on the present ECG (Fig. 4).

Other arguments from the Vereckei algorithm supporting the diagnosis of ventricular tachycar-

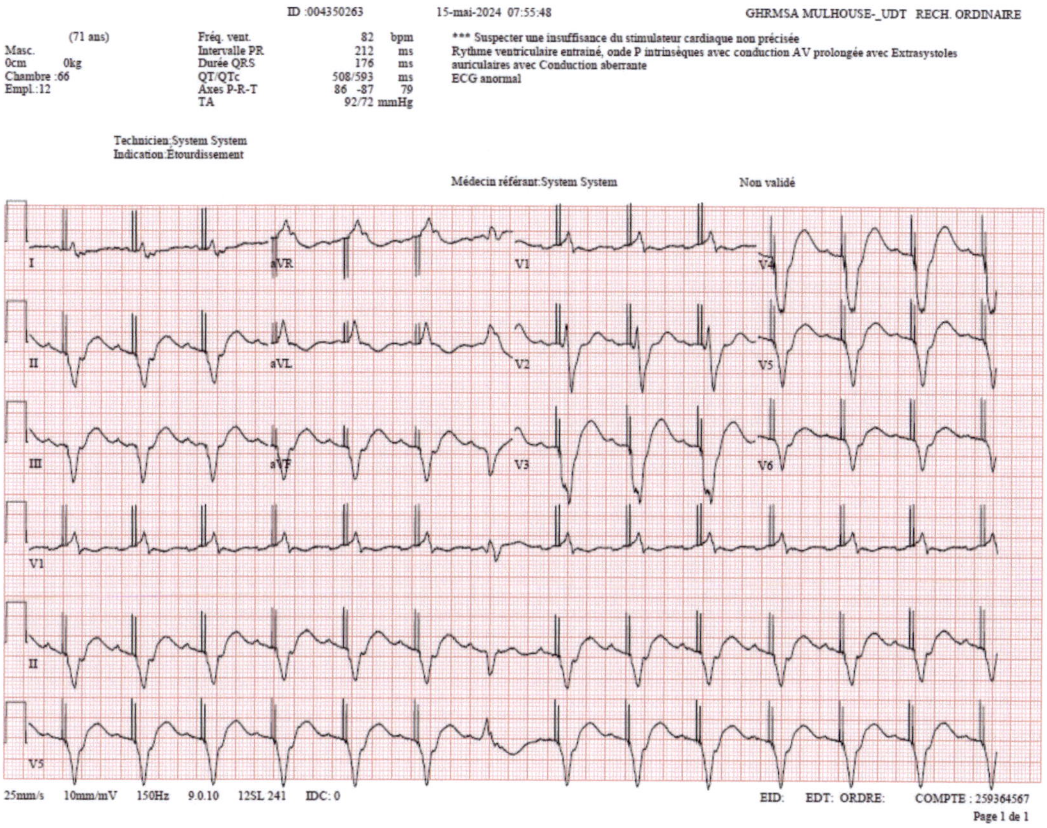

Fig. 2 Twelve-lead ECG recorded after the end of the episode of palpitations

Fig. 3 Lead V2 recorded during the wide QRS complex tachycardia from Fig. 1 demonstrating an R to S interval of 125 ms, criterion in favor of ventricular tachycardia

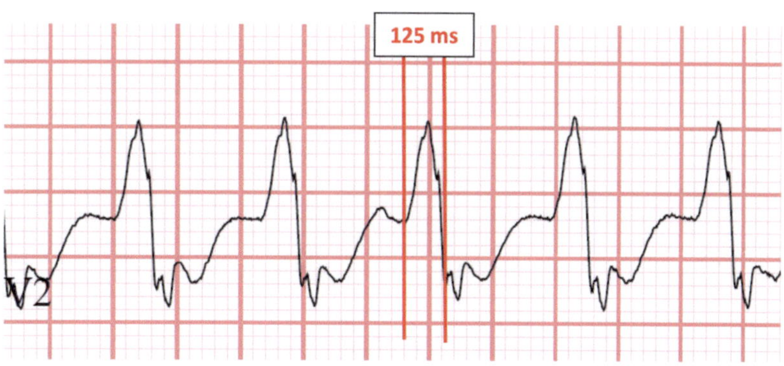

dia are: the presence of an initial predominant R wave in lead aVR (Fig. 6) and the morphology of the QRS not being in favor of a typical RBBB.

The Basel algorithm [4] is also in favor of ventricular tachycardia as the right answer. According to this algorithm, a positive diagnosis of VT is established if at least two out of three criteria are present: (1) Structural heart disease (history of myocardial infarction, congestive heart failure (LVEF <35%), and the presence of an ICD and CRT), which the present patient has; (2) the time to first peak in lead II > 40 ms (Fig. 7); and (3) the time to first peak in lead aVR > 40 ms (Fig. 8) [4].

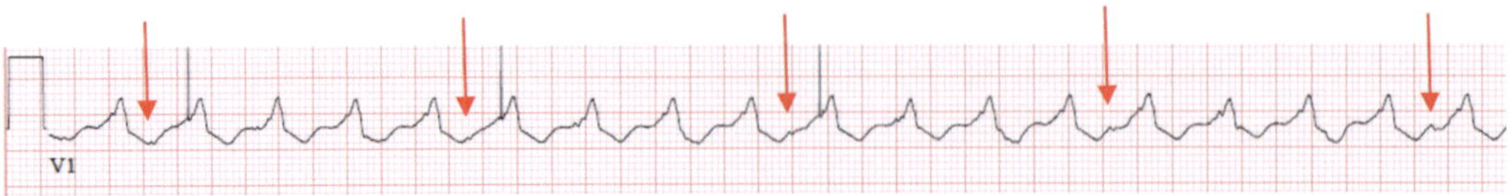

Fig. 4 Lead V1 recorded during the wide QRS complex tachycardia from Fig. 1 demonstrating atrioventricular dissociation, criterion in favor of ventricular tachycardia. The red arrows point to the P waves

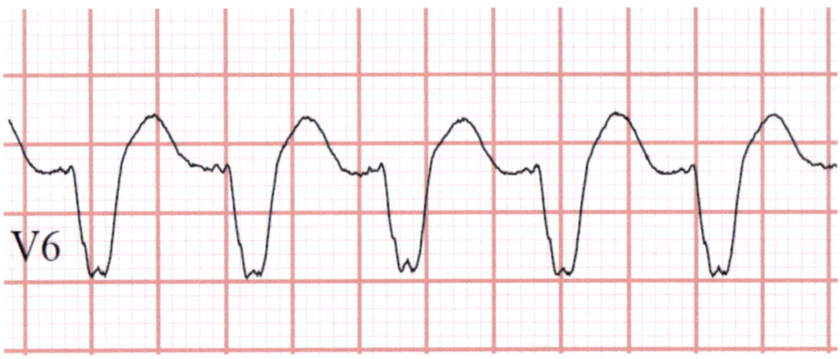

Fig. 5 Lead V6 recorded during the wide QRS complex tachycardia from Fig. 1 demonstrating an R to S ratio > 1, criterion in favor of ventricular tachycardia

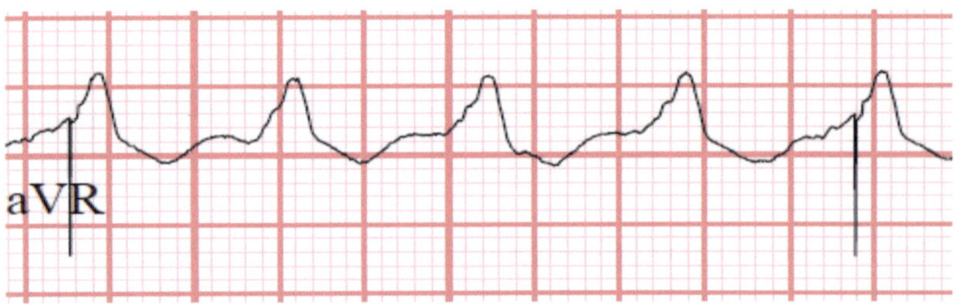

Fig. 6 Lead aVR from the tachycardia presented in Fig. 1, showing the presence of an initial positive tall R wave, criterion in favor of ventricular tachycardia

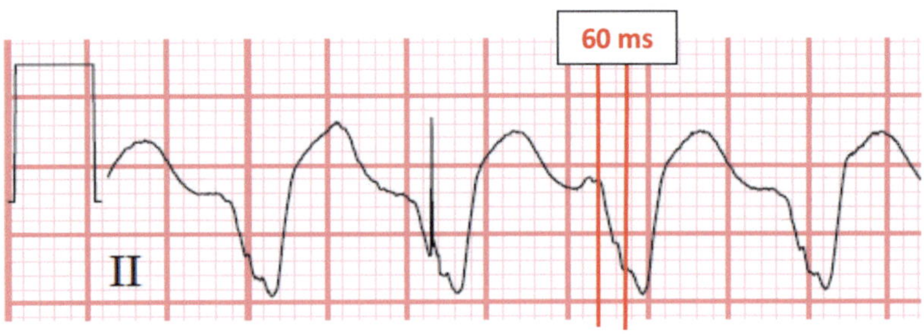

Fig. 7 Lead II from the ECG from Fig. 1 showing the time to first peak of 60 ms, criterion in favor of ventricular tachycardia

Therefore, according to the Basel algorithm, the diagnosis of ventricular tachycardia can be retained.

The origin of the ventricular tachycardia is: at the level of the left ventricle (RBBB morphology), at the level of the inferior LV wall (negative QRS complexes in leads II, III, and aVF), and at the level of the septal wall (positive QRS complexes in lead I and aVL).

The patient underwent an electrophysiological study, which confirmed the diagnosis, and a catheter ablation procedure.

Observation: How does one explain the pacing spikes visible sporadically during the wide QRS complex tachycardia?

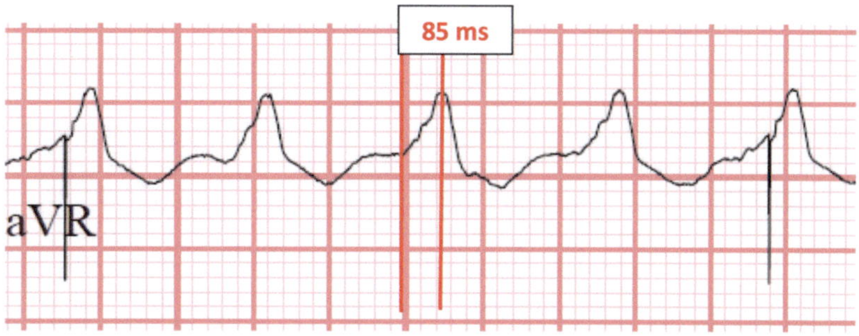

Fig. 8 Lead aVR from the ECG from Fig. 1 showing the time to the first peak of 85 ms, criterion in favor of ventricular tachycardia

As (better) seen in Fig. 4, each pacing spike is present after a P wave (indicated by the red arrows). Each of the first three P waves seen in lead V1 initiates an A–V interval, and the ICD delivers a pacing spike at the end of this interval, in the absence of a detected spontaneous ventricular activity. For the last two P waves indicated in Fig. 4, it is likely that the R wave of the QRS complex is detected just at the end of the sAV interval, and the ICD does not deliver a pacing spike.

References

1. Surawicz B, Childers R, Deal BJ, Gettes LS, Bailey JJ, Gorgels A, et al. AHA/ACCF/HRS recommendations for the standardization and interpretation of the electrocardiogram: part III: intraventricular conduction disturbances: a scientific statement from the American Heart Association Electrocardiography and Arrhythmias Committee, Council on Clinical Cardiology; the American College of Cardiology Foundation; and the Heart Rhythm Society. Endorsed by the International Society for Computerized Electrocardiology. J Am Coll Cardiol. 2009;53(11):976–81.
2. Brugada P, Brugada J, Mont L, Smeets J, Andries EW. A new approach to the differential diagnosis of a regular tachycardia with a wide QRS complex. Circulation. 1991;83(5):1649–59.
3. Vereckei A, Duray G, Szenasi G, Altemose GT, Miller JM. Application of a new algorithm in the differential diagnosis of wide QRS complex tachycardia. Eur Heart J. 2007;28(5):589–600.
4. Moccetti F, Yadava M, Latifi Y, Strebel I, Pavlovic N, Knecht S, et al. Simplified integrated clinical and electrocardiographic algorithm for differentiation of wide QRS complex tachycardia: the Basel algorithm. JACC Clin Electrophysiol. 2022;8(7):831–9.

ECG 4

Charline Daval

1 Case Presentation

A 74-year-old male patient with a history of ischemic heart disease, persistent atrial fibrillation treated with a catheter ablation procedure 7 years prior, arterial hypertension, obesity, and dyslipidemia is admitted to the hospital for an episode of malaise accompanied by palpitations and dyspnea that had started 1 h prior to his presentation to the hospital. His ECG recorded at the arrival to the Cardiology Department is presented in Fig. 1.

Question: What is the nature of the tachycardia presented in the ECG?

(a) Intrafascicular re-entry ventricular tachycardia (posterior fascicle)
(b) Intrafascicular re-entry ventricular tachycardia (anterior fascicle)
(c) Pre-excited atrial fibrillation
(d) Antidromic tachycardia using a left-sided bypass tract
(e) Atrial fibrillation with bifascicular block (RBBB + LAFB)

Hint: An ECG recorded after amiodarone administration is presented in Fig. 2.

C. Daval (✉)
Department of Cardiology, Emile Muller Hospital, Mulhouse, France
e-mail: charline.daval@ghrmsa.fr

Correct answer: a. Atrial fibrillation with a bifascicular block (RBBB + LAFB)

Explanation: The ECG in Fig. 1 shows an irregular wide QRS complex tachycardia with a heart rate of 154 bpm and RBBB morphology. The width of the QRS complex is 126 ms. The QRS axis is at −75°. The differential diagnosis of this irregular wide QRS complex tachycardia with RBBB morphology includes: ventricular tachycardia (myocardial-related VT and fascicular ventricular tachycardia), supraventricular tachycardia (atrial fibrillation, atrial flutter, atrial tachycardia, AVNRT, and AVRT) with a functional or pre-existing bundle branch block. Antidromic tachycardia (in pre-excitation syndromes) is usually regular and unlikely present in this case.

The morphology of the right bundle branch block of the QRS complex during tachycardia from Fig. 1 is that of a typical one [1]: the QRS duration is >120 ms; the QRS morphology is "RSR'" in lead V1, and there is an RS pattern in lead I, aVL, and in V5 and V6. The R-to-S ratio in lead V6 is <1. Therefore, at this point of the analysis, we cannot say whether this is SVT with RBBB or VT.

The ECG from Fig. 2 shows a sinus rhythm with a heart rate of 66 bpm, QRS axis at −20°, absence of LV hypertrophy, and absence of ischemia, with first-degree AV block and with no

L. Muresan (ed.), *ECG Interpretation of Wide QRS Complex Tachycardia*,
https://doi.org/10.1007/978-3-031-97030-6_5

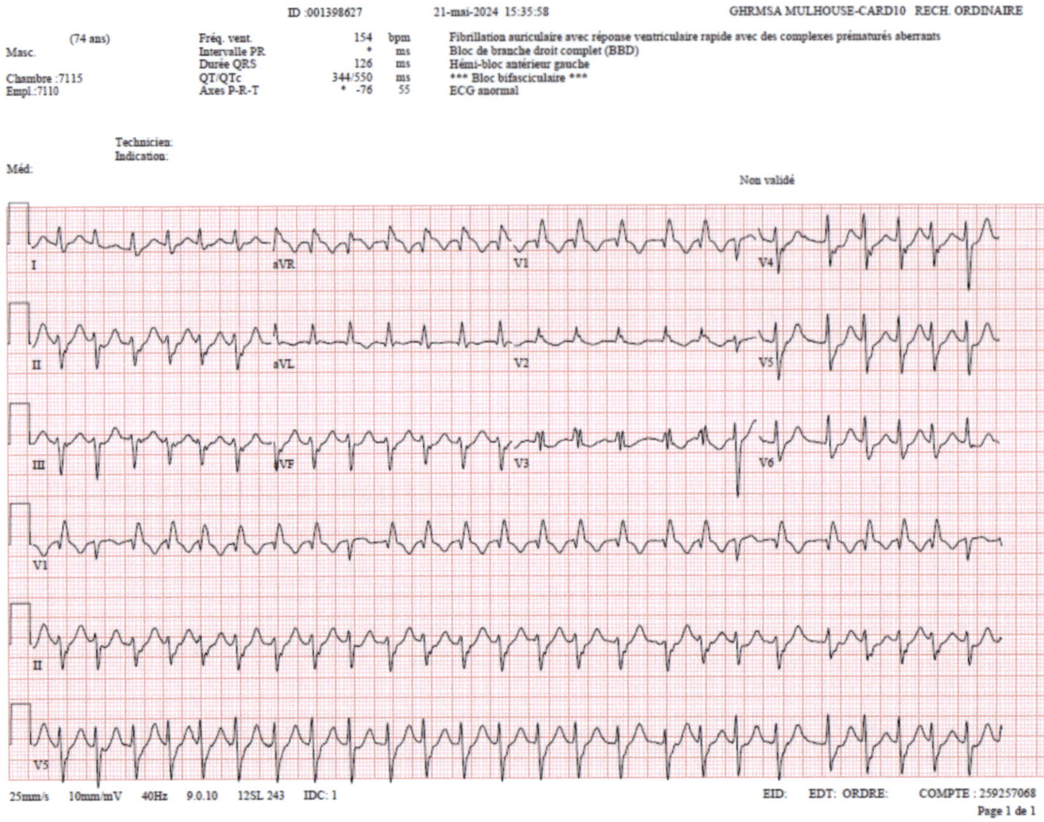

Fig. 1 Twelve-lead ECG recorded at admittance to the Cardiology Department

signs of ventricular pre-excitation (no short PR interval and no delta waves). This makes antidromic tachycardia unlikely.

Applying the Brugada algorithm [2] to the tachycardia from Fig. 2, it can be seen that: 1. There is no absence of an RS complex in the precordial leads (otherwise said, there are rS complexes in leads V4–V6) (Fig. 3); we therefore move to the second step of the algorithm.

The second step analyzes the presence of an R to S interval > 100 ms in any precordial lead. This is not the case (Fig. 4).

Step 3 of the algorithm looks for A–V dissociation. If we analyze the atrial activity, there are no P waves visible, and the rhythm is irregular. This is actually atrial fibrillation. Therefore, we cannot say if there is AV dissociation. We therefore need to move to step 4 of the algorithm.

For an RBBB morphology wide QRS complex tachycardia, an argument in favor of VT would be the presence of a taller left peak of the QRS complex in lead V1 (the rabbit ear sign), or for biphasic RS or QR complexes, which is not the case (Fig. 5). Next, in lead V6, an argument in favor of VT would be the presence of an "rS" complex, which is also not the case (Fig. 3). Therefore, there are no arguments in favor of VT according to the Brugada algorithm.

The Vereckei algorithm [3] for the differential diagnosis of wide QRS complex tachycardias also finds no arguments in favor of VT. The first step of the algorithm looks for A–V dissociation, which is not seen on the present ECG. The second step of the algorithm looks for an initial predominant R wave in lead aVR, which is not the case (Fig. 6).

The third step "QRS morphology unlike BBB or fascicular block" suggests SVT with RBBB, based on the arguments exposed above.

These findings, together with the irregularity of the rhythm, are in favor of atrial fibrillation with RBBB. A closer inspection of the ECG from

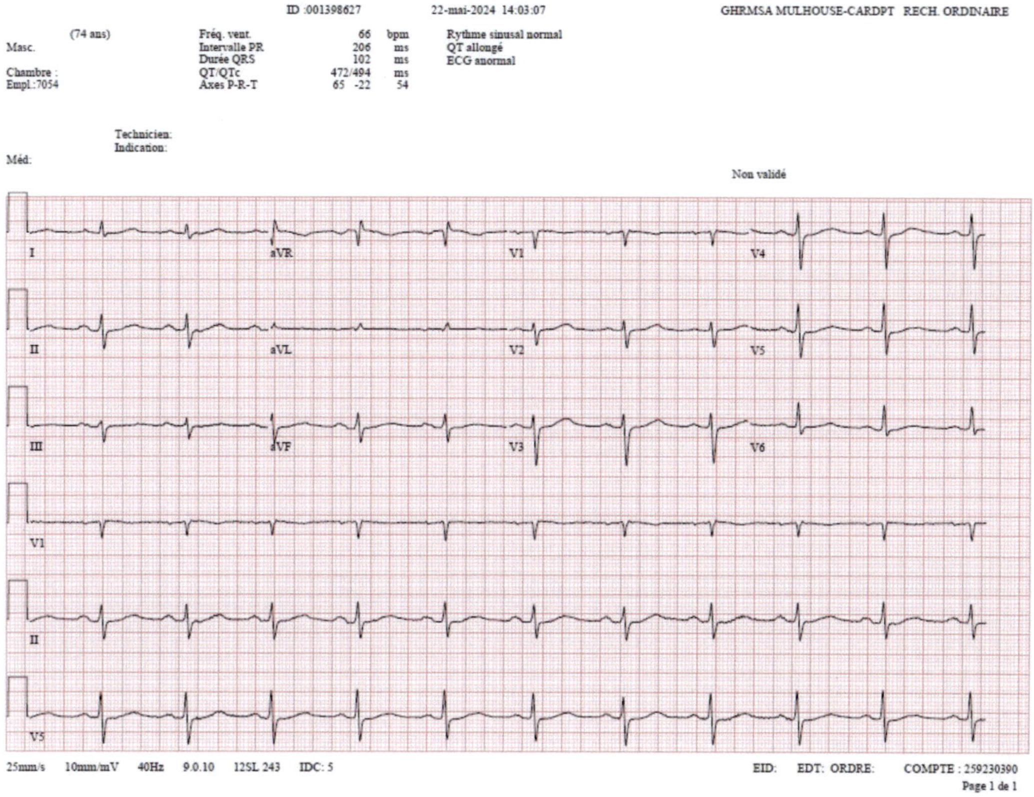

Fig. 2 Twelve-lead ECG recorded after the end of the episode of palpitations

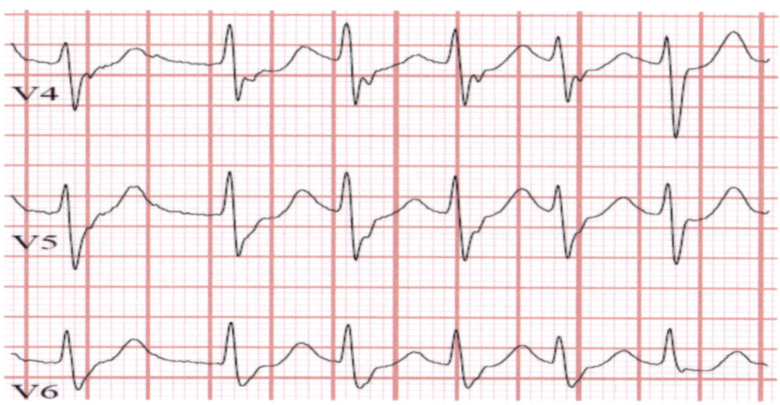

Fig. 3 Leads V4–V6 recorded during the wide QRS complex tachycardia from Fig. 1 demonstrating the presence of RS complexes, criterion not in favor of ventricular tachycardia (but not excluding it either)

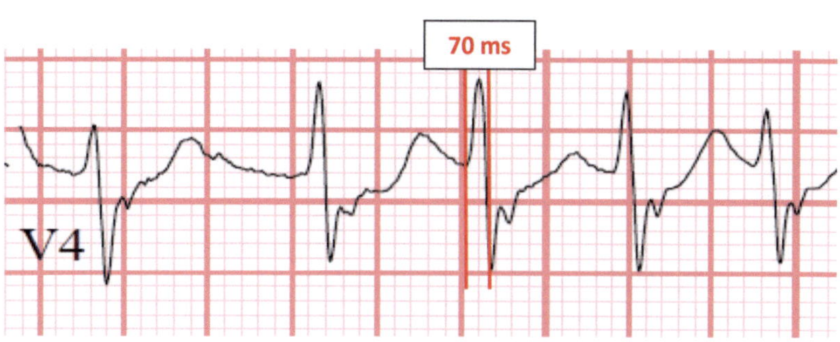

Fig. 4 Lead V4 from the tachycardia from Fig. 1 demonstrating an R to S interval of 70 ms, argument not in favor of ventricular tachycardia (but not excluding it either)

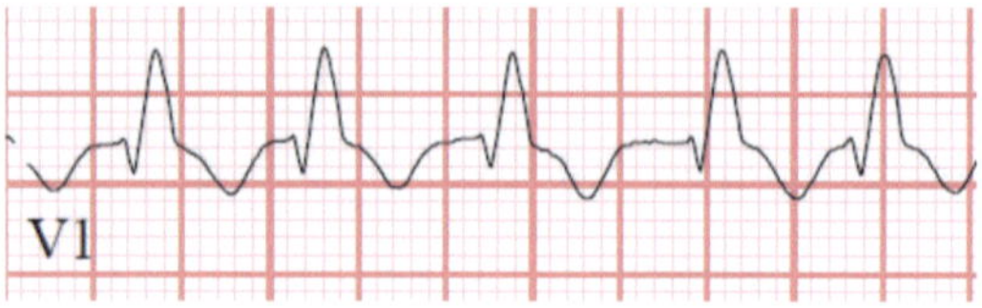

Fig. 5 Lead V1 from the tachycardia from Fig. 1 demonstrating an "rsR'" morphology, argument not in favor of ventricular tachycardia (but not excluding it either)

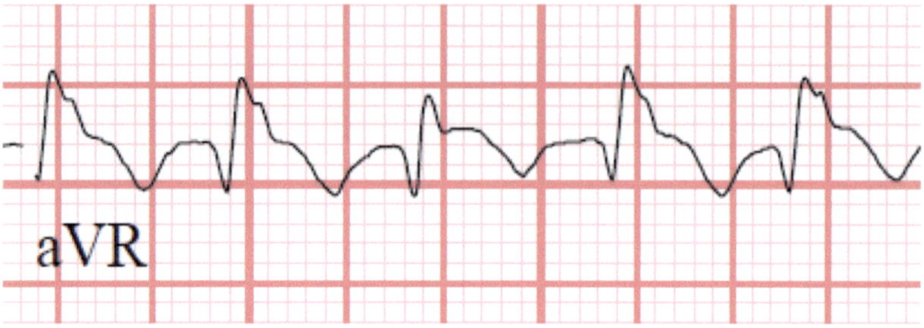

Fig. 6 Lead aVR from the tachycardia from Fig. 1 demonstrating the absence of a tall initial R wave in lead aVR, argument not in favor of ventricular tachycardia (but not excluding it either)

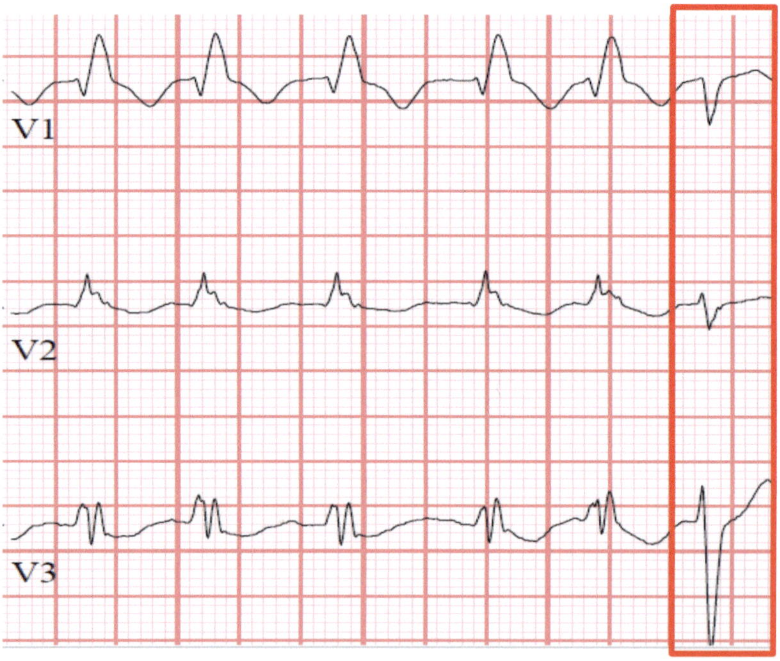

Fig. 7 Leads V1–V3 from the tachycardia from Fig. 1 demonstrating the presence of a narrow QRS complex, identical to the one from Fig. 2. This is compatible with AV conduction over the AV node

Fig. 1 finds the presence of 4 narrow QRS complexes, identical to the ones from the ECG 2 (Fig. 7). These are compatible with atrioventricular conduction over the atrioventricular node and the His–Purkinje system. The large QRS complexes with RBBB are compatible with aberrant conduction.

Therefore, this is atrial fibrillation with functional RBBB. There is left axis deviation; therefore, there is an associated LAFHB. The correct answer is e. "Atrial fibrillation with bifascicular block (RBBB and LAFB)". The differential diagnosis of this tachycardia includes left anterior fascicular re-entry ventricular tachycardia.

However, this type of VT is usually regular, and the "rabbit ear sign" is usually present in lead V1 (which is not the case for the present patient). The narrow QRS complexes should not be mistaken for capture beats during VT, since they represent normal conduction using the His–Purkinje system during atrial fibrillation.

References

1. Surawicz B, Childers R, Deal BJ, Gettes LS, Bailey JJ, Gorgels A, et al. AHA/ACCF/HRS recommendations for the standardization and interpretation of the electrocardiogram: part III: intraventricular conduction disturbances: a scientific statement from the American Heart Association Electrocardiography and Arrhythmias Committee, Council on Clinical Cardiology; the American College of Cardiology Foundation; and the Heart Rhythm Society. Endorsed by the International Society for Computerized Electrocardiology. J Am Coll Cardiol. 2009;53(11):976–81.
2. Brugada P, Brugada J, Mont L, Smeets J, Andries EW. A new approach to the differential diagnosis of a regular tachycardia with a wide QRS complex. Circulation. 1991;83(5):1649–59.
3. Vereckei A, Duray G, Szenasi G, Altemose GT, Miller JM. Application of a new algorithm in the differential diagnosis of wide QRS complex tachycardia. Eur Heart J. 2007;28(5):589–600.

ECG 5

Serban Schiau

1 Case Presentation

A 77-year-old male patient with no significant past medical history is admitted to the Cardiology Department for an episode of palpitations with a sudden onset and regular rhythm, accompanied by pre-syncope, dyspnea, lightheadedness, and chest pain that had started 45 min prior to his presentation to the hospital. His ECG recorded at admittance to the Cardiology Department is presented in Fig. 1.

Question: What is the nature of the rhythm presented in Fig. 1?

(a) Ventricular tachycardia originating from the moderator band (right ventricle)
(b) Ventricular tachycardia originating from the anterior septal LV wall
(c) Upper septal fascicular ventricular tachycardia
(d) Antidromic tachycardia using a right-sided bypass tract
(e) AVNRT with 1:1 atrioventricular conduction and left bundle branch block

Hint: A second ECG recorded several minutes later is presented in Fig. 2.

S. Schiau (✉)
Department of Cardiology, Emile Muller Hospital, Mulhouse, France
e-mail: serban.schiau@ghrmsa.fr

Correct answer: a. Ventricular tachycardia originating from the moderator band (right ventricle)

Explanation: The ECG in Fig. 1 shows a regular wide QRS complex tachycardia with a heart rate of 223 bpm and LBBB morphology. The width of the QRS complex is 125 ms (contrary to what is automatically showed of 96 ms). The QRS axis is at +65°. The differential diagnosis of this regular wide QRS complex tachycardia with LBBB morphology includes: ventricular tachycardia (myocardial-related VT and fascicular ventricular tachycardia) and supraventricular tachycardia (atrial flutter, atrial tachycardia, AVNRT, and AVRT) with functional or pre-existing bundle branch block and antidromic tachycardia (in pre-excitation syndromes).

The morphology of the left bundle branch block of the QRS complex during tachycardia from Fig. 1 is compatible with that of a typical one [1]: the QRS duration is >120 ms; the QRS has a "QS'" morphology in lead V1 and a unique notched R wave in leads V5, V6, and lead I; the QRS transition takes place in lead V5; there are repolarization abnormalities (positive T waves from V1 to V3 and negative T waves from V4 to V6), compatible with those encountered in patients with typical LBBB. Therefore, at this

L. Muresan (ed.), *ECG Interpretation of Wide QRS Complex Tachycardia*,
https://doi.org/10.1007/978-3-031-97030-6_6

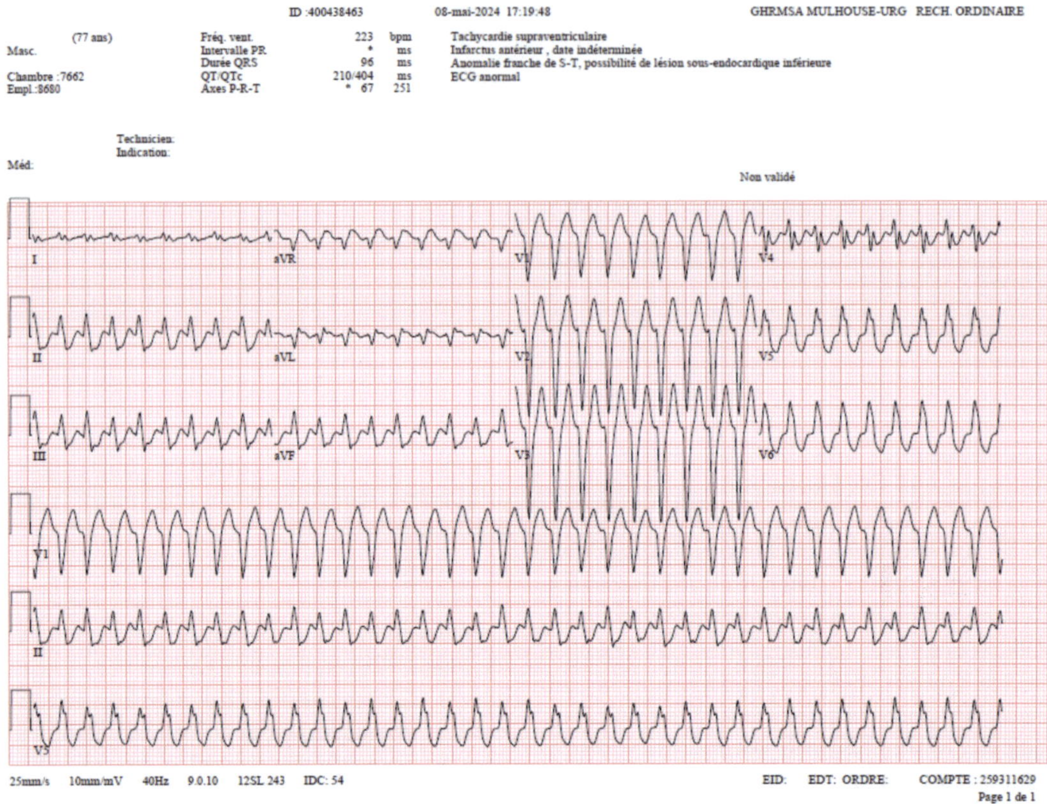

Fig. 1 Twelve-lead ECG recorded at admittance to the Cardiology Department

point of the analysis, one cannot say whether this is VT or SVT with a bundle branch block.

The ECG from Fig. 2 shows a sinus rhythm with a heart rate of 55 bpm, QRS axis at +60°, absence of LV hypertrophy, and absence of ischemia; there are no signs of ventricular preexcitation (no short PR interval and no delta waves). This makes antidromic tachycardia unlikely as the correct diagnosis for the tachycardia from Fig. 1.

Applying the Brugada algorithm [2] to the tachycardia from Fig. 1, it can be seen that: (1) There is no absence of an RS complex in the precordial leads (otherwise said, there are rS complexes in leads V2 to V4); we therefore move to the second step of the algorithm: (2) This step analyzes the absence of an R to S interval > 100 ms in any precordial lead. This is not the case (Fig. 3). We therefore continue to step 3 of the algorithm.

Step 3 looks for atrioventricular dissociation. No P waves are visible on the ECG recorded during tachycardia; therefore, one cannot say whether atrioventricular dissociation is present. One needs to proceed to step 4 of the algorithm.

Step 4 analyzes morphological elements of the QRS complex. For a wide QRS complex tachycardia with LBBB, arguments in favor of VT are: the presence of an “r wave” > 0.04 s in lead V1 or V2, which is not the case, or the presence of a “QS” pattern in lead V6, which is also not the case [3].

Other arguments in favor of ventricular tachycardia are: (1) For an LBBB QRS morphology, a QRS duration of over 160 ms, which is also not the case [4]. (2) A duration of >60 ms from the onset of the QRS to the nadir of the S wave in lead V1, which is also not the case (Fig. 4) (3). Therefore, according to the Brugada algorithm, there are no elements in favor of ventricular tachcyardia.

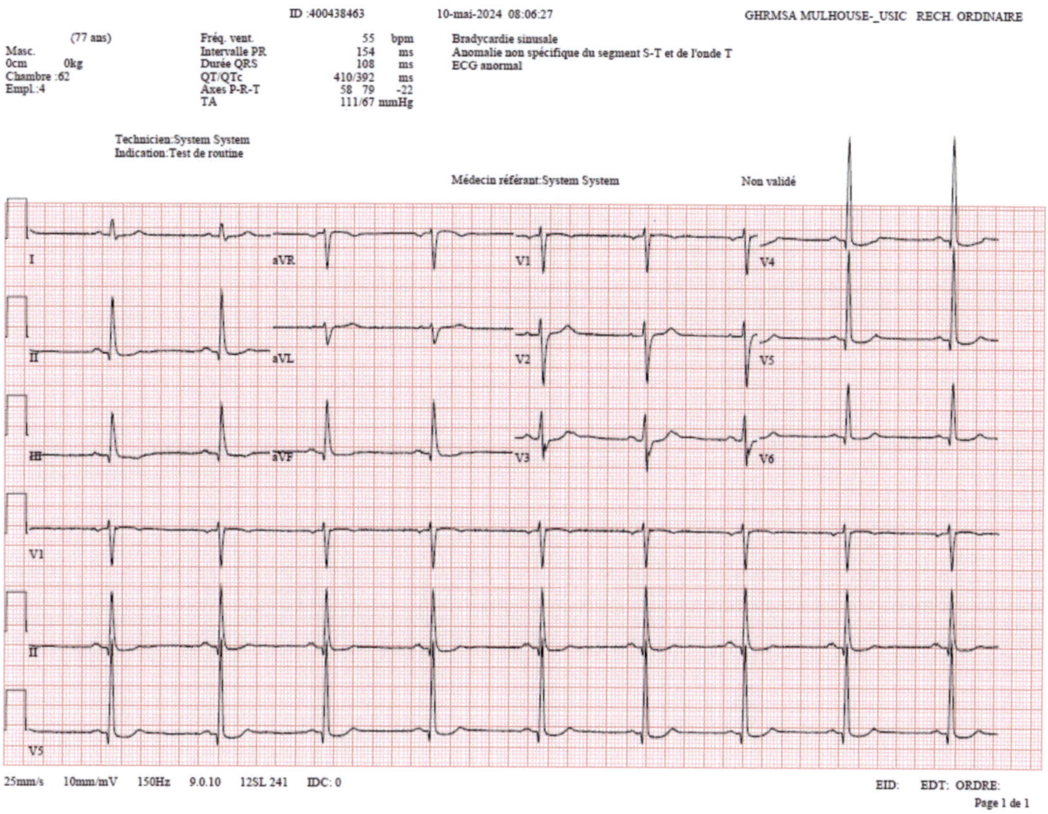

Fig. 2 Twelve-lead ECG recorded after the end of the episode of palpitations

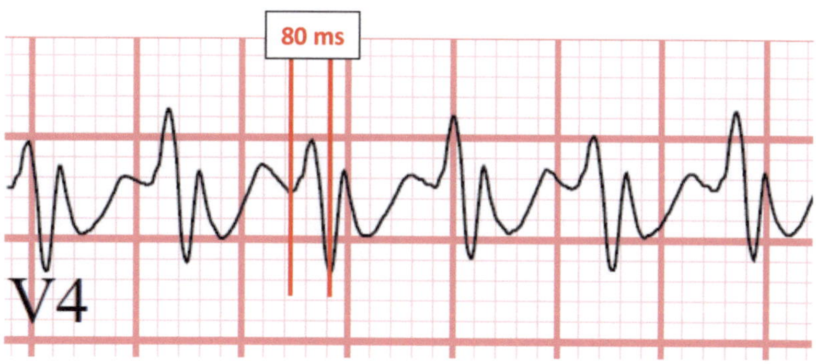

Fig. 3 Detailed analysis of the QRS morphology in lead V4 during the wide QRS complex tachycardia. The RS interval measures 80 ms. This is not diagnostic of ventricular tachycardia (but it does not exclude it either)

The Vereckei algorithm [5] for the differential diagnosis of wide QRS complex tachycardia also suggests SVT as the correct answer. The first step of the algorithm looks for A–V dissociation, which is not seen on the present ECG. The second step of the algorithm looks for an initial predominant R wave in lead aVR, which is also not the case (Fig. 5).

The third step of the algorithm "QRS morphology unlike BBB or fascicular block" actually suggests SVT with LBBB, based on the arguments exposed above. Therefore, according to the Vereckei algorithm, the diagnosis is that of supraventricular tachycardia with LBBB.

The Basel algorithm [6] is also in favor of supraventricular tachycardia as the right answer.

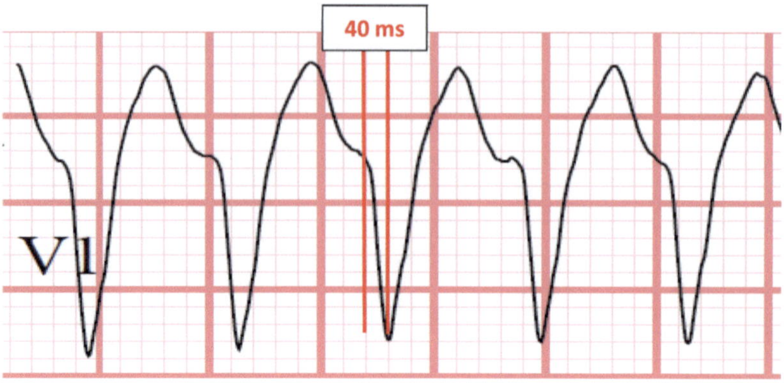

Fig. 4 Detailed analysis of the QRS morphology in lead V1 during the wide QRS complex tachycardia. The RS interval measures 40 ms, criterion not in favor of ventricular tachycardia (but not excluding it either)

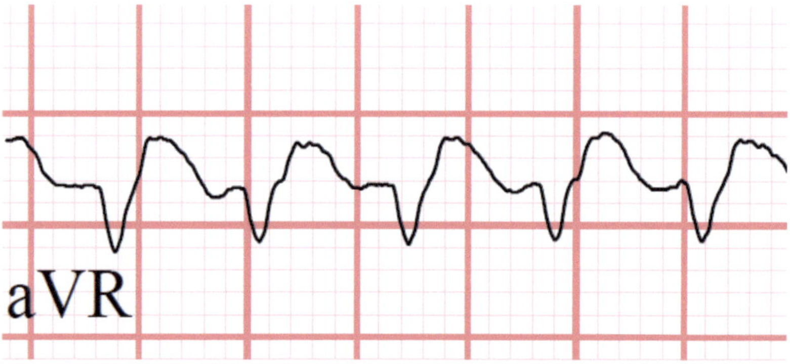

Fig. 5 Lead aVR from the tachycardia presented in Fig. 1, showing the absence of an initial positive tall R wave, criterion not in favor of ventricular tachycardia (but not excluding it either)

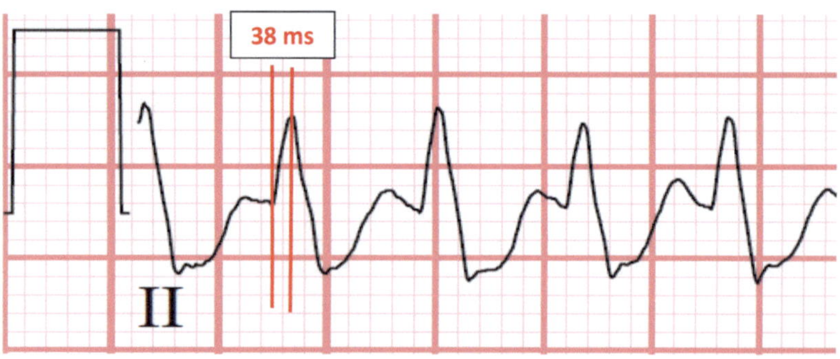

Fig. 6 Lead II from the ECG from Fig. 1 showing the time to first peak of 38 ms, criterion not in favor of ventricular tachycardia (but not excluding it either)

According to this algorithm, a positive diagnosis of VT is established if at least two out of three criteria are present: (1) Structural heart disease (history of myocardial infarction, congestive heart failure (LVEF <35%), the presence of an ICD, and CRT), which is not found in the present patient; (2) the time to first peak in lead II > 40 ms (Fig. 6); and (3) the time to first peak in lead aVR > 40 ms (Fig. 7) [6].

The patient received 20 mg of iv adenosine triphosphate, with no effect on the tachycardia. Carotid sinus massage was also performed, with no effect on the heart rate or on the rhythm. Sinus rhythm was restored by external electrical cardioversion.

The patient underwent an electrophysiological study with programmed ventricular stimulation. The nature of the tachycardia was ventricular. Its origin was found at the insertion of the moderator band at the level of the septal RV wall. Catheter ablation was successfully performed, and the patient did not present any arrhythmia during the

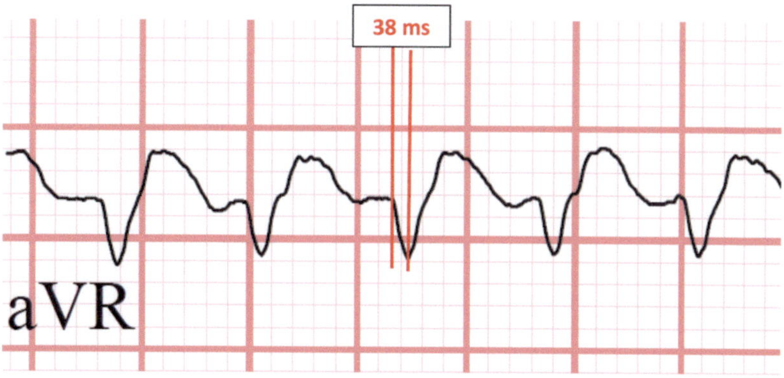

Fig. 7 Lead aVR from the ECG from Fig. 1 showing the time to first peak of 38 ms, criterion not in favor of ventricular tachycardia (but not excluding it either)

follow-up period in the hospital. He was later discharged on no antiarrhythmic drugs.

Ventricular arrhythmias originating from the moderator are a well-known entity [6, 7]. They can manifest as PVC or NSVT and sustained VT. Sustained monomorphic VT is usually characterized by an LBBB morphology and left superior axis, with positive QRS in leads I and aVL. The QRS complexes are relatively narrow. Transition in the precordial leads usually takes place in lead V4 or later and always later than the QRS transition during the sinus rhythm. Treatment of these arrhythmias comprises antiarrhythmic drugs and catheter ablation.

This case underlines the fact that algorithms used for the differential diagnosis between several types of wide QRS complex tachycardia are not always correct and that clinical judgment remains a cornerstone of patients' management.

References

1. Surawicz B, Childers R, Deal BJ, Gettes LS, Bailey JJ, Gorgels A, et al. AHA/ACCF/HRS recommendations for the standardization and interpretation of the electrocardiogram: part III: intraventricular conduction disturbances: a scientific statement from the American Heart Association Electrocardiography and Arrhythmias Committee, Council on Clinical Cardiology; the American College of Cardiology Foundation; and the Heart Rhythm Society. Endorsed by the International Society for Computerized Electrocardiology. J Am Coll Cardiol. 2009;53(11):976–81.
2. Brugada P, Brugada J, Mont L, Smeets J, Andries EW. A new approach to the differential diagnosis of a regular tachycardia with a wide QRS complex. Circulation. 1991;83(5):1649–59.
3. Kindwall KE, Brown J, Josephson ME. Electrocardiographic criteria for ventricular tachycardia in wide complex left bundle branch block morphology tachycardias. Am J Cardiol. 1988;61(15):1279–83.
4. Eckardt L, Breithardt G, Kirchhof P. Approach to wide complex tachycardias in patients without structural heart disease. Heart. 2006;92(5):704–11.
5. Vereckei A, Duray G, Szenasi G, Altemose GT, Miller JM. Application of a new algorithm in the differential diagnosis of wide QRS complex tachycardia. Eur Heart J. 2007;28(5):589–600.
6. Moccetti F, Yadava M, Latifi Y, Strebel I, Pavlovic N, Knecht S, et al. Simplified integrated clinical and electrocardiographic algorithm for differentiation of wide QRS complex tachycardia: the Basel algorithm. JACC Clin Electrophysiol. 2022;8(7):831–9.
7. Barber M, Chinitz J, John R. Arrhythmias from the right ventricular moderator band: diagnosis and management. Arrhythm Electrophysiol Rev. 2019;8(4):294–9.

ECG 6

Lucien Diene

1 Case Presentation

A 39-year-old male patient presents to the Cardiology Department for repeated episodes of palpitations occurring several times per week, which had appeared several weeks prior. There was no associated syncope or chest pain. He had undergone a thorough cardiovascular examination with a 12-lead ECG, TTE, a 24-h Holter ECG monitoring, and cardiac MRI. Based on the results of these investigations, the implantation of an ICD was suggested. An ECG recorded during an episode of palpitations is presented in Fig. 1.

Question 1: What is the nature of the tachycardia presented in Fig. 1?

(a) Accelerated idioventricular rhythm originating from the right ventricle
(b) Atrial tachycardia with 2: 1 atrioventricular conduction with left bundle branch block
(c) Antidromic tachycardia using a right-sided bypass tract
(d) Monomorphic ventricular tachycardia originating from the right ventricle
(e) AVNRT with functional LBBB

L. Diene (✉)
Department of Cardiology, Clinique Le Noirmont, Le Noirmont, Switzerland

Question 2: What is the most likely underlying heart disease?

(a) Remote inferior myocardial infarction
(b) Familial dilated cardiomyopathy
(c) Hypertrophic cardiomyopathy
(d) Left ventricular noncompaction
(e) Arrhythmogenic cardiomyopathy (formerly known as right ventricular dysplasia)

Hint: An ECG during the sinus rhythm is presented in Fig. 2.

Answer to Q1: d. Sustained monomorphic ventricular tachycardia originating from the right ventricle

Answer to Q2: e. Arrhythmogenic cardiomyopathy (formerly known as arrhythmogenic right ventricular dysplasia)

Explanation: The first ECG shows a regular wide QRS complex tachycardia with LBBB morphology with a heart rate of 110 bpm. The QRS axis is in the normal quadrant.

The differential diagnosis of this wide QRS complex tachycardia with LBBB morphology includes: ventricular tachycardia (myocardial-related VT and bundle branch re-entry VT), supraventricular tachycardia (atrial flutter, atrial

L. Muresan (ed.), *ECG Interpretation of Wide QRS Complex Tachycardia*,
https://doi.org/10.1007/978-3-031-97030-6_7

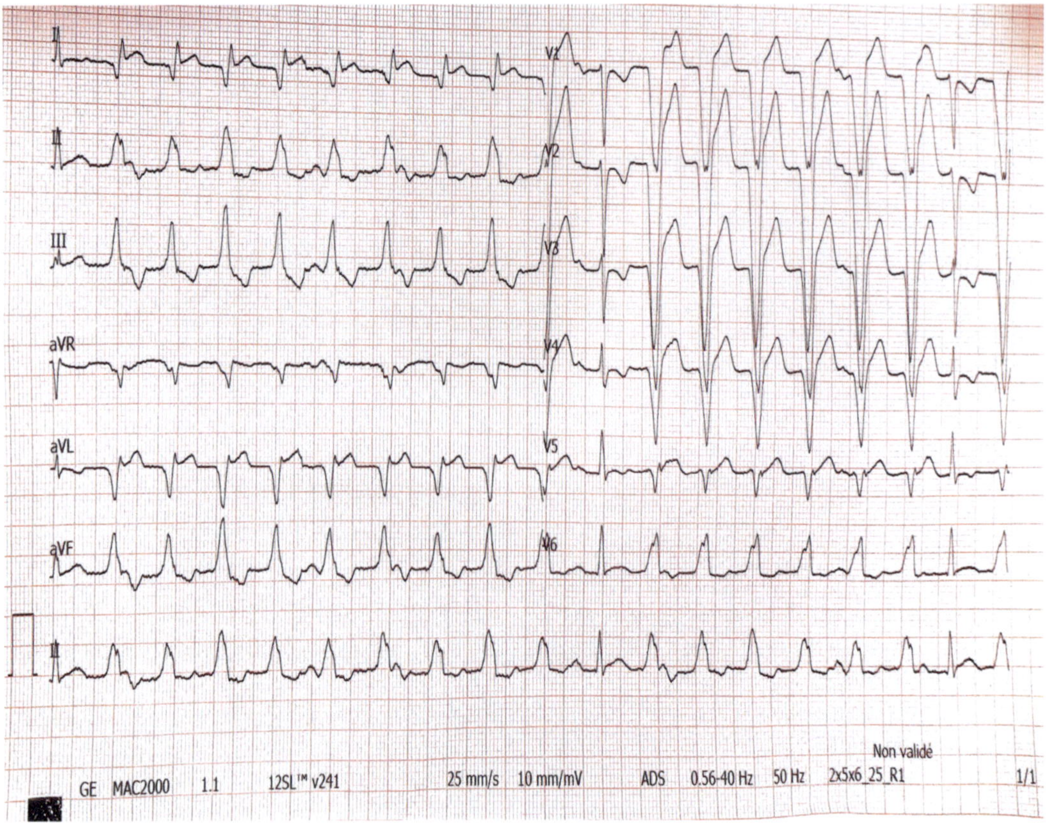

Fig. 1 Twelve-lead ECG recorded during an episode of palpitations

tachycardia, AVNRT, and AVRT) with functional or pre-existing bundle branch block, and antidromic tachycardia (in pre-excitation syndromes).

The morphology of the left bundle branch block of the QRS complex during tachycardia from Fig. 1 might be that of a typical one: the QRS duration is >120 ms; there is a "QS'" pattern in leads V1–V5, with a QRS transition in lead V6; there is an "RSR'" pattern in lead V6; and there is an ST segment and T wave modification opposite to the major deflection of the QRS complex: positive T waves in leads V1–V4. However, there is a "QR" pattern in leads DI and aVL, which is not characteristic of a typical LBBB.

A careful analysis identifies several arguments in favor of a ventricular origin: (1) there is A–V dissociation, best seen in lead II (Fig. 3); (2) there are capture beats (marked with a red star in the ECG explained below: the first, 11th, and 18th QRS complexes); (3) the tachycardia has an LBBB morphology, and the QRS duration is over 160 ms (174 ms) [1]; (4) the QRS complex during tachycardia has deep "Q" waves in leads I and aVL, which is atypical for an SVT with LBBB [2] (Fig. 4); (5) R wave to peak time > 40 ms in lead II and in lead aVR (Fig. 5); and (6) R wave to peak time is greater than 50 ms in lead II [3] (Fig. 5).

Concerning the presence of A–V dissociation during tachycardia, the atrial rate during tachycardia is 64 bpm. Therefore, answer b—"Atrial tachycardia with 2: 1 atrioventricular conduction with left bundle branch block"—can be excluded. This also excludes answer c—"Antidromic tachycardia using a right-sided bypass tract"—since this type of tachycardia requires an A:V relationship of 1:1. AVNRT can exist with an A:V relationship different from 1:1. However, during

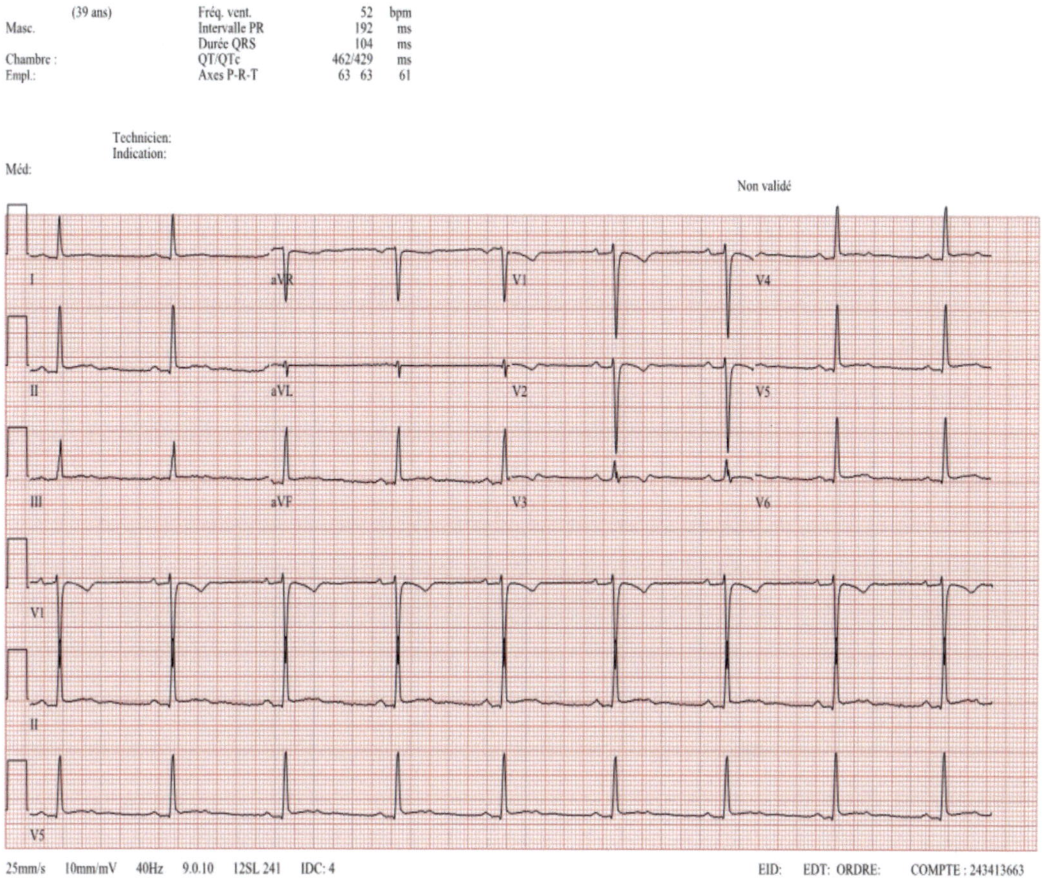

Fig. 2 Twelve-lead ECG recorded in the Cardiology Department after the end of palpitations

AVNRT, the atria are activated from the AV node region, and the P waves on the surface ECG, when visible, are negative. This is not the case for the above-presented ECG, where positive P waves are visible during tachycardia, best seen in lead II. Therefore, answer e—"AVNRT with functional LBBB"—can also be excluded. The heart rate of the tachycardia is 110–120 bpm, which is slightly more than that of an accelerated idioventricular rhythm.

All these arguments point toward answer d—"Monomorphic ventricular tachycardia originating from the right ventricle".

Concerning the second question, related to the underlying heart disease, the second ECG shows a sinus rhythm with a heart rate of 52 bpm; the QRS axis is at +60° (in the normal quadrant). There are negative T waves in leads V1–V3, and the QRS complexes are slightly enlarged (duration of 104 ms). There is no sign in favor of acute ischemia (ST segment elevation or depression) and no sign of myocardial infarction (no pathological Q waves). There is also no sign of left or right ventricular enlargement.

The origin of the tachycardia is most likely compatible with an anterior apical RV origin (the QRS axis is inferior: positive QRS complexes in leads II, III, and aVF, in favor of an origin at the anterior ventricular wall; there is LBBB morphology, in favor of an origin in the right ventricle; there is late QRS transition in the precordial leads – V6, in favor of an origine close to the ventricular apex.) [4]. This element, together with the presence of negative T waves in leads V1–V3, is in favor of arrhythmogenic cardiomyopathy as the underlying disease [5, 6]. Indeed, the patient's

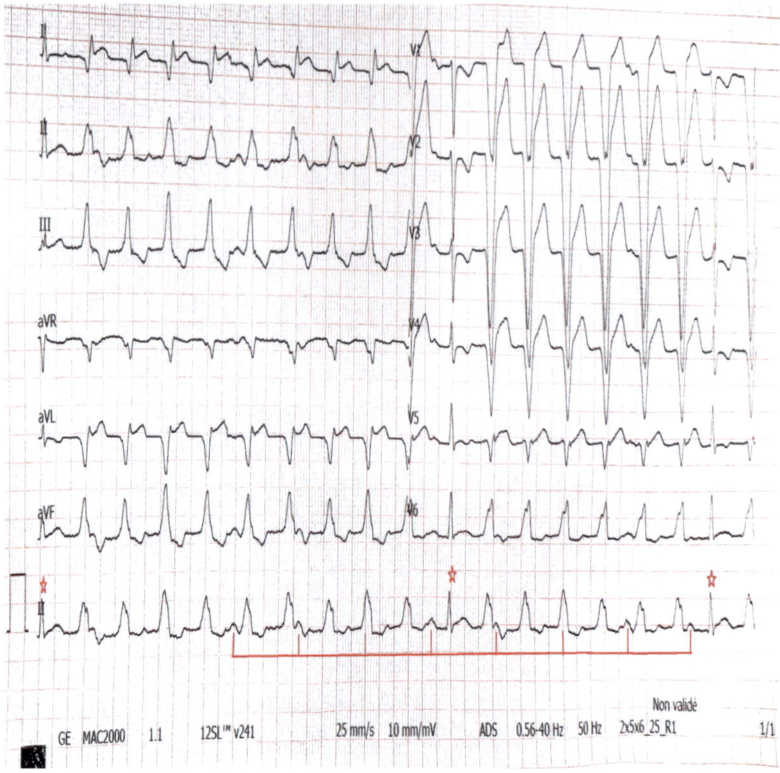

Fig. 3 Twelve-lead ECG (the same from Fig. 1) demonstrating atrioventricular dissociation shown by the red vertical lines in lead II and capture beats indicated by the red star, arguments in favor of ventricular tachycardia

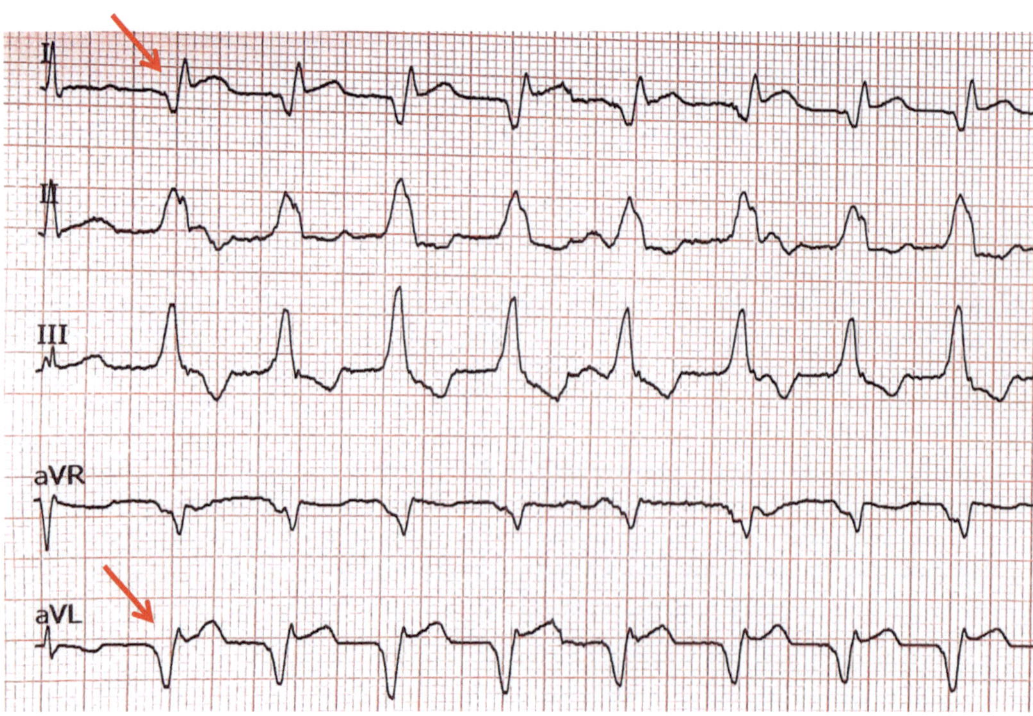

Fig. 4 Leads I, II, III, aVR, and aVL from the ECG from Fig. 1, showing a "QR" pattern in leads I and aVL (red arrows), which is not characteristic for a typical LBBB

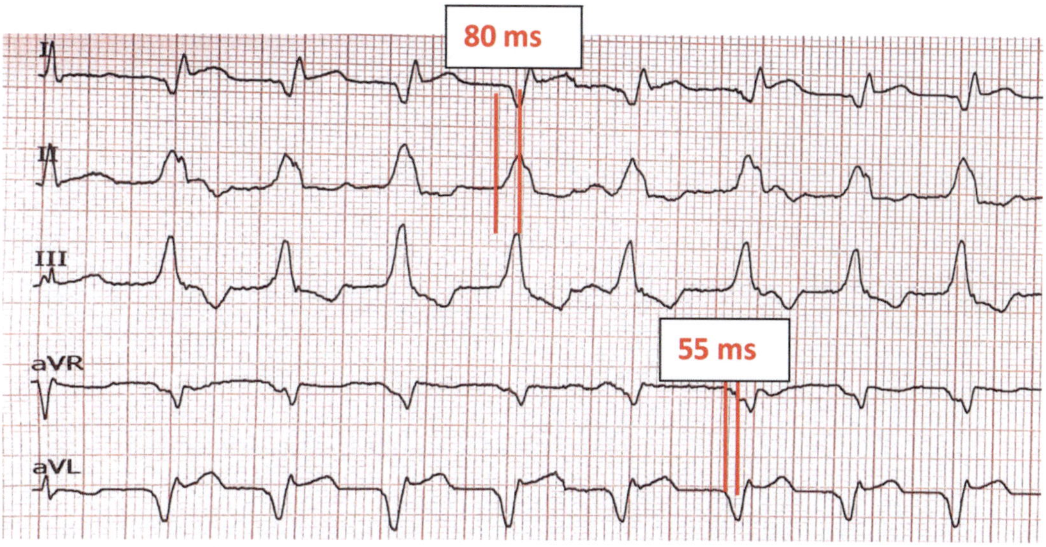

Fig. 5 Leads I, II, III, aVR, and aVL from the ECG from Fig. 1, showing the time to peak of 80 ms in lead II and of 55 ms in lead aVR, argument in favor of ventricular tachycardia

cardiac MRI had shown the presence of a localized aneurysm and dyskinesia in the RVOT and the presence of late gadolinium enhancement at this level, as well as at the level of the RV apex [7]. The patient underwent a catheter ablation procedure of his ventricular tachycardia.

References

1. Wellens HJ, Bar FW, Lie KI. The value of the electrocardiogram in the differential diagnosis of a tachycardia with a widened QRS complex. Am J Med. 1978;64(1):27–33.
2. Surawicz B, Childers R, Deal BJ, Gettes LS, Bailey JJ, Gorgels A, et al. AHA/ACCF/HRS recommendations for the standardization and interpretation of the electrocardiogram: part III: intraventricular conduction disturbances: a scientific statement from the American Heart Association Electrocardiography and Arrhythmias Committee, Council on Clinical Cardiology; the American College of Cardiology Foundation; and the Heart Rhythm Society. Endorsed by the International Society for Computerized Electrocardiology. J Am Coll Cardiol. 2009;53(11):976–81.
3. Pava LF, Perafan P, Badiel M, Arango JJ, Mont L, Morillo CA, et al. R-wave peak time at DII: a new criterion for differentiating between wide complex QRS tachycardias. Heart Rhythm. 2010;7(7):922–6.
4. Mariani MV, Piro A, Della Rocca DG, Forleo GB, Pothineni NV, Romero J, et al. Electrocardiographic criteria for differentiating left from right idiopathic outflow tract ventricular arrhythmias. Arrhythmia Electrophysiol Rev. 2021;10(1):10–6.
5. Haugaa KH, Haland TF, Leren IS, Saberniak J, Edvardsen T. Arrhythmogenic right ventricular cardiomyopathy, clinical manifestations, and diagnosis. Europace. 2016;18(7):965–72.
6. Marcus FI, McKenna WJ, Sherrill D, Basso C, Bauce B, Bluemke DA, et al. Diagnosis of arrhythmogenic right ventricular cardiomyopathy/dysplasia: proposed modification of the Task Force Criteria. Eur Heart J. 2010;31(7):806–14.
7. Corrado D, Zorzi A, Cipriani A, Bauce B, Bariani R, Beffagna G, et al. Evolving diagnostic criteria for arrhythmogenic cardiomyopathy. J Am Heart Assoc. 2021;10(18):e021987.

ECG 7

Gabriel Gusetu

1 Case Presentation

A 58-year-old male patient with a history of ischemic cardiomyopathy with severe LV systolic dysfunction (LVEF of 21%), remote anterior myocardial infarction (2007), implanted with a CRT-D device for the primary prevention of sudden cardiac death, paroxysmal atrial fibrillation, and type 2 diabetes mellitus, presents to the Emergency Department for dyspnea on exertion, bilateral peripheral edema suggesting an episode of decompensated heart failure. His ECG at admittance is presented in Fig. 1.

Question: What is the nature of the tachycardia presented in Fig. 1?

(a) Sinus tachycardia with left bundle branch block
(b) Atrial fibrillation with left bundle branch block
(c) Atrial flutter with left bundle branch block
(d) Bundle branch re-entry ventricular tachycardia
(e) Ventricular tachycardia originating from the inferoseptal LV

Hint: Look at the atrial activity in leads II, III, and aVF.

G. Gusetu (✉)
Department of Cardiology, Hôpital Emile Muller, Mulhouse, France

Correct answer: c. Atrial flutter with left bundle branch block

Explanation: The ECG in Fig. 1 shows an irregular wide QRS complex tachycardia with a heart rate around 120 bpm and LBBB morphology. The width of the QRS complex is 160 ms. The QRS axis is at −30°. The differential diagnosis of this irregular wide QRS complex tachycardia with LBBB morphology includes: ventricular tachycardia (myocardial-related VT, bundle branch re-entry VT) and supraventricular tachycardia (atrial fibrillation, atrial flutter, atrial tachycardia, AVNRT, and AVRT) with functional or pre-existing left bundle branch block. Antidromic tachycardia (in pre-excitation syndromes) is generally regular and is less likely present in this case.

The morphology of the left bundle branch block of the QRS complex during tachycardia from Fig. 1 is a typical one: the QRS duration is >120 ms; there is a monomorphic R wave in leads I, aVL, and V6; there are no q waves in lead V6; and there is ST segment and T wave modification opposite to the major deflection of the QRS complex: ST segment elevation with positive T waves in leads V1 to V4. The aspect in lead V1 is "QS", with an "rS" morphology in leads V2 and V3, with an r wave amplitude of <0.04 ms

L. Muresan (ed.), *ECG Interpretation of Wide QRS Complex Tachycardia*,
https://doi.org/10.1007/978-3-031-97030-6_8

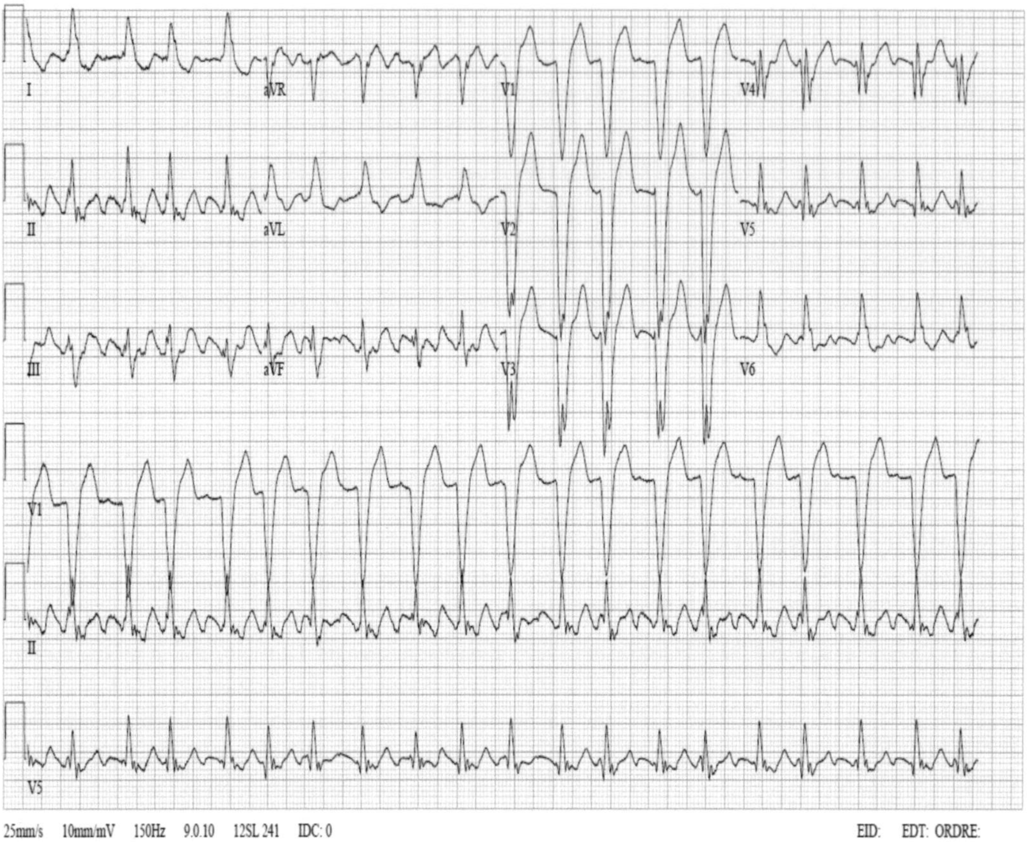

Fig. 1 Twelve-lead ECG recorded at admittance to the Cardiology Department

[1]. This suggests that the tachycardia is likely an SVT with LBBB.

Applying the Brugada algorithm [2] to the tachycardia from Fig. 1, it can be seen that: (1) There is no absence of an RS complex in the precordial leads (otherwise said, there are rS complexes in leads V2 to V4); we therefore move to the second step of the algorithm: (2) This step analyzes the absence of an R to S interval > 100 ms in any precordial lead. This is not the case. Step 3 of the algorithm looks for A–V dissociation. If we analyze the atrial activity, we can see that the atrial rhythm is actually atrial flutter, with negative F waves being present in leads II, III, and aVF (see Fig. 2). The A:V conduction is variable, which explains the variable RR interval. Therefore, answer a—"Sinus tachycardia with left bundle branch block"—and answer b—"Atrial fibrillation with left bundle branch block"—are not correct.

For a wide QRS complex tachycardia with LBBB, arguments in favor of VT are: the presence of an "r wave" > 0.04 s in lead V1 or V2, which is not the case in the ECG presented in Fig. 1. The presence of a notch on the downside of the S wave in lead V1 or V2 is also not the case (see Fig. 3). And the presence of a delayed S nadir >0.06 s in lead V1 or V2 is not the case [3] (see Fig. 4).

Another argument in favor of ventricular tachycardia for an LBBB QRS morphology would be a QRS duration of over 160 ms [4], which is not the case.

Therefore, according to the Brugada algorithm, there are no criteria in favor of VT, and the diagnosis is SVT with LBBB.

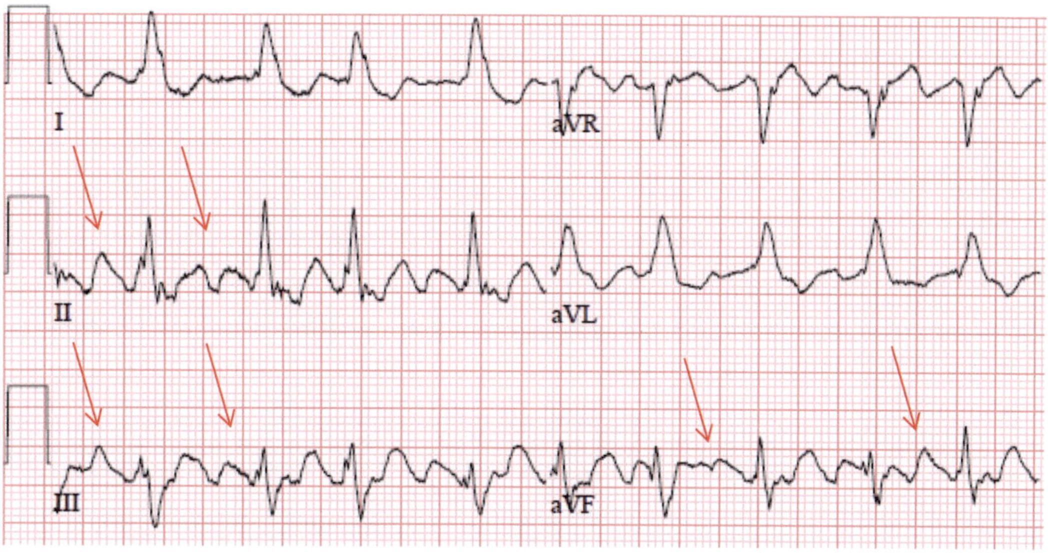

Fig. 2 Limb leads from the ECG in Fig. 1 demonstrating atrial flutter (red arrows point to the negative F waves from leads II, III, and aVF)

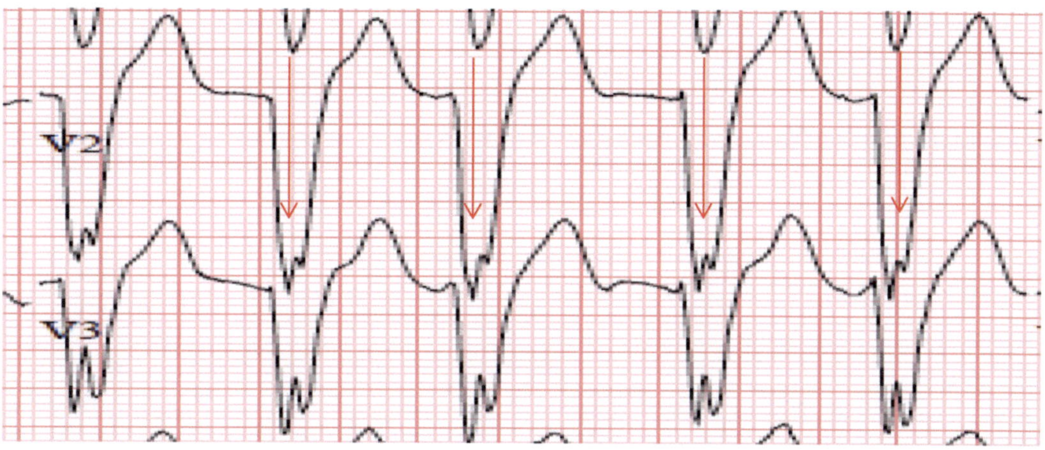

Fig. 3 Leads V2 and V3 from the ECG from Fig. 1 showing the presence of a notch on the ascending part of the S wave of the QRS complex in V2 (not to be mistaken with Josephson's sign, which is a notch on the descending part of the S wave), criterion not favoring ventricular tachycardia

The Vereckei algorithm [5] for the differential diagnosis of wide QRS complex tachycardias also suggests SVT with BBB as the correct answer. The first step of the algorithm looks for A–V dissociation, which is not evaluable on the present ECG since the atrial rhythm is atrial flutter. The second step of the algorithm looks for an initial predominant R wave in lead aVR, which, again, is not the case. The third step "QRS morphology unlike BBB or fascicular block" suggests SVT (atrial flutter) with BBB, based on the arguments explained above.

The Basel algorithm [6] also suggests SVT with BBB as the correct answer. There is only one criterion present in favor of the ventricular origin of the wide QRS complex tachycardia: clinical high-risk features (a history of myocardial infarction and an LVEF of <35%). The other criteria: the time to first peak in lead II of >40 ms (Fig. 5) and the time to first peak in lead aVR of

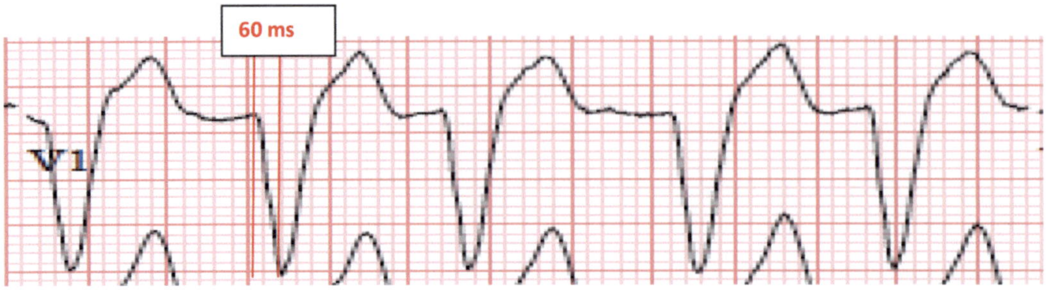

Fig. 4 Lead V1 from the ECG from Fig. 1 showing the presence of a delayed S nadir > 0.06 s in lead V1, argument in favor of ventricular tachycardia

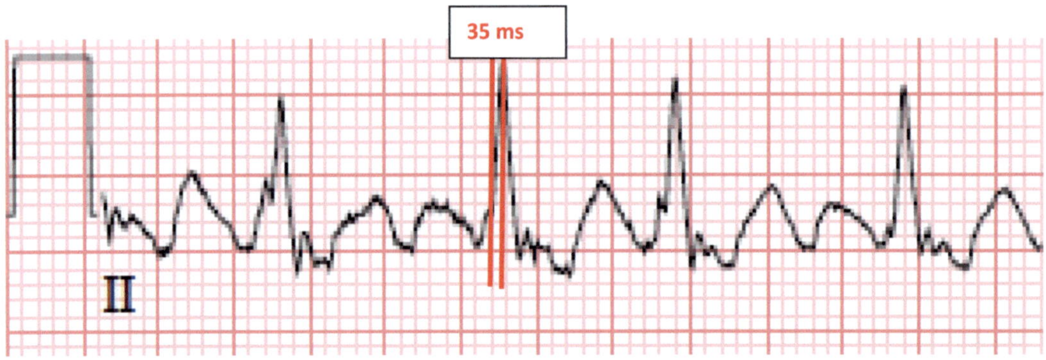

Fig. 5 Lead II from the ECG from Fig. 1 showing the time to first peak of 35 ms, argument not in favor of ventricular tachycardia

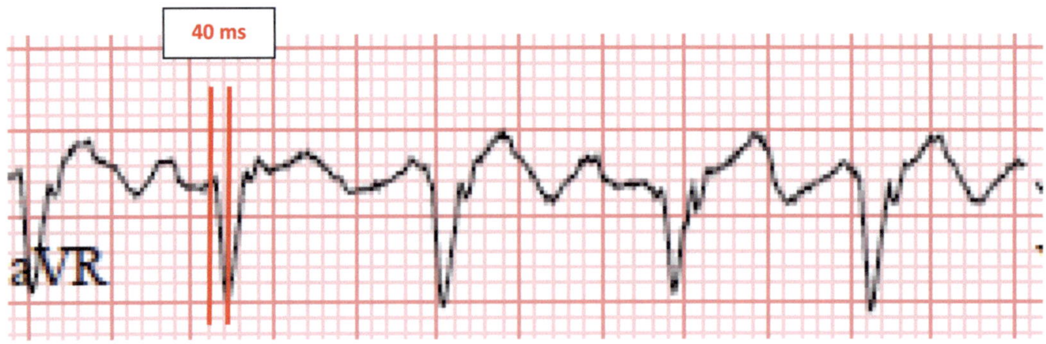

Fig. 6 Lead aVR from the ECG from Fig. 1 showing the time to first peak of 40 ms, argument not in favor of ventricular tachycardia

>40 ms (Fig. 6) are not present on the ECG from Fig. 1. In the Basel algorithm, the diagnosis of ventricular tachycardia can be established if at least two criteria are present, which is not the present case.

Therefore, all the three algorithms (Brugada, Vereckei, and the Basel) favor the diagnosis of atrial flutter with variable A:V conduction and LBBB.

The patient underwent an electrophysiological study which confirmed the diagnosis of typical counterclockwise atrial flutter with left bundle branch block. Catheter ablation of the cavo-tricuspid isthmus was successfully performed,

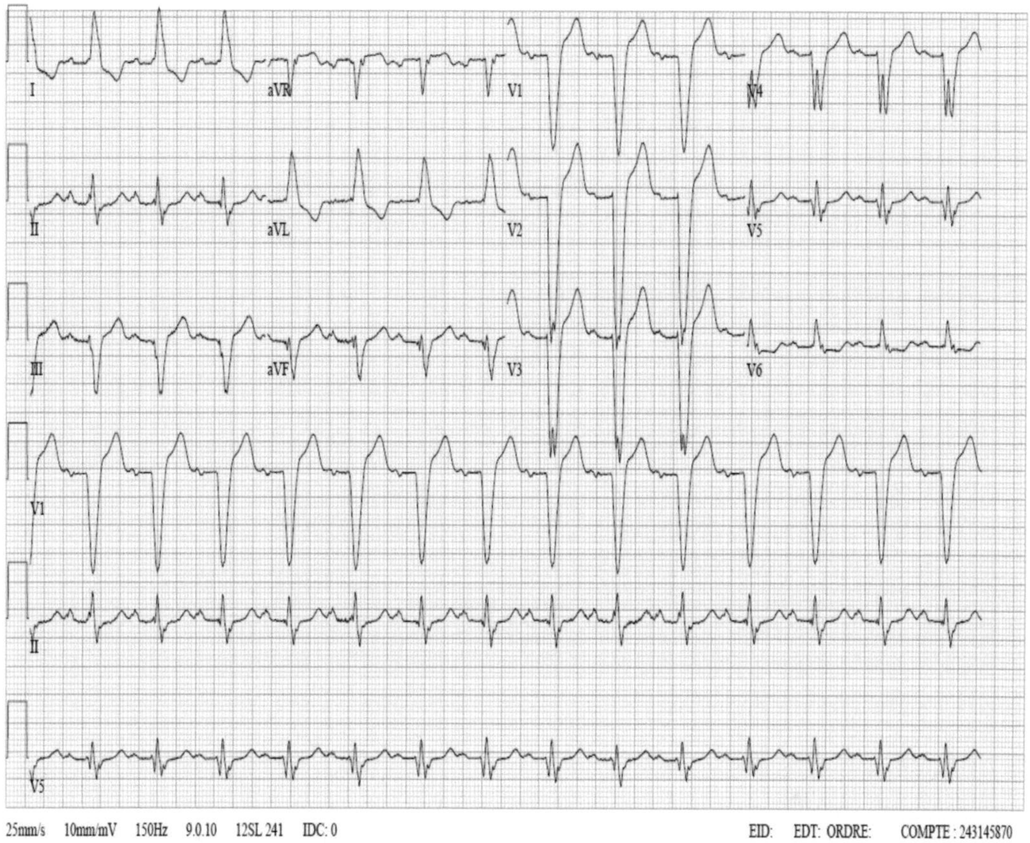

Fig. 7 Twelve-lead ECG recorded after catheter ablation of atrial flutter showing sinus rhythm with LBBB and first-degree AV block. The morphology of the QRS complex is identical to the one from Fig. 1

and the sinus rhythm was restored. An ECG of the patient after catheter ablation of atrial flutter is presented in Fig. 7.

References

1. Surawicz B, Childers R, Deal BJ, Gettes LS, Bailey JJ, Gorgels A, et al. AHA/ACCF/HRS recommendations for the standardization and interpretation of the electrocardiogram: part III: intraventricular conduction disturbances: a scientific statement from the American Heart Association Electrocardiography and Arrhythmias Committee, Council on Clinical Cardiology; the American College of Cardiology Foundation; and the Heart Rhythm Society. Endorsed by the International Society for Computerized Electrocardiology. J Am Coll Cardiol. 2009;53(11):976–81.
2. Brugada P, Brugada J, Mont L, Smeets J, Andries EW. A new approach to the differential diagnosis of a regular tachycardia with a wide QRS complex. Circulation. 1991;83(5):1649–59.
3. Kindwall KE, Brown J, Josephson ME. Electrocardiographic criteria for ventricular tachycardia in wide complex left bundle branch block morphology tachycardias. Am J Cardiol. 1988;61(15):1279–83.
4. Eckardt L, Breithardt G, Kirchhof P. Approach to wide complex tachycardias in patients without structural heart disease. Heart. 2006;92(5):704–11.
5. Vereckei A, Duray G, Szenasi G, Altemose GT, Miller JM. Application of a new algorithm in the differential diagnosis of wide QRS complex tachycardia. Eur Heart J. 2007;28(5):589–600.
6. Moccetti F, Yadava M, Latifi Y, Strebel I, Pavlovic N, Knecht S, et al. Simplified integrated clinical and electrocardiographic algorithm for differentiation of wide QRS complex tachycardia: the Basel algorithm. JACC Clin Electrophysiol. 2022;8(7):831–9.

ECG 8

Gabriel Cismaru

1 Case Presentation

An 82-year-old male patient with a history of ischemic dilated cardiomyopathy with severe LV dysfunction (LVEF of 22%), remote anterior myocardial infarction, implanted with a dual chamber ICD for the primary prevention of sudden cardiac death, severe degenerative aortic stenosis treated with surgical aortic valve replacement (bioprothesis), and ischemic stroke is admitted to the Emergency Department for palpitations and pre-syncope. A 12-lead ECG was recorded at admittance and is presented in Fig. 1. An ECG after the termination of the tachycardia is presented in Fig. 2.

Question What is the nature of the tachycardia presented in Fig. 1?

(a) Atrial fibrillation with right bundle branch block
(b) Ventricular tachycardia originating from the anterolateral wall of the left ventricle
(c) Ventricular tachycardia originating from the inferolateral wall of the left ventricle
(d) Antidromic tachycardia using a left-sided by-pass tract
(e) Orthodromic reciprocating tachycardia with functional right bundle branch block

Correct answer c. Ventricular tachycardia originating from the inferolateral wall of the left ventricle.

Explanation The ECG during tachycardia shows an irregular wide QRS complex tachycardia with a heart rate of 142 bpm. The width of the QRS complex is 204 ms. There is an extreme (north-west) axis deviation. The differential diagnosis of this wide QRS complex tachycardia with RBBB morphology includes: ventricular tachycardia (myocardial-related VT, bundle branch reentry VT), supraventricular tachycardia (atrial fibrillation, atrial flutter, atrial tachycardia, AVNRT, and AVRT) with functional or pre-existing bundle branch block and antidromic tachycardia (in pre-excitation syndromes).

The ECG in Fig. 2 shows atrial and ventricular paced rhythms, with a heart rate of 70 bpm (small pacing spikes can be observed preceding P waves and QRS complexes, best seen in lead V1). There is no short PR interval in favor of ventricular pre-excitation.

The morphology of the right bundle branch block of the QRS complex during tachycardia from Figs. 1 and 2 is not that of a typical one: the QRS duration is indeed of 120 ms, and the QRS

G. Cismaru (✉)
Department of Cardiology, Rehabilitation Hospital, Cluj-Napoca, Romania

L. Muresan (ed.), *ECG Interpretation of Wide QRS Complex Tachycardia*,
https://doi.org/10.1007/978-3-031-97030-6_9

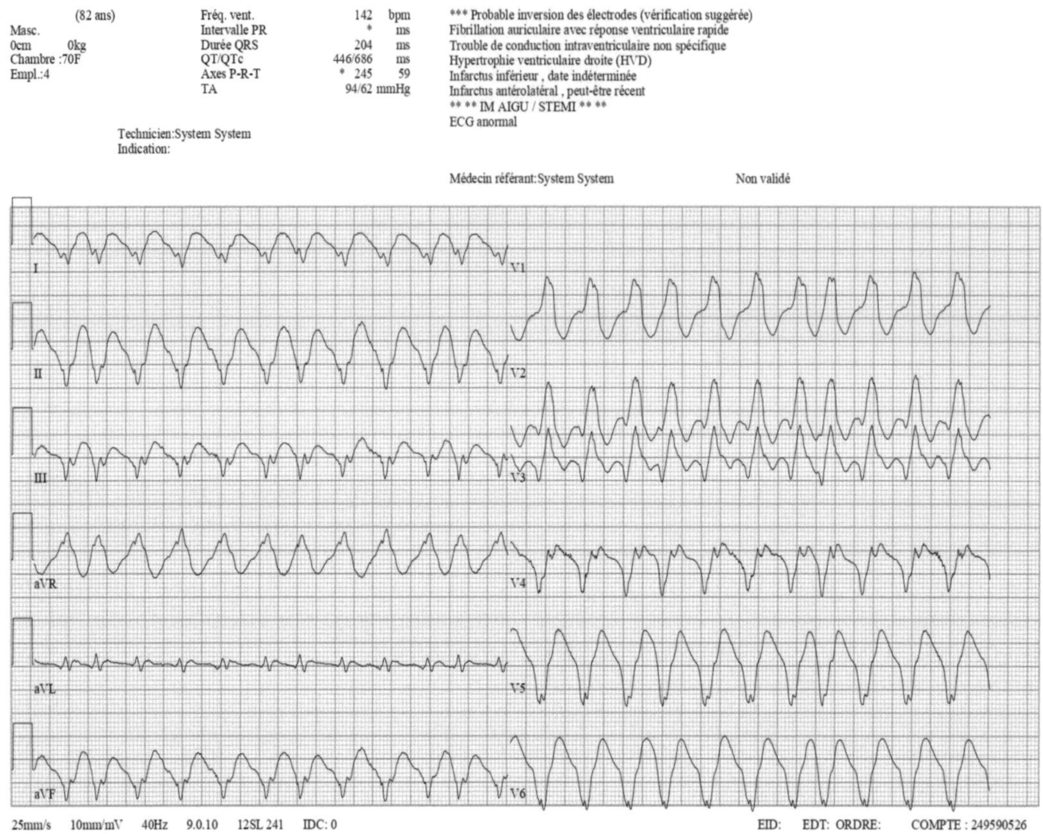

Fig. 1 ECG recorded at admittance to the Emergency Department

complex is clearly positive in lead V1. However, the QRS complex has a "QS" morphology in leads V4 to V6, and especially in leads I and aVL, elements which are not in favor of a typical right bundle branch block. This makes SVT with RBBB highly unlikely.

Applying the Brugada algorithm [1] for the tachycardia presented in the first ECG, it can be seen that: 1. There are no RS complexes in any of the precordial leads, which strongly suggests the diagnosis of ventricular tachycardia.

The Vereckei algorithm [2] for the differential diagnosis of wide QRS complex tachycardias also suggests VT as the correct answer. The first step of the algorithm looks for A–V dissociation, which is not seen on the present ECG. The second step of the algorithm looks for an initial predominant R wave in lead aVR, which is clearly the case (Fig. 3).

The simplified Vereckei algorithm also suggests VT as the correct diagnosis, based on the presence of a positive initial R wave in lead aVR [3] (Fig. 3).

The Basel algorithm [4] is also in favor of ventricular tachycardia as the right answer. According to this algorithm, a positive diagnosis of VT is established if at least two out of three criteria are present: 1. structural heart disease (history of myocardial infarction, congestive heart failure (LVEF <35%)), the presence of an ICD and CRT, which the patient has (ischemic cardiomyopathy, history of myocardial infarction, with LVEF of 22%), and is an ICD carrier; 2. the time to first peak in lead II > 40 ms (Fig. 4); and 3. the time to first peak in lead aVR > 40 ms (Fig. 5) [4].

Other arguments in favor of a ventricular origin of the tachycardia are: 1. The fact that the QRS morphology during tachycardia is not compatible with a typical right bundle branch block, making SVT with RBBB unlikely [5]. 2. The QRS width of 204 ms (more than 140 ms) for

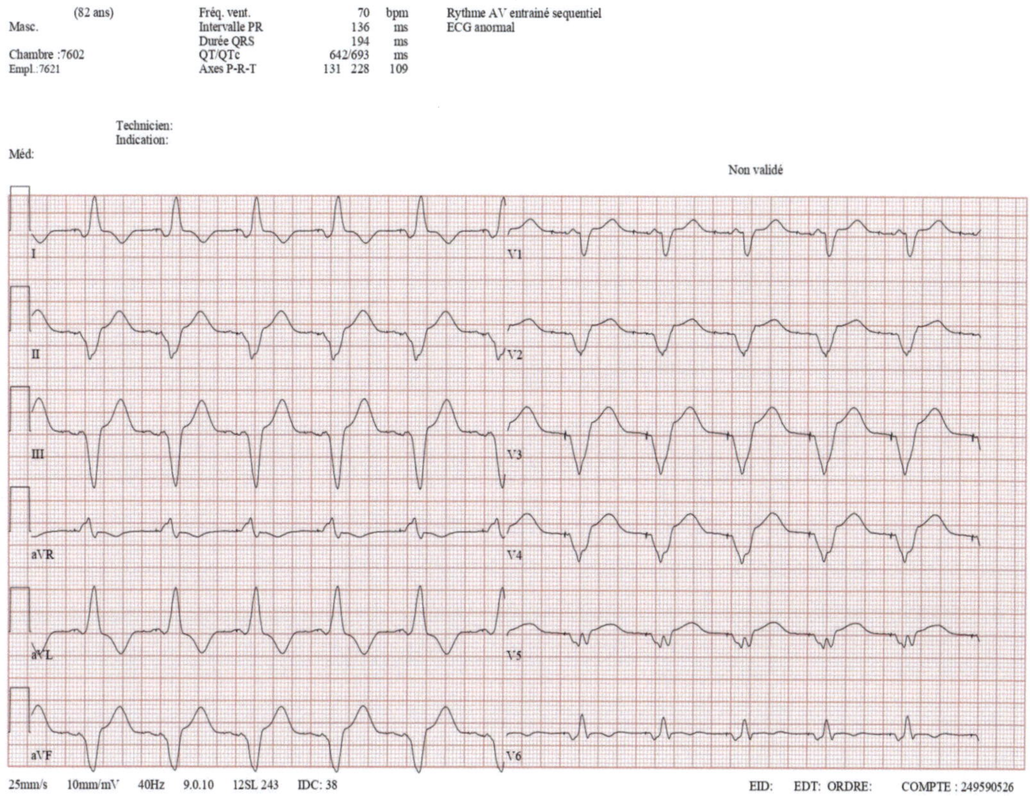

Fig. 2 ECG recorded after the end of the tachycardia

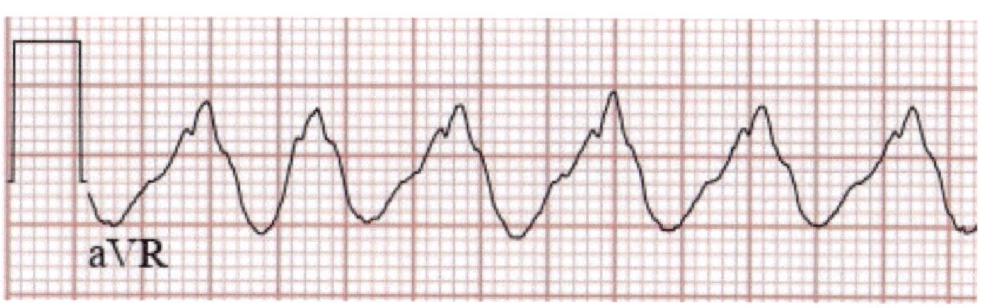

Fig. 3 Lead aVR from the ECG from Fig. 1 showing the presence of a tall initial R wave, criterion in favor of ventricular tachycardia

an RBBB tachycardia [6]. 3. Extreme (northwest) axis deviation [7]; 3. the presence of a "QS" pattern in lead V6 for an RBBB tachycardia [1]. 4. The rabbit ear sign [1]: in lead V1, the amplitude of the initial R wave is greater than that of the R' wave (Fig. 6). 5. Brugada's sign: the time from the onset of QRS to the nadir (the deepest point) of S wave >100 ms, best seen in lead V6 (Fig. 7).

Based on all these observations, the tachycardia presented in Fig. 1 is therefore ventricular tachycardia.

An interesting observation is the fact that the ventricular tachycardia from Fig. 1 is irregular, possibly suggesting atrial fibrillation with RBBB. However, all the abovementioned criteria favor the diagnosis of VT, and, as it is well known, VT can sometimes be irregular [8].

The origin of the ventricular tachycardia is most likely at the level of: 1. The LV: the tachycardia has an RBBB morphology; 2. The inferior wall of the LV: "QS" aspect in leads II, III, and aVF; 3. The lateral wall of the LV: "QS" aspect in leads I and aVL; 4. The middle segment of the

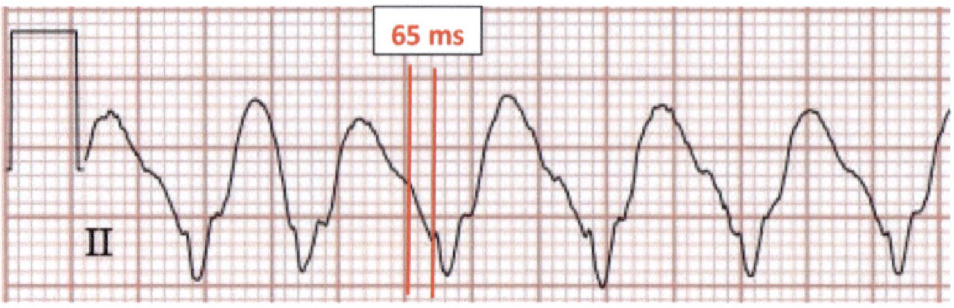

Fig. 4 Lead II from the ECG from Fig. 1 showing the time to first peak of 65 ms, criterion in favor of ventricular tachycardia

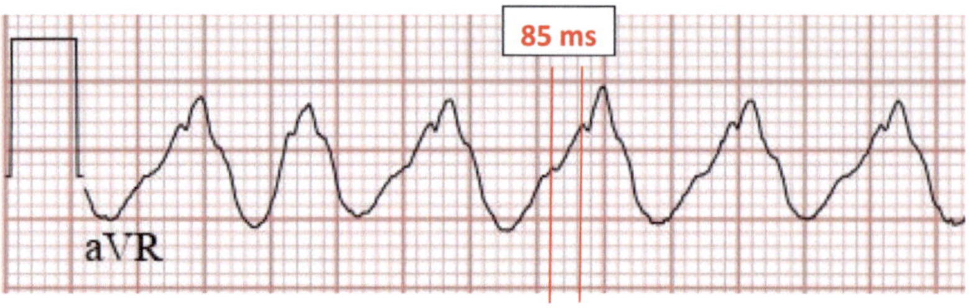

Fig. 5 Lead aVR from the ECG from Fig. 1 showing the time to first peak of 85 ms, criterion in favor of ventricular tachycardia

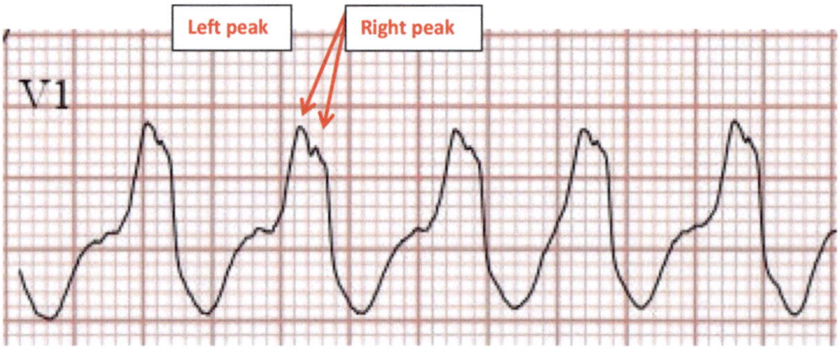

Fig. 6 Lead V1 from the ECG from Fig. 1 showing the "rabbit ear" sign, argument in favor of ventricular tachycardia

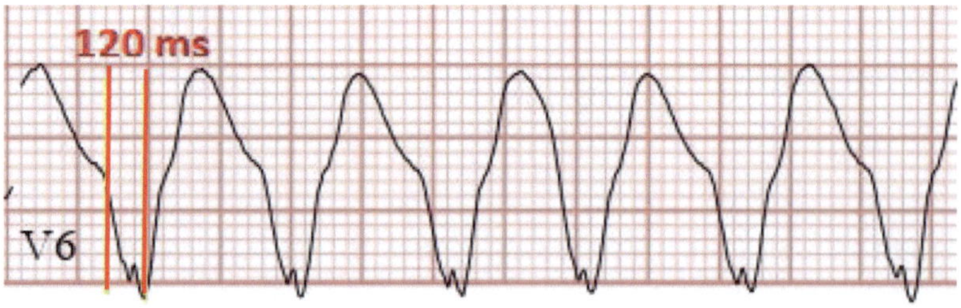

Fig. 7 Lead V6 during the wide QRS complex tachycardia, showing Brugada's sign (see text for explanation), an argument in favor of ventricular tachycardia

lateral LV wall: tall R waves from V1 to V3, with an abrupt transition in V4. Putting this information together, the origin is at the level of the inferolateral middle area of the LV wall.

The patient underwent an electrophysiological study which confirmed the diagnosis of VT and a catheter ablation procedure was subsequently performed.

References

1. Brugada P, Brugada J, Mont L, Smeets J, Andries EW. A new approach to the differential diagnosis of a regular tachycardia with a wide QRS complex. Circulation. 1991;83(5):1649–59.
2. Vereckei A, Duray G, Szenasi G, Altemose GT, Miller JM. Application of a new algorithm in the differential diagnosis of wide QRS complex tachycardia. Eur Heart J. 2007;28(5):589–600.

3. Vereckei A, Duray G, Szenasi G, Altemose GT, Miller JM. New algorithm using only lead aVR for differential diagnosis of wide QRS complex tachycardia. Heart Rhythm. 2008;5(1):89–98.
4. Moccetti F, Yadava M, Latifi Y, Strebel I, Pavlovic N, Knecht S, et al. Simplified integrated clinical and electrocardiographic algorithm for differentiation of wide QRS complex tachycardia: the Basel algorithm. JACC Clin Electrophysiol. 2022;8(7):831–9.
5. Surawicz B, Childers R, Deal BJ, Gettes LS, Bailey JJ, Gorgels A, et al. AHA/ACCF/HRS recommendations for the standardization and interpretation of the electrocardiogram: part III: intraventricular conduction disturbances: a scientific statement from the American Heart Association Electrocardiography and Arrhythmias Committee, Council on Clinical Cardiology; the American College of Cardiology Foundation; and the Heart Rhythm Society. Endorsed by the International Society for Computerized Electrocardiology. J Am Coll Cardiol. 2009;53(11):976–81.
6. Eckardt L, Breithardt G, Kirchhof P. Approach to wide complex tachycardias in patients without structural heart disease. Heart. 2006;92(5):704–11.
7. Wellens HJ. Electrophysiology: ventricular tachycardia: diagnosis of broad QRS complex tachycardia. Heart. 2001;86(5):579–85.
8. Oreto G, Satullo G, Luzza F, Donato A, Scimone IM, Cavalli A. Irregular ventricular tachycardia: a possible manifestation of longitudinal dissociation within the reentry pathway. Am Heart J. 1992;124(6):1506–11.

ECG 9

Radu Rosu

1 Case Presentation

A 51-year-old male patient presents to the Cardiology Department for three episodes of palpitations with sudden onset accompanied by nausea and vomiting, the last occurring during a 3 h flight that took place on the day of presentation to the hospital. He had no significant past medical history, and he was not on any chronic medication. A 12-lead ECG was recorded (Fig. 1).

Question: What is the nature of the tachycardia presented in Fig. 1?

(a) Ventricular tachycardia originating from the superolateral wall of the left ventricle
(b) Atrial flutter with 1: 1 atrioventricular conduction and right bundle branch block
(c) Antidromic tachycardia using a left-sided by-pass tract
(d) Orthodromic reciprocating tachycardia with functional right bundle branch block
(e) Ventricular tachycardia originating from the inferolateral wall of the left ventricle

Continuation: Adenosine triphosphate was repeatedly administered (up to 30 mg iv), without any effect. Amiodarone 300 mg iv was then administered and Lidocaine 80 mg iv bolus, but the tachycardia persisted. Electrical cardioversion was then subsequently performed. The ECG post-cardioversion is presented in Fig. 2. A transthoracic echocardiography was then performed, showing moderate left ventricular dysfunction (LVEF of 45%) and moderate global hypokinesia.

Correct answer: e. Ventricular tachycardia originating from the inferolateral wall of the left ventricle.

Explanation: The first ECG shows a regular wide QRS complex tachycardia with a heart rate of 210 bpm. The width of the QRS complex is 160 ms (Fig. 3).

The differential diagnosis of this wide QRS complex tachycardia with RBBB includes: ventricular tachycardia (myocardial-related VT, bundle branch re-entry VT, and fascicular VT), supraventricular tachycardia (atrial fibrillation, atrial flutter, atrial tachycardia, AVNRT, and AVRT) with functional bundle branch block, and antidromic tachycardia (in pre-excitation syndromes).

The ECG in sinus rhythm can sometimes provide valuable clues concerning the most likely and the most unlikely nature of the tachycardia.

R. Rosu (✉)
Department of Cardiology, Rehabilitation Hospital, Cluj-Napoca, Romania

L. Muresan (ed.), *ECG Interpretation of Wide QRS Complex Tachycardia*,
https://doi.org/10.1007/978-3-031-97030-6_10

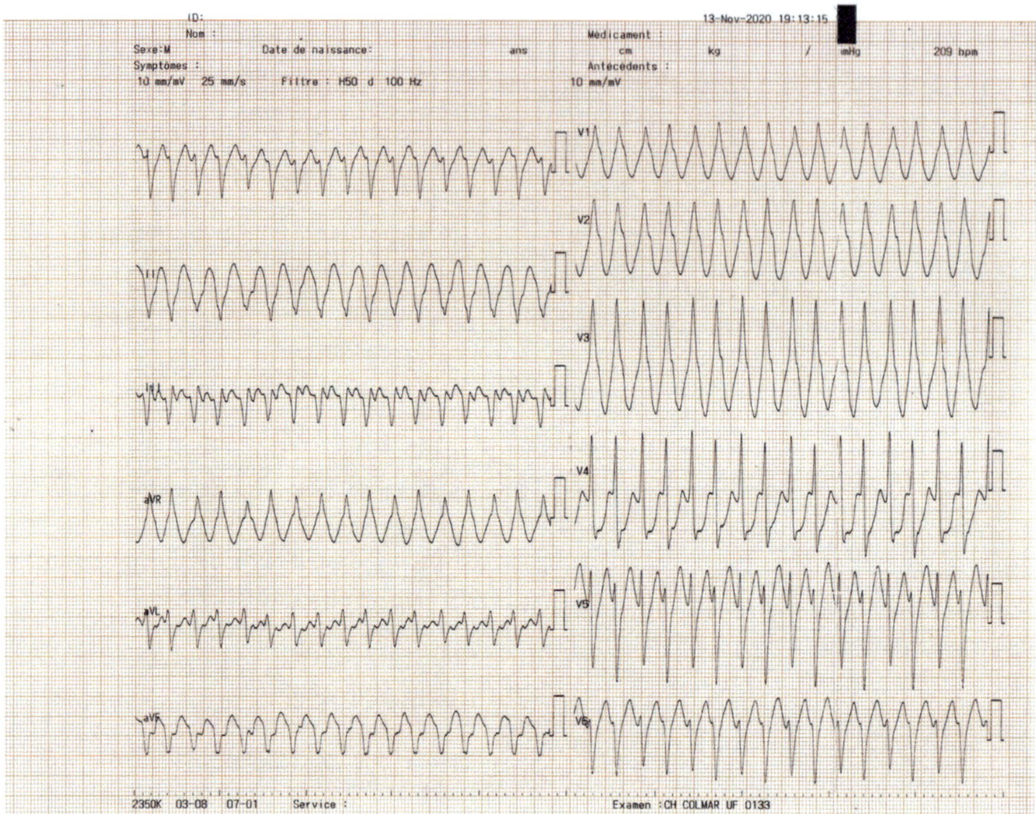

Fig. 1 ECG recorded during the wide QRS complex tachycardia

In the present case, the ECG in Fig. 2 shows sinus rhythm with a heart rate of 54 bpm (sinus bradycardia), QRS axis at +60°, absence of hypertrophy, biphasic T waves in lead V4, negative T waves in leads V5 and V6, DII, DIII, and aVF in favor of myocardial ischemia. There are no pathological Q waves in favor of an old myocardial infarction and no elements in favor of ventricular pre-excitation (short PR interval and delta waves). The absence of ventricular pre-excitation makes antidromic tachycardia less likely (but not impossible, since transient pre-excitation not recorded on this ECG could still be the case). There is also no RBBB, in favor of an SVT with pre-existing RBBB.

The morphology of the right bundle branch block of the QRS complex during tachycardia from Figs. 1 and 2 is not that of a typical one: the QRS duration is indeed >120 ms, and the QRS complex is clearly positive in lead V1. However, the QRS complex has an "rS" morphology in lead V6, which is not in favor of a typical right bundle branch block. This makes SVT with RBBB unlikely.

Applying the Brugada algorithm [1] to the ECG from Fig. 1, it can be seen that: 1. There is no absence of an RS complex in the precordial leads (otherwise said, there are RS complexes in leads V4 to V6). 2. There is no R to S interval > 100 ms in any precordial lead (Fig. 4). 3. There is no AV dissociation visible. Therefore, we need to move to the fourth step of the algorithm and analyze the morphology of the QRS complexes during tachycardia.

For an RBBB morphology wide QRS complex tachycardia, an argument in favor of VT would be the presence of a taller left peak of the QRS complex in lead V1 (the rabbit ear sign) or for biphasic RS or QR complexes, which is not the case. Next, in lead V6, an argument in favor

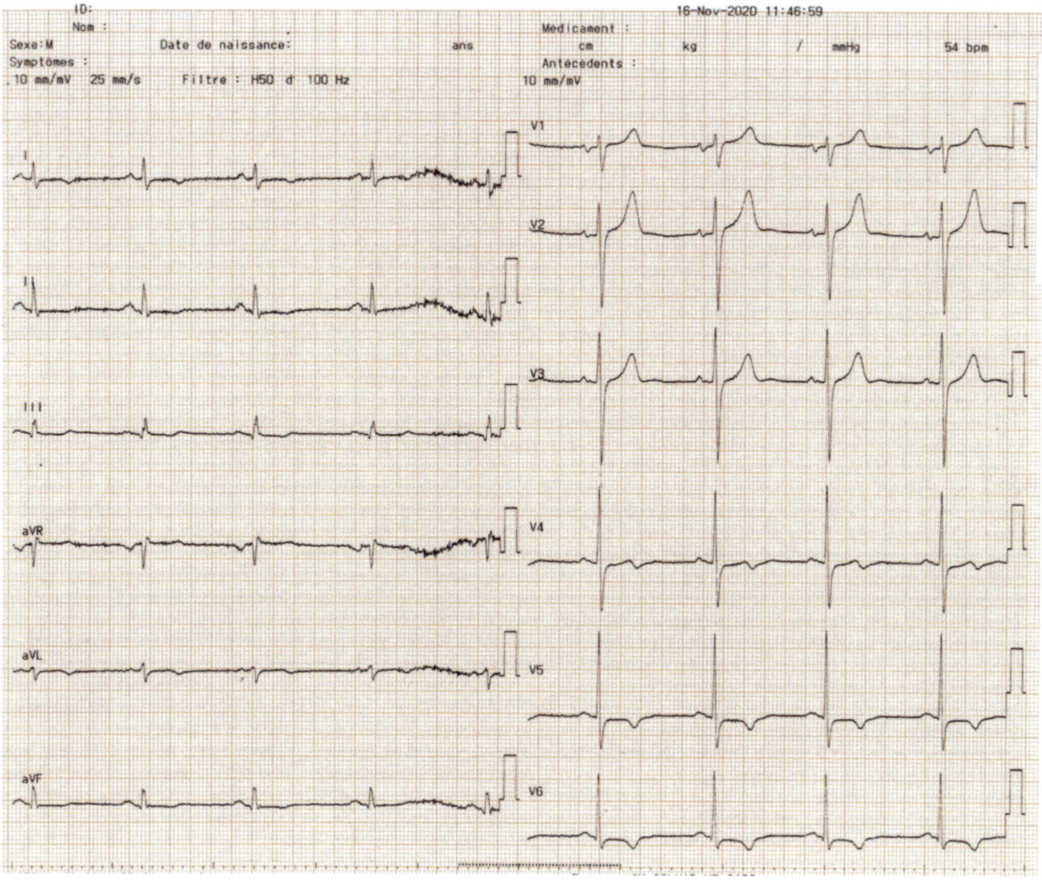

Fig. 2 ECG recorded during sinus rhythm, after electrical cardioversion

of VT would be the presence of an "rS" complex, which is actually the case (Fig. 5). This is therefore an argument in favor of VT. This can also be expressed as a ratio of R/S < 1 in lead V6.

The simplified Vereckei algorithm also suggests VT as the correct diagnosis, based on the presence of a positive initial R wave in lead aVR [2] (Fig. 6).

The Basel algorithm [3] is also in favor of ventricular tachycardia as the right answer. According to this algorithm, a positive diagnosis of VT is established if at least two out of three criteria are present: 1. structural heart disease (history of myocardial infarction, congestive heart failure (LVEF <35%), the presence of an ICD and CRT), which is not found in the present patient; 2. the time to first peak in lead II > 40 ms (Fig. 7); and 3. the time to first peak in lead aVR > 40 ms (Fig. 8) [3].

Other arguments in favor of ventricular tachycardia are: 1. The fact that the QRS morphology during tachycardia is not compatible with the typical right bundle branch block [4], making SVT with RBBB unlikely. 2. A QRS duration >140 ms for a wide QRS complex tachycardia with RBBB. Based on all these observations, the tachycardia presented in Fig. 1 is therefore ventricular tachycardia.

Atrial fibrillation with RBBB would demonstrate an irregular rhythm, which is not the case. Atrial flutter with 1:1 atrioventricular conduction would have a heart rate of around 260–280 bpm. An argument against any SVT with RBBB, as mentioned above, is the fact that the morphology

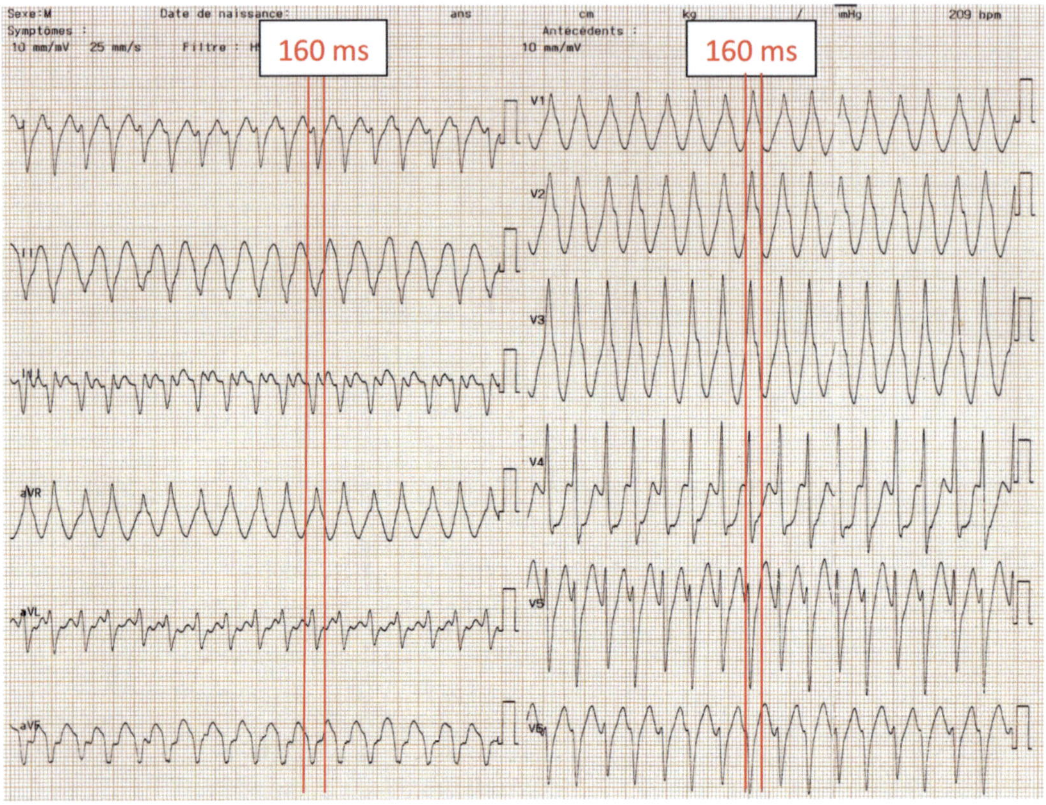

Fig. 3 ECG recorded during the wide QRS complex tachycardia showing the QRS duration of 160 ms

of the wide QRS complex tachycardia is not that of a typical RBBB, making any SVT with functional BBB unlikely.

The origin of the ventricular tachycardia is most likely at the level of: 1. The LV: the tachycardia has an RBBB morphology. 2. The inferior wall of the LV: "QS" aspect in leads II and aVF. 3. The lateral wall of the LV: "rS" aspect in lead I and aVL. 4. The middle segment of the lateral LV wall: tall R waves from V1 to V3 with a transition in V4. Putting this information together, the origin is at the level of the inferolateral LV wall, in its middle third.

The patient underwent coronary angiography, which showed the absence of any significant stenosis at the level of the epicardial coronary arteries. A cardiac MRI demonstrated the absence of myocardial necrosis but the presence of subepicardial zones of late gadolinium enhancement, compatible the with sequelae of myocarditis.

The patient underwent an electrophysiological study which demonstrated the ventricular nature of the tachycardia and successful radiofrequency catheter ablation (epicardial ablation was necessary to terminate the tachycardia and render it noninducible).

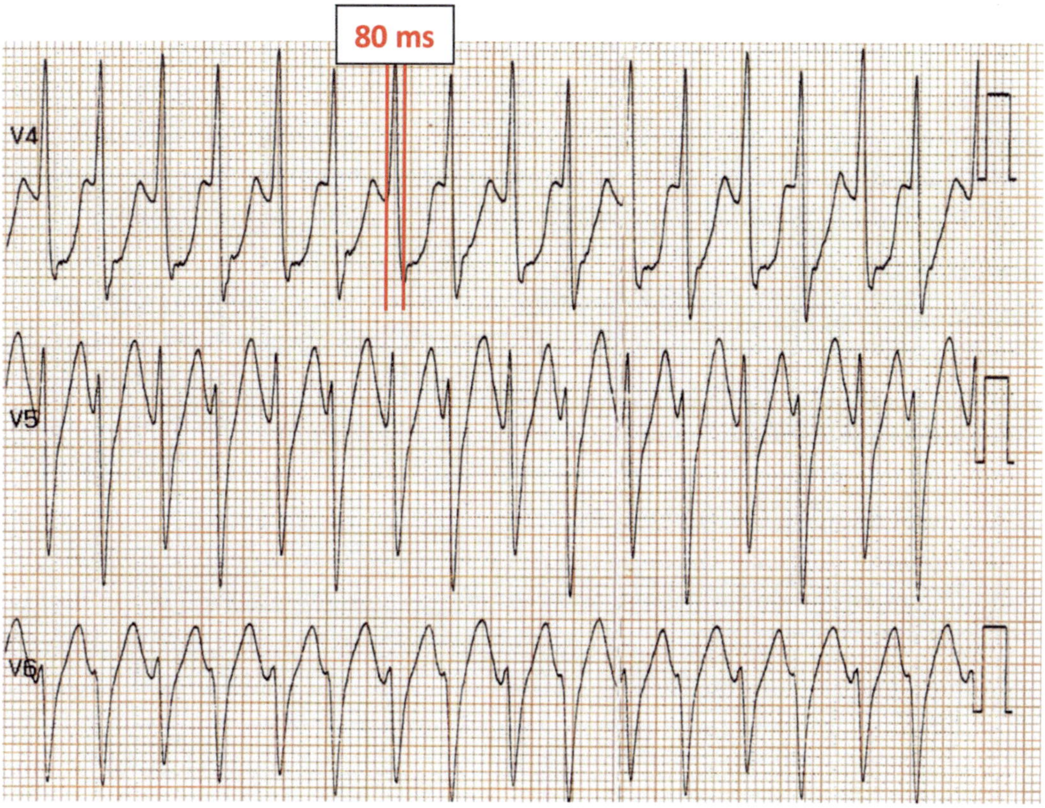

Fig. 4 Precordial leads V4, V5, and V6 showing the presence of an RS interval of 80 ms, not in favor of ventricular tachycardia (but not excluding it either)

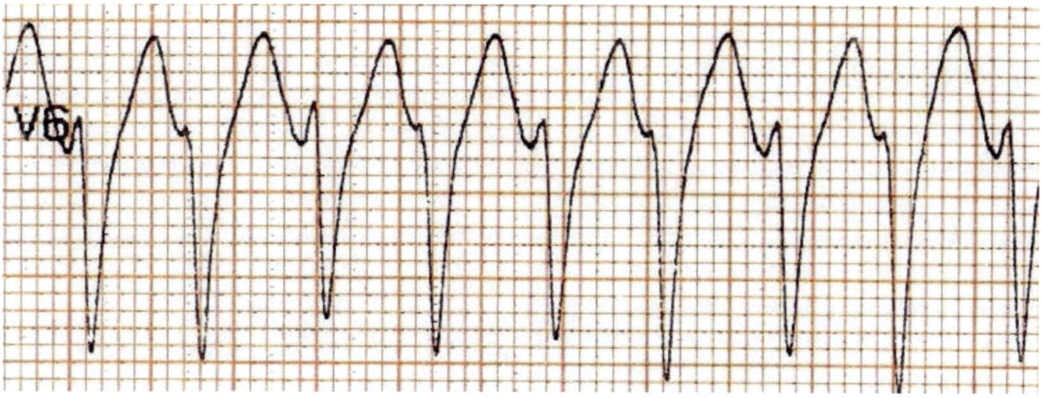

Fig. 5 Lead V6 from the wide QRS tachycardia from Fig. 1 showing an R-to-S ratio < 1, criterion in favor of ventricular tachycardia

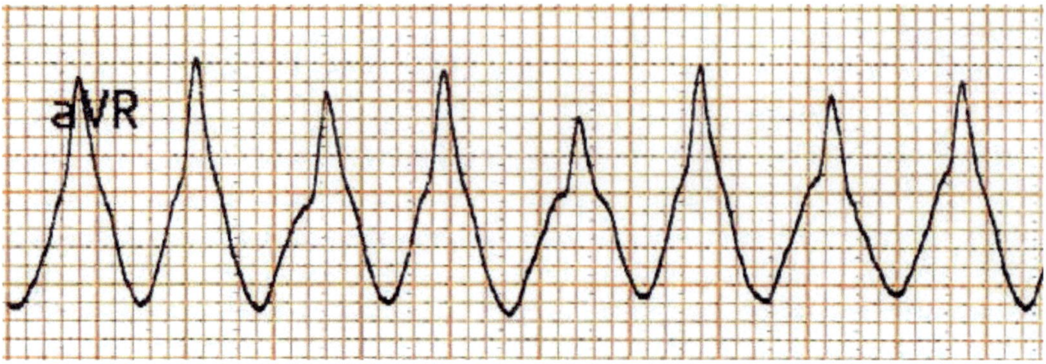

Fig. 6 Lead aVR from the ECG from Fig. 1 showing the presence of an initial positive R wave, criterion in favor of ventricular tachycardia

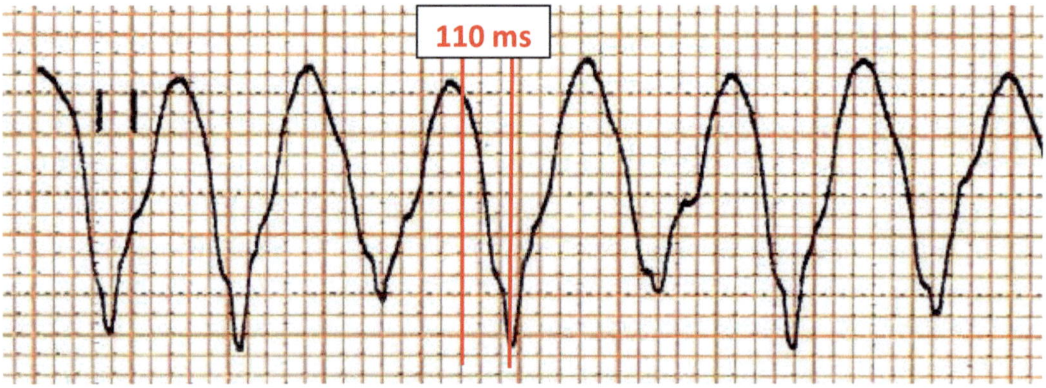

Fig. 7 Lead II from the ECG from Fig. 1 showing the time to first peak of 110 ms, criterion in favor of ventricular tachycardia

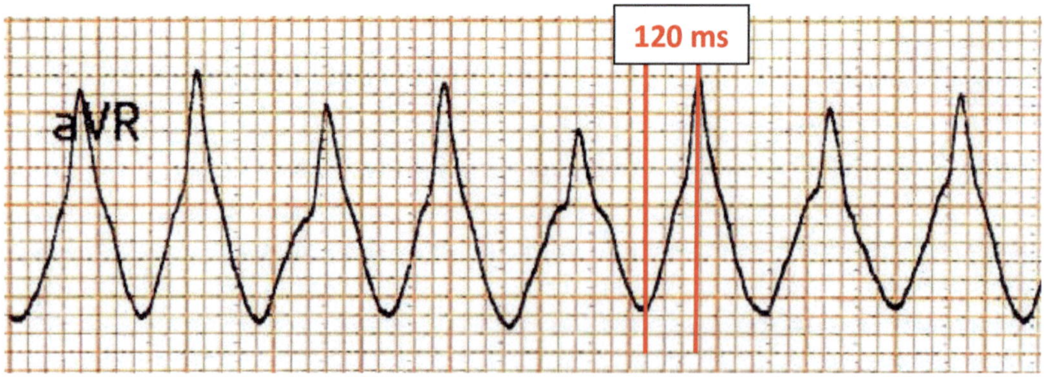

Fig. 8 Lead aVR from the ECG from Fig. 1 showing the time to the first peak of 120 ms, criterion in favor of ventricular tachycardia

References

1. Brugada P, Brugada J, Mont L, Smeets J, Andries EW. A new approach to the differential diagnosis of a regular tachycardia with a wide QRS complex. Circulation. 1991;83(5):1649–59.
2. Vereckei A, Duray G, Szenasi G, Altemose GT, Miller JM. New algorithm using only lead aVR for differential diagnosis of wide QRS complex tachycardia. Heart Rhythm. 2008;5(1):89–98.
3. Moccetti F, Yadava M, Latifi Y, Strebel I, Pavlovic N, Knecht S, et al. Simplified integrated clinical and electrocardiographic algorithm for differentiation of wide QRS complex tachycardia: the Basel algorithm. JACC Clin Electrophysiol. 2022;8(7):831–9.
4. Surawicz B, Childers R, Deal BJ, Gettes LS, Bailey JJ, Gorgels A, et al. AHA/ACCF/HRS recommendations for the standardization and interpretation of the electrocardiogram: part III: intraventricular conduction disturbances: a scientific statement from the American Heart Association Electrocardiography and Arrhythmias Committee, Council on Clinical Cardiology; the American College of Cardiology Foundation; and the Heart Rhythm Society. Endorsed by the International Society for Computerized Electrocardiology. J Am Coll Cardiol. 2009;53(11):976–81.

ECG 10

Mihai Puiu

1 Case Presentation

A 78-year-old male patient with a history of long-standing persistent atrial fibrillation, implanted with a single-chamber pacemaker for tachycardia–bradycardia syndrome (before atrial fibrillation became permanent), is admitted to the Cardiology Department due to an episode of palpitations with a sudden onset and regular rhythm, accompanied by dyspnea, lightheadedness, and chest pain, which had started 20 min before arriving at the Emergency Department. His ECG recorded at admittance to the Cardiology Department is presented in Fig. 1.

Question: What is the nature of the rhythm presented in Fig. 1?

(a) Ventricular tachycardia originating from the inferior lateral and apical LV wall
(b) Ventricular tachycardia originating from the anterior lateral and apical LV wall
(c) Ventricular tachycardia originating from the inferior septal and apical LV wall
(d) Antidromic tachycardia using a right-sided bypass tract
(e) Atrial tachycardia with 1:1 atrioventricular conduction and left bundle branch block

M. Puiu (✉)
Department of Cardiology, Rehabilitation Hospital, Cluj-Napoca, Romania

Hint: A second ECG recorded several minutes later is presented in Fig. 2.

Correct answer: c. Ventricular tachycardia originating from the inferior septal and apical LV walls.

Explanation: The ECG in Fig. 1 shows a regular wide QRS complex tachycardia with a heart rate of 181 bpm and LBBB morphology. The width of the QRS complex is 134 ms. The QRS axis is at −60°. The differential diagnosis of this regular wide QRS complex tachycardia with LBBB morphology includes: ventricular tachycardia (myocardial-related VT, bundle branch reentry VT, and fascicular tachycardia), supraventricular tachycardia (atrial flutter, atrial tachycardia, AVNRT, and AVRT) with functional or pre-existing bundle branch block, and antidromic tachycardia (in pre-excitation syndromes).

The morphology of the left bundle branch block of the QRS complex during tachycardia from Fig. 1 is not that of a typical one: the QRS duration is indeed >120 ms, and the QRS has a "QS'" morphology in lead V1 and a unique notched R wave in leads I and aVL. However, the QRS complex does not have a unique notched R wave morphology in V5 and V6, element which is not in favor of a typical left bundle branch block. This makes SVT with LBBB unlikely.

L. Muresan (ed.), *ECG Interpretation of Wide QRS Complex Tachycardia*,
https://doi.org/10.1007/978-3-031-97030-6_11

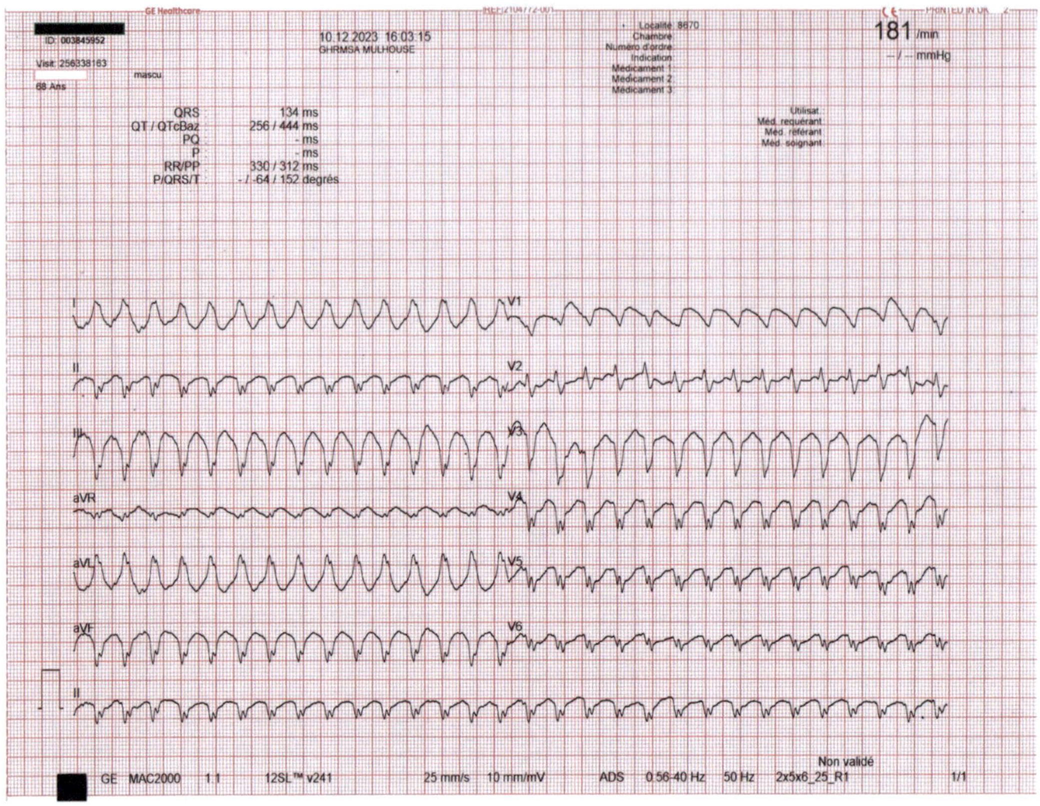

Fig. 1 Twelve-lead ECG recorded at admittance to the Cardiology Department

The ECG from Fig. 2 shows atrial tachycardia with a ventricular rate of 60 bpm and paced QRS complexes; there are no signs of ventricular preexcitation (no short PR interval and no delta waves). This makes antidromic tachycardia unlikely as the correct diagnosis for the tachycardia from Fig. 1.

Applying the Brugada algorithm [1] to the tachycardia from Fig. 1, it can be seen that: 1. There is no absence of an RS complex in the precordial leads (otherwise said, there are rS complexes in lead V2) (Fig. 3); we therefore move to the second step of the algorithm.

The second step analyzes the absence of an R to S interval > 100 ms in any precordial lead. This is not the case, since the only lead which displays an "RS pattern" is lead V2, where the RS interval is of 80 ms (Fig. 4).

For a wide QRS complex tachycardia with LBBB, arguments in favor of VT are: the presence of an "r wave" > 0.04 s in lead V1 or V2, which is actually the case for lead V2 [2] (Fig. 5).

Other arguments in favor of ventricular tachycardia are: 1. For an LBBB QRS morphology, a QRS duration of over 160 ms [3]. 2. A duration of >60 ms from the onset of the QRS to the nadir of the S wave in lead V1 (Fig. 6) [2].

The Vereckei algorithm [4] for the differential diagnosis of wide QRS complex tachycardias also suggests VT as the correct answer. The first step of the algorithm looks for A–V dissociation, which is not seen on the present ECG (ECG 2 shows that the atrial rhythm is actually atrial fibrillation). The second step of the algorithm looks for an initial predominant R wave in lead aVR, which is also not the case (Fig. 7).

The third step of the algorithm "QRS morphology unlike BBB or fascicular block" does not suggest SVT with RBBB, based on the

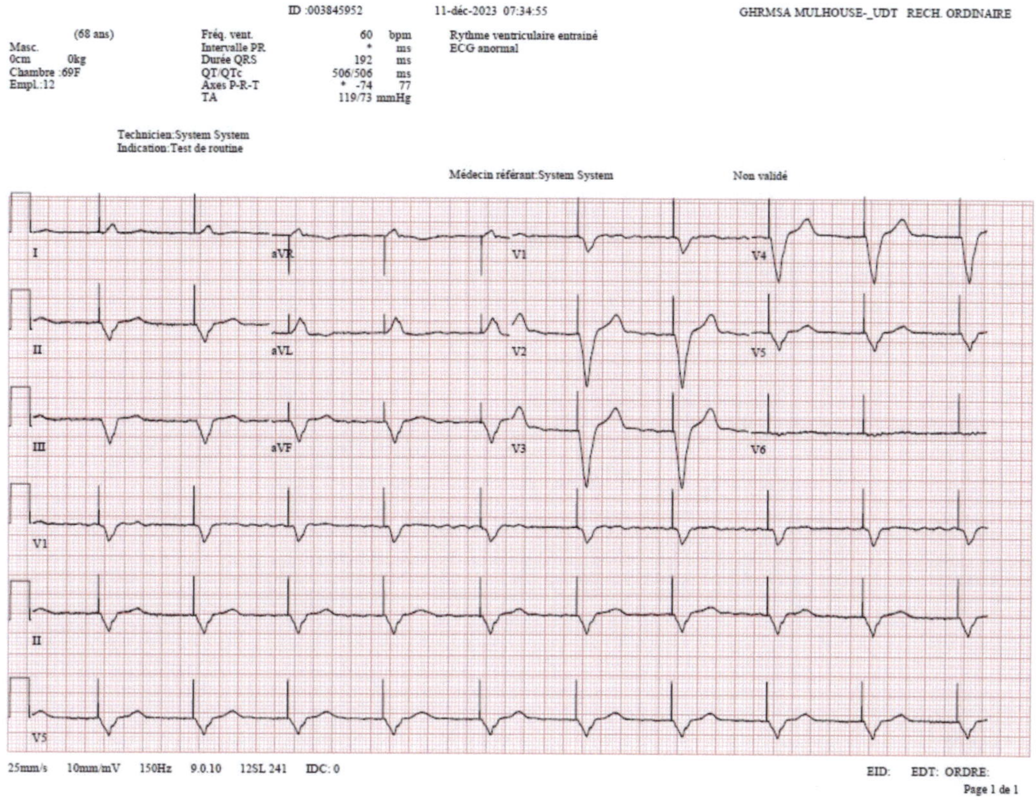

Fig. 2 Twelve-lead ECG recorded after the end of the episode of palpitations

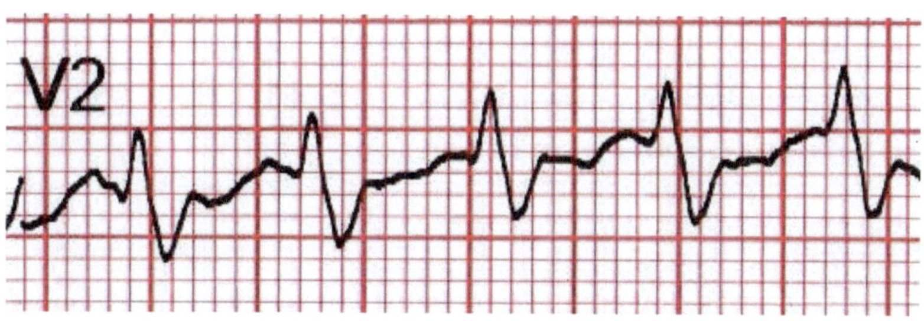

Fig. 3 LeadV2 from the ECG presented in Fig. 1 showing the presence of RS complexes, argument not in favor of VT (but not excluding it either)

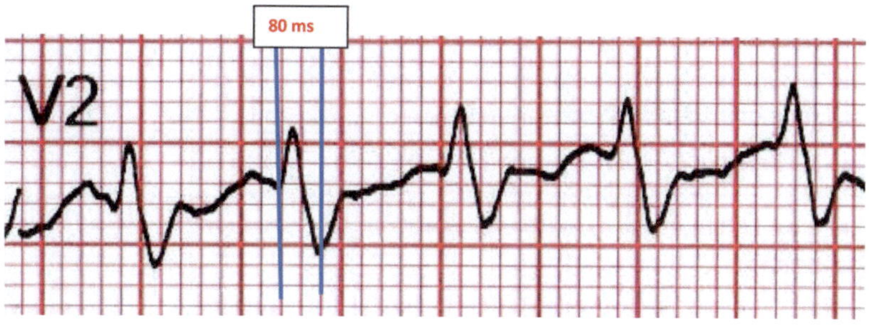

Fig. 4 Detailed analysis of the QRS morphology in lead V2 during the wide QRS complex tachycardia. The RS interval measures 80 ms. This is not diagnostic of ventricular tachycardia

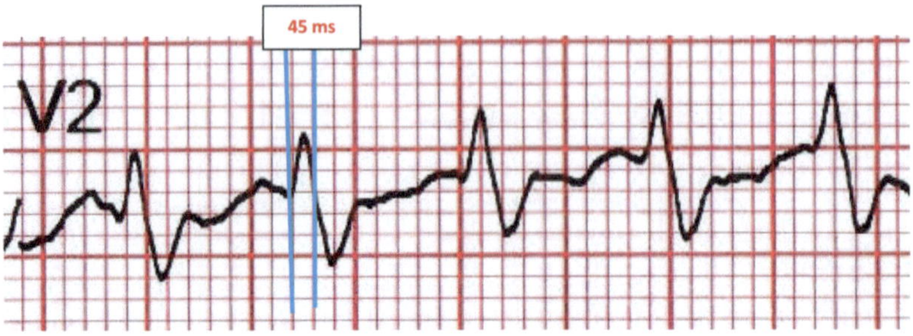

Fig. 5 Detailed analysis of the QRS morphology in lead V2 during the wide QRS complex tachycardia. The R wave measures 45 ms. This is a criterion in favor of ventricular tachycardia

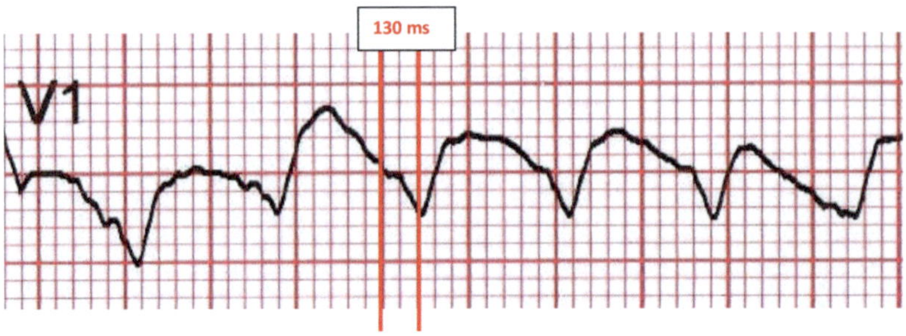

Fig. 6 Detailed analysis of the QRS morphology in lead V1 during the wide QRS complex tachycardia. The RS interval measures 80 ms, criterion in favor of ventricular tachycardia

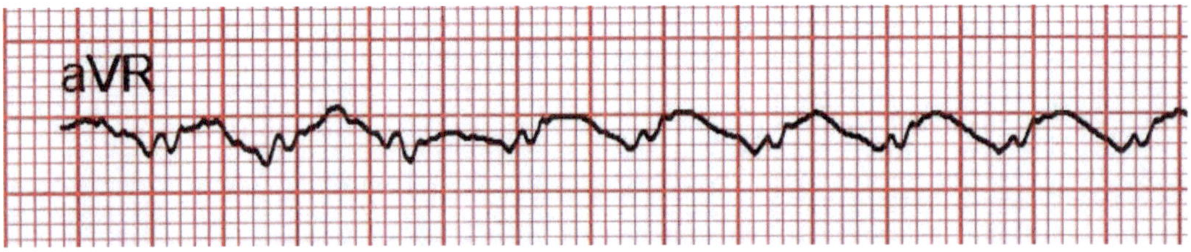

Fig. 7 Lead aVR from the tachycardia presented in Fig. 1, showing the absence of an initial positive tall R wave, criterion not in favor of ventricular tachycardia (but not excluding it either)

arguments exposed above. Therefore, the diagnosis is that of ventricular tachycardia.

Its origin is at the level of the left ventricle (even though the tachycardia has an LBBB morphology, there is anteroseptal necrosis of the LV wall seen on the ECG from Fig. 2, which represents the substrate of the VT), inferior LV wall (negative QRS complexes in leads III and aVF), and at the level of the septall wall (positive QRS complex in leads I and aVL).

The patient underwent an electrophysiological study which confirmed the diagnosis of VT and a catheter ablation procedure was subsequently performed.

References

1. Brugada P, Brugada J, Mont L, Smeets J, Andries EW. A new approach to the differential diagnosis of a regular tachycardia with a wide QRS complex. Circulation. 1991;83(5):1649–59.
2. Kindwall KE, Brown J, Josephson ME. Electrocardiographic criteria for ventricular tachycardia in wide complex left bundle branch block morphology tachycardias. Am J Cardiol. 1988;61(15):1279–83.
3. Eckardt L, Breithardt G, Kirchhof P. Approach to wide complex tachycardias in patients without structural heart disease. Heart. 2006;92(5):704–11.
4. Vereckei A, Duray G, Szenasi G, Altemose GT, Miller JM. Application of a new algorithm in the differential diagnosis of wide QRS complex tachycardia. Eur Heart J. 2007;28(5):589–600.

ECG 11

Stefan-Lucian Popa

1 Case Presentation

A 76-year-old male patient with a history of moderate aortic stenosis, moderate systolic dysfunction (LVEF of 40–45%), mild pulmonary hypertension (sPAP of 45 mmHg), COPD, and active hepatic carcinoma presents to the Emergency Department for dyspnea and palpitations that had begun 3 days prior to his presentation at the hospital. A 12-lead ECG was recorded and is presented in Fig. 1.

Question: What is the nature of the tachycardia presented in Fig. 1?

(a) Bundle branch re-entry ventricular tachycardia
(b) Atrial fibrillation with right bundle branch block
(c) Antidromic tachycardia using a left-sided by-pass tract
(d) Pre-excited atrial fibrillation
(e) Fascicular ventricular tachycardia (re-entry in the left posterior fascicle)

Hint: A second ECG recorded after the administration of 5 mg of iv Atenolol is presented at the end of this case presentation.

S.-L. Popa (✉)
Department of Internal Medicine, Second Medical Clinic, Cluj-Napoca, Romania
e-mail: popa.stefan@umfcluj.ro

Correct answer: b. Atrial fibrillation with right bundle branch block

Explanation: The ECG in Fig. 1 shows an irregular wide QRS complex tachycardia with a heart rate of 125 bpm with RBBB morphology. The width of the QRS complex is 138 ms. The QRS axis is at +25°. The differential diagnosis of this wide QRS complex tachycardia with RBBB morphology includes: ventricular tachycardia (myocardial-related VT, bundle branch re-entry VT, and fascicular VT), supraventricular tachycardia (atrial fibrillation, atrial flutter, atrial tachycardia, AVNRT, and AVRT) with functional or pre-existing bundle branch block, and antidromic tachycardia (in pre-excitation syndromes).

The morphology of the right bundle branch block is that of a typical one: QRS duration >120 ms, an "RSR'" pattern in lead V1, an "RS" pattern in leads I, aVL, V5, and V6, and a duration of the S wave >40 ms in lead V6 [1].

Applying the Brugada algorithm [2] to the tachycardia from Fig. 1, it can be seen that: 1. There is no absence of an RS complex in the precordial leads (otherwise said, there are RS complexes in leads V4 to V6). 2. There is no R to S interval > 100 ms in any precordial lead (see Fig. 2). 3. There is no AV dissociation visible (actually there are no P waves visible). Therefore,

L. Muresan (ed.), *ECG Interpretation of Wide QRS Complex Tachycardia*,
https://doi.org/10.1007/978-3-031-97030-6_12

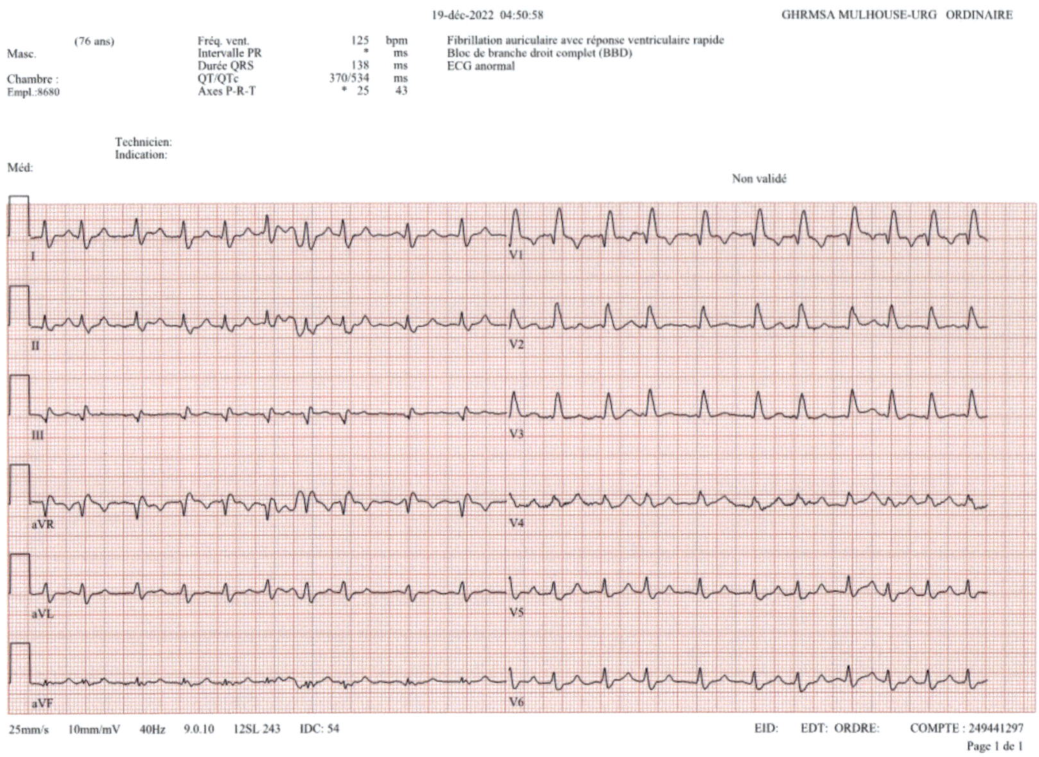

Fig. 1 ECG recorded at admittance to the Emergency Department

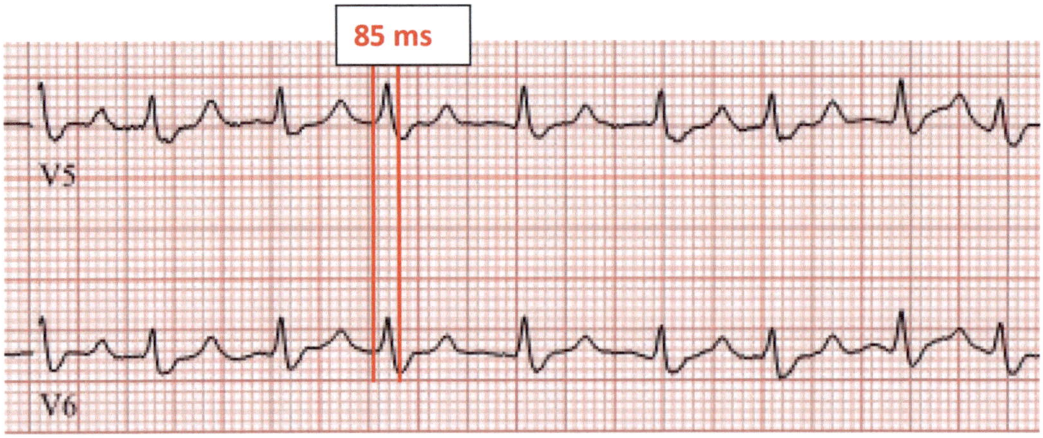

Fig. 2 Leads V5 and V6 from the wide QRS complex tachycardia presented in Fig. 1 showing an R to S interval of 85 ms (<100 ms), argument not favoring the diagnosis of ventricular tachycardia (but not excluding it either)

we need to move to the fourth step of the algorithm and analyze the morphology of the QRS complexes during tachycardia.

For an RBBB morphology wide QRS complex tachycardia, an argument in favor of VT would be the presence of taller left peak of the QRS complex in lead V1 (the rabbit ear sign) or for biphasic RS or QR complexes, which is not the case (the aspect is RSR', with the amplitude of the first R wave being smaller than the amplitude of the R' wave) (Fig. 3).

Next, in lead V6, an argument in favor of VT would be the presence of an "rS" complex (a ratio of R/S < 1), which is not the case either (Fig. 4).

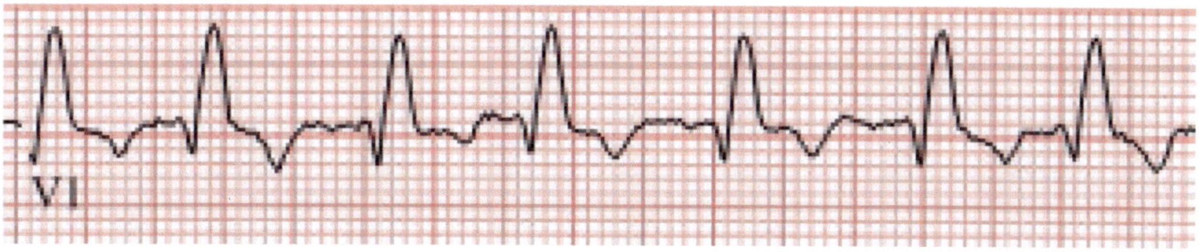

Fig. 3 Lead V1 from the wide QRS complex tachycardia presented in Fig. 1 showing an "rSR'" pattern, argument not favoring the diagnosis of ventricular tachycardia (but not excluding it either)

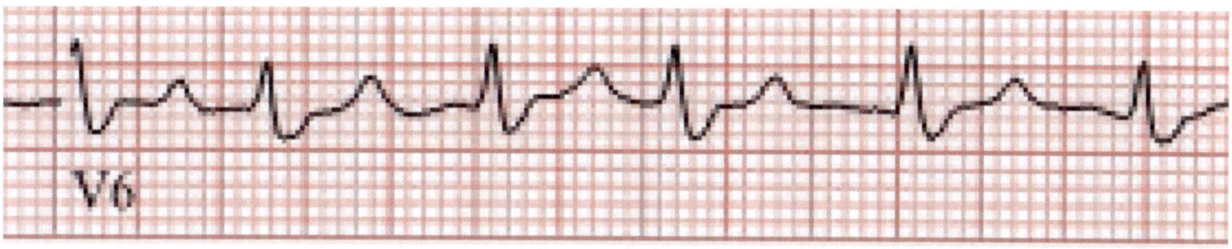

Fig. 4 Lead V6 from the wide QRS complex tachycardia presented in Fig. 1 showing an R-to-S ratio of >1, argument not favoring the diagnosis of ventricular tachycardia (but not excluding it either)

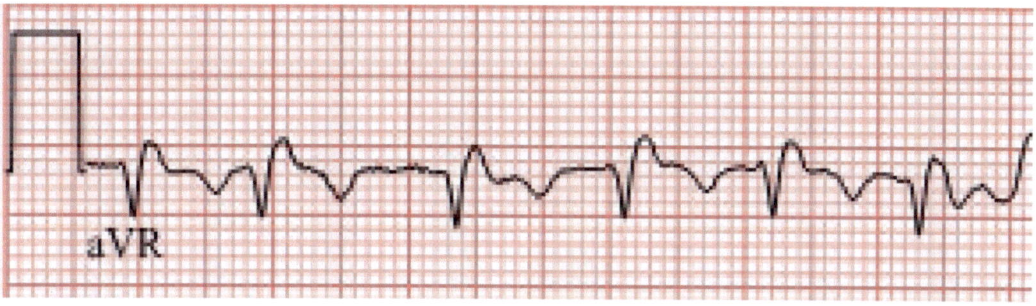

Fig. 5 Lead aVR from the wide QRS complex tachycardia presented in Fig. 1 showing the "rSr'" pattern or the absence of an initial tall R wave, argument not favoring the diagnosis of ventricular tachycardia (but not excluding it either)

Therefore, we have no argument in favor of VT and, according to this algorithm, the tachycardia can therefore be classified as SVT with RBBB.

The Vereckei algorithm [3] for the differential diagnosis of wide QRS complex tachycardias also suggests SVT with RBBB as the correct answer. The first step of the algorithm looks for A–V dissociation, which is not seen on the present ECG. The second step of the algorithm looks for an initial predominant R wave in lead aVR, which, again, is not the case (Fig. 5).

The third step "QRS morphology unlike BBB or fascicular block" is in fact in favor of SVT (atrial fibrillation) with typical BBB: the presence of an irregular rhythm, with no visible P waves and a large QRS complex with typical RBBB morphology.

Therefore, the correct answer is: "b. Atrial fibrillation with right bundle branch block".

Answer e is not correct since intrafascicular re-entry in the left posterior fascicle has an RBBB morphology but superior axis. Answers c and d are also not correct, since there is no ventricular pre-excitation present. Answer a is also not correct since bundle branch re-entry ventricular tachycardia (with RBBB morphology in this case) usually has a wider QRS complex, is regular rather than irregular, and has a higher heart

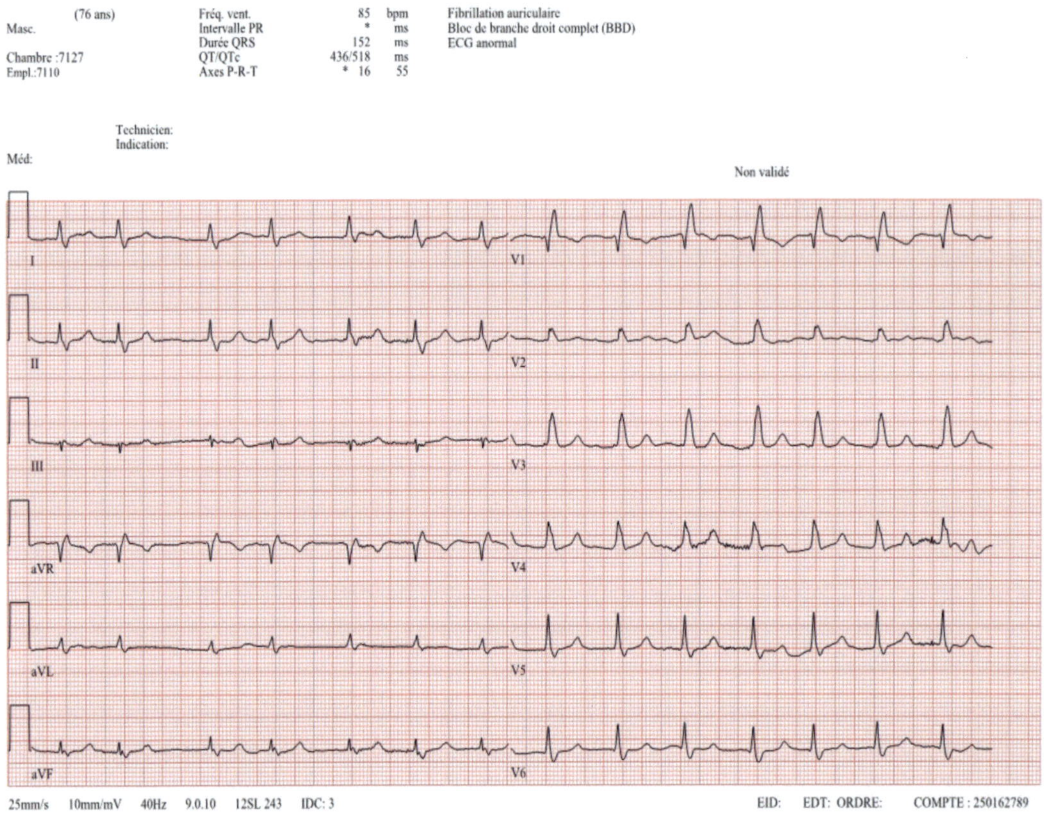

Fig. 6 Twelve-lead ECG showing atrial fibrillation with a heart rate of 85 bpm and complete right bundle branch block

rate [4, 5]. The ECG of these patients during sinus rhythm usually shows a prolonged PR interval and advanced intraventricular conduction disorder.

The patient received an anticoagulant treatment, beta-blockers, and was scheduled for an electrical cardioversion after 3 weeks of full anticoagulation treatment (Fig. 6).

References

1. Wellens HJ, Bar FW, Lie KI. The value of the electrocardiogram in the differential diagnosis of a tachycardia with a widened QRS complex. Am J Med. 1978;64(1):27–33.
2. Brugada P, Brugada J, Mont L, Smeets J, Andries EW. A new approach to the differential diagnosis of a regular tachycardia with a wide QRS complex. Circulation. 1991;83(5):1649–59.
3. Vereckei A, Duray G, Szenasi G, Altemose GT, Miller JM. Application of a new algorithm in the differential diagnosis of wide QRS complex tachycardia. Eur Heart J. 2007;28(5):589–600.
4. Kusa S, Taniguchi H, Hachiya H, Miyazaki S, Nakamura H, Uchiyama T, et al. Bundle branch reentrant ventricular tachycardia with wide and narrow QRS morphology. Circ Arrhythm Electrophysiol. 2013;6(6):e87–91.
5. Mizusawa Y, Sakurada H, Nishizaki M, Ueda-Tatsumoto A, Fukamizu S, Hiraoka M. Characteristics of bundle branch reentrant ventricular tachycardia with a right bundle branch block configuration: feasibility of atrial pacing. Europace. 2009;11(9):1208–13.

ECG 12

Razvan Mada

1 Case Presentation

A 69-year-old female patient with a history of ischemic cardiomyopathy with severe LV systolic dysfunction (LVEF of 25%), remote anterior myocardial infarction, and ischemic stroke due to embolism from an LV apical thrombus is admitted to the Cardiology Department for an episode of palpitations accompanied by chest pain, dyspnea, anxiety, and lightheadedness that had occurred 2 h prior to her presentation to the hospital. Her ECG recorded at admittance to the Cardiology Department is presented in Fig. 1.

Question: What is the nature of the tachycardia presented in Fig. 1?

(a) Ventricular tachycardia originating from the inferior lateral LV wall
(b) Ventricular tachycardia originating from the inferior septal LV wall
(c) Bundle branch re-entry ventricular tachycardia
(d) Antidromic tachycardia using a left-sided bypass tract
(e) AVNRT with right bundle branch block

Hint: A second ECG recorded several minutes later is presented in Fig. 2.

R. Mada (✉)
Department of Cardiology, "Niculae Stancioiu" Heart Institute, Cluj-Napoca, Romania

Correct answer: a. Ventricular tachycardia originating from the inferior lateral LV wall

Explanation The ECG in Fig. 1 shows a regular wide QRS complex tachycardia with a heart rate of 102 bpm and RBBB morphology. The width of the QRS complex is 160 ms (contrary to what the automatic interpretation of the ECG shows: 208 ms). There is extreme (north-west) axis deviation, the QRS axis being at −160°. The differential diagnosis of this wide QRS complex tachycardia with RBBB morphology includes: ventricular tachycardia (myocardial-related VT and bundle branch re-entry VT), supraventricular tachycardia (atrial tachycardia, AVNRT, and AVRT) with functional or pre-existing bundle branch block, and antidromic tachycardia (in pre-excitation syndromes).

Analyzing the ECG from Fig. 2, it can be observed that there is sinus rhythm with a heart rate of 81 bpm, the QRS axis is at +90°, there is no LV hypertrophy, and there is a QS aspect in leads V1 and V2, compatible with anteroseptal myocardial necrosis and pathological Q waves in leads I and aVL, in favor of necrosis of the lateral LV wall. There are no elements in favor of ventricular pre-excitation (no short PR interval and no delta waves). Therefore, answer d—"Antidromic tachycardia using a left-sided bypass tract"—is highly unlikely. There is also

L. Muresan (ed.), *ECG Interpretation of Wide QRS Complex Tachycardia*,
https://doi.org/10.1007/978-3-031-97030-6_13

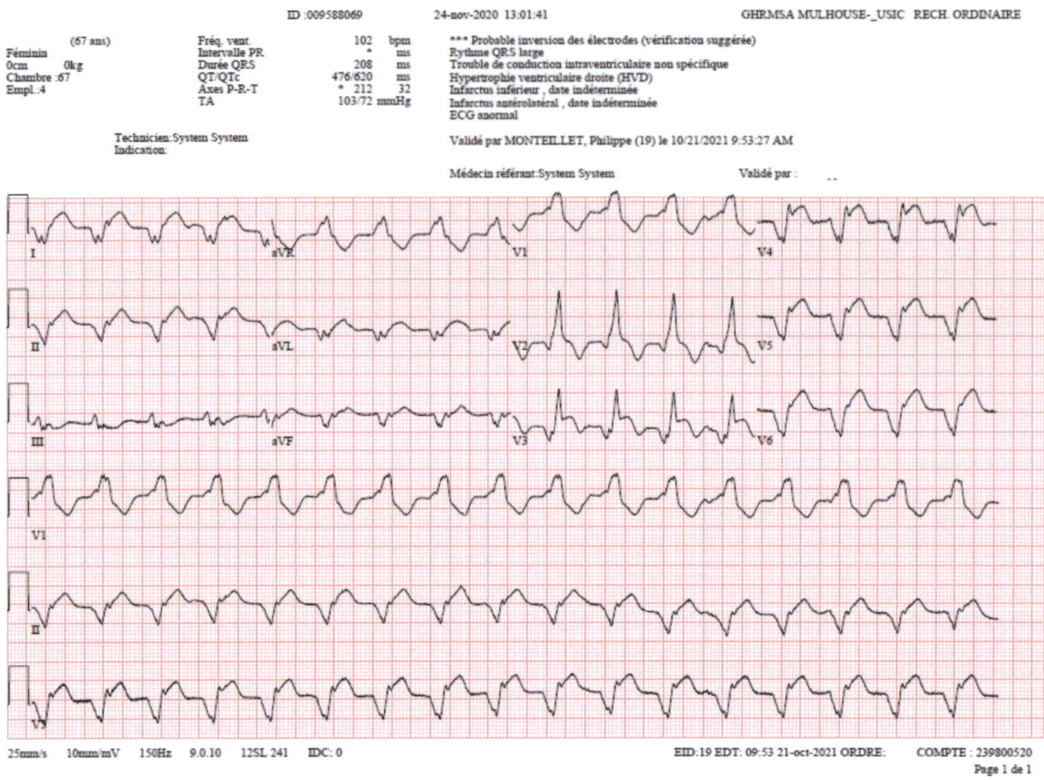

Fig. 1 Twelve-lead ECG recorded at admittance to the Cardiology Department

ST segment elevation in leads V1 and V2, compatible with the aneurysm of the anterior wall (confirmed by transthoracic echocardiography).

The morphology of the right bundle branch block of the QRS complex during tachycardia from Fig. 1 is not that of a typical one [1]: the QRS duration is indeed >120 ms; there is an "RSR'" pattern in lead I, but not in lead aVL, and in lead V6, where there is a "QS" morphology; the R-to-S ratio is <1 in lead V6; and there is ST segment and T wave modification opposite to the major deflection of the QRS complex: ST segment elevation with positive T waves in leads V3 to V5, which is not at all common for a typical RBBB. Therefore, answer e—"AVNRT with right bundle branch block"—is highly unlikely.

Applying the Brugada algorithm [2] to the tachycardia from Fig. 2, it can be seen that there is an absence of "RS" complexes in the precordial leads (Fig. 3). This is an argument in favor of ventricular tachycardia.

The Vereckei algorithm [3] for the differential diagnosis of wide QRS complex tachycardias also suggests VT as the correct answer. The first step of the algorithm looks for A–V dissociation, which is not seen on the present ECG. The second step of the algorithm looks for an initial predominant R wave in lead aVR, which is actually the case (Fig. 4).

The simplified Vereckei algorithm also suggests VT as the correct diagnosis, based on the presence of a positive initial R wave in lead aVR [4] (Fig. 4).

The Basel algorithm [5] is also in favor of ventricular tachycardia as the right answer. According to this algorithm, a positive diagnosis of VT is established if at least two out of three criteria are present: 1. structural heart disease (history of myocardial infarction, congestive heart failure (LVEF <35%), the presence of an ICD, and CRT), which the patient has (ischemic cardiomyopathy, history of myocardial infarction, and

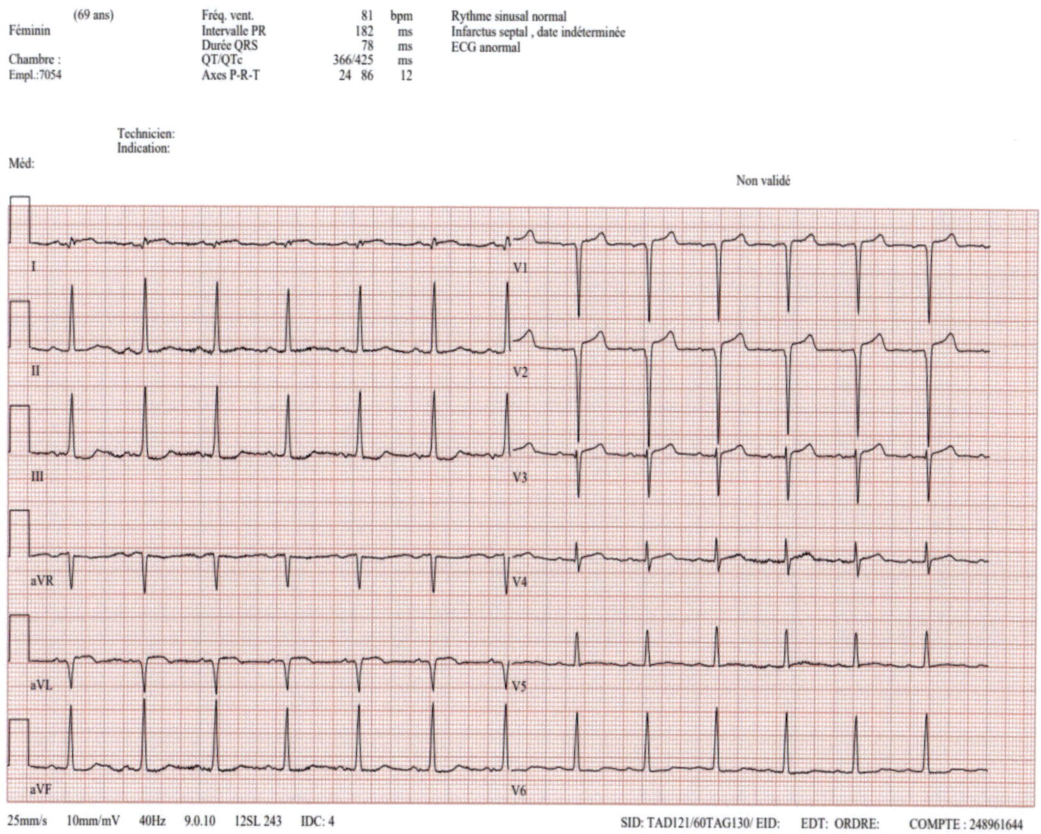

Fig. 2 Twelve-lead ECG recorded after administration of 300 mg of iv amiodarone

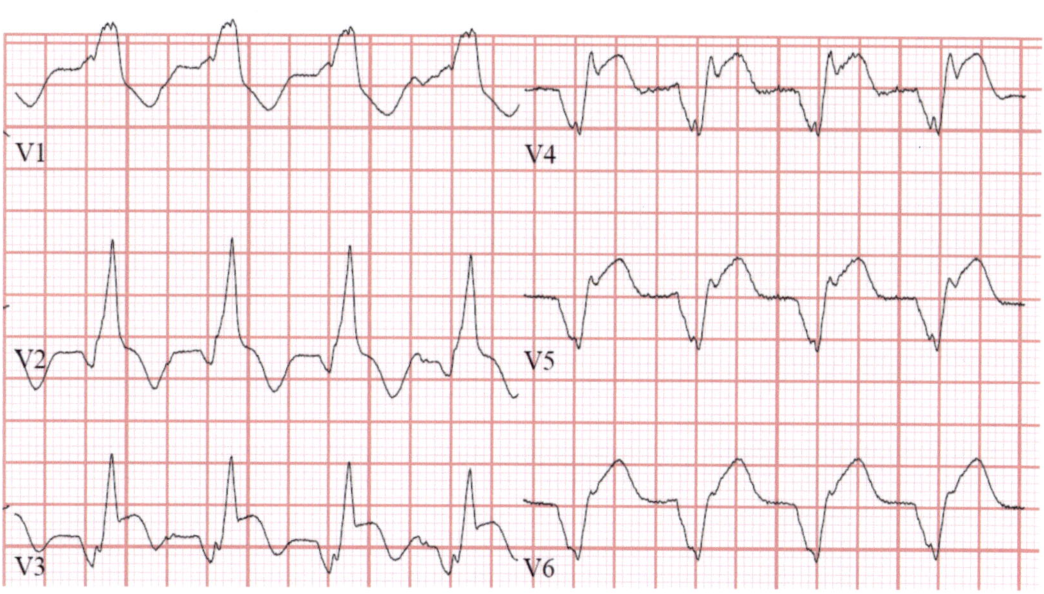

Fig. 3 Precordial leads from the ECG from Fig. 1 demonstrating the absence of an "RS" complex, argument in favor of ventricular tachycardia

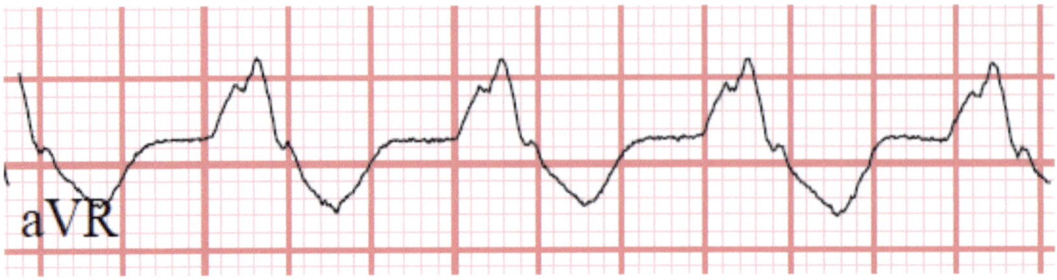

Fig. 4 Lead aVR from the ECG presented in Fig. 1, showing a tall initial R wave, argument in favor of ventricular tachycardia

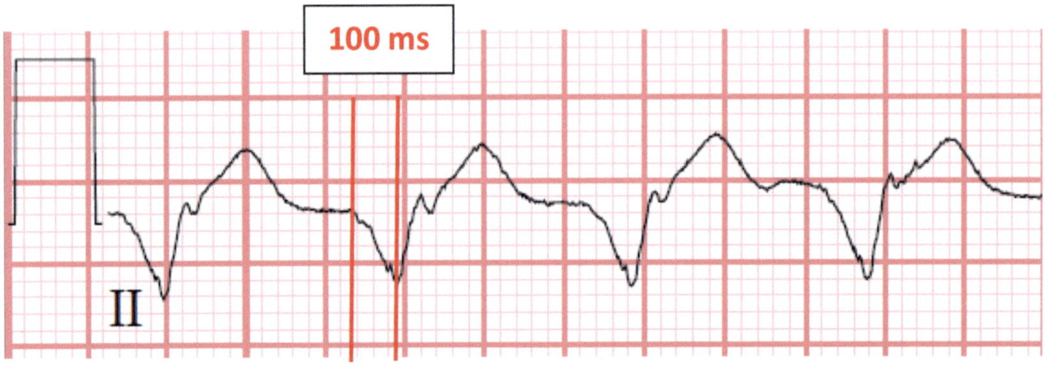

Fig. 5 Lead II from the ECG from Fig. 1 showing the time to the first peak of 100 ms, criterion in favor of ventricular tachycardia

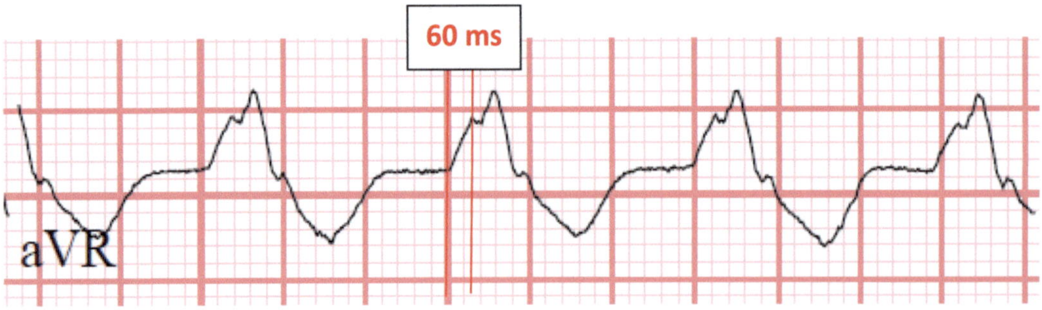

Fig. 6 Lead aVR from the ECG from Fig. 1 showing the time to the first peak of 60 ms, criterion in favor of ventricular tachycardia

LVEF of 25%); 2. the time to first peak in lead II > 40 ms (Fig. 5); and 3. the time to first peak in lead aVR > 40 ms (Fig. 6) [5].

Another argument in favor of ventricular tachycardia for a RBBB QRS morphology would be a QRS duration of over 140 ms [6], which is also the case, and extreme (north-west) axis deviation.

Concerning the origin of the VT, this is situated in the left ventricle (right bundle branch block pattern), at the level of the inferior wall (negative QRS complexes in leads II, III, and aVF) and the level of the lateral wall (negative QRS complexes in leads I and aVL).

Based on these arguments, the diagnosis of ventricular tachycardia was retained.

The patient underwent an ICD implantation. A catheter ablation procedure was also scheduled.

References

1. Surawicz B, Childers R, Deal BJ, Gettes LS, Bailey JJ, Gorgels A, et al. AHA/ACCF/HRS recommendations for the standardization and interpretation of the electrocardiogram: part III: intraventricular conduction disturbances: a scientific statement from the American Heart Association Electrocardiography and Arrhythmias Committee, Council on Clinical Cardiology; the American College of Cardiology Foundation; and the Heart Rhythm Society. Endorsed by the International Society for Computerized Electrocardiology. J Am Coll Cardiol. 2009;53(11):976–81.
2. Brugada P, Brugada J, Mont L, Smeets J, Andries EW. A new approach to the differential diagnosis of a regular tachycardia with a wide QRS complex. Circulation. 1991;83(5):1649–59.
3. Vereckei A, Duray G, Szenasi G, Altemose GT, Miller JM. Application of a new algorithm in the differential diagnosis of wide QRS complex tachycardia. Eur Heart J. 2007;28(5):589–600.
4. Vereckei A, Duray G, Szenasi G, Altemose GT, Miller JM. New algorithm using only lead aVR for differential diagnosis of wide QRS complex tachycardia. Heart Rhythm. 2008;5(1):89–98.
5. Moccetti F, Yadava M, Latifi Y, Strebel I, Pavlovic N, Knecht S, et al. Simplified integrated clinical and electrocardiographic algorithm for differentiation of wide QRS complex tachycardia: the Basel algorithm. JACC Clin Electrophysiol. 2022;8(7):831–9.
6. Eckardt L, Breithardt G, Kirchhof P. Approach to wide complex tachycardias in patients without structural heart disease. Heart. 2006;92(5):704–11.

ECG 13

Ronan Le Bouar

1 Case Presentation

A 53-year-old male patient with a history of alcoholism, ruptured abdominal aortic aneurysm complicated with hemorrhagic shock, treated with urgent surgery is transferred to the Cardiac Care Unit for repeated episodes of wide QRS complex tachycardia recorded while in the Post-Surgical Intensive Care Unit. His ECG recorded at admittance to the Cardiology Department is presented in Fig. 1.

Question: What is the nature of the tachycardia presented in Fig. 1?

(a) Ventricular tachycardia originating from the superior septal LV wall
(b) Ventricular tachycardia originating from the inferior septal LV wall
(c) Atypical AVNRT with LBBB
(d) Antidromic tachycardia using a right-sided bypass tract
(e) Sinus tachycardia with ventricular pre-excitation

Hint: A second ECG recorded several minutes later is presented in Fig. 2.

R. Le Bouar (✉)
Department of Cardiology, Emile Muller Hospital, Mulhouse, France
e-mail: LEBOUARR@ghrmsa.fr

Correct answer: c. Sinus tachycardia with ventricular pre-excitation

Explanation: The ECG in Fig. 1 shows a regular wide QRS complex tachycardia with a heart rate of 107 bpm and LBBB morphology. The width of the QRS complex is 140 ms. The QRS axis is at +10°. The differential diagnosis of this regular wide QRS complex tachycardia with LBBB morphology includes: ventricular tachycardia (myocardial-related VT, bundle branch reentry VT, and fascicular VT), supraventricular tachycardia (atrial tachycardia, AVNRT, and AVRT) with functional or pre-existing bundle branch block, and ventricular pre-excitation (antidromic tachycardia or supraventricular tachycardia conducted over an accessory pathway).

The morphology of the left bundle branch block of the QRS complex during tachycardia from Fig. 1 might be that of a typical one [1]: the QRS duration is >120 ms, there is a monomorphic R wave in leads I, aVL, V5, and V6; and there is ST segment and T wave modification opposite to the major deflection of the QRS complex: ST segment elevation with positive T waves in leads V1 to V3. However, the QRS transition in the precordial leads takes place in lead V3, which is not common for a typical LBBB.

L. Muresan (ed.), *ECG Interpretation of Wide QRS Complex Tachycardia*,
https://doi.org/10.1007/978-3-031-97030-6_14

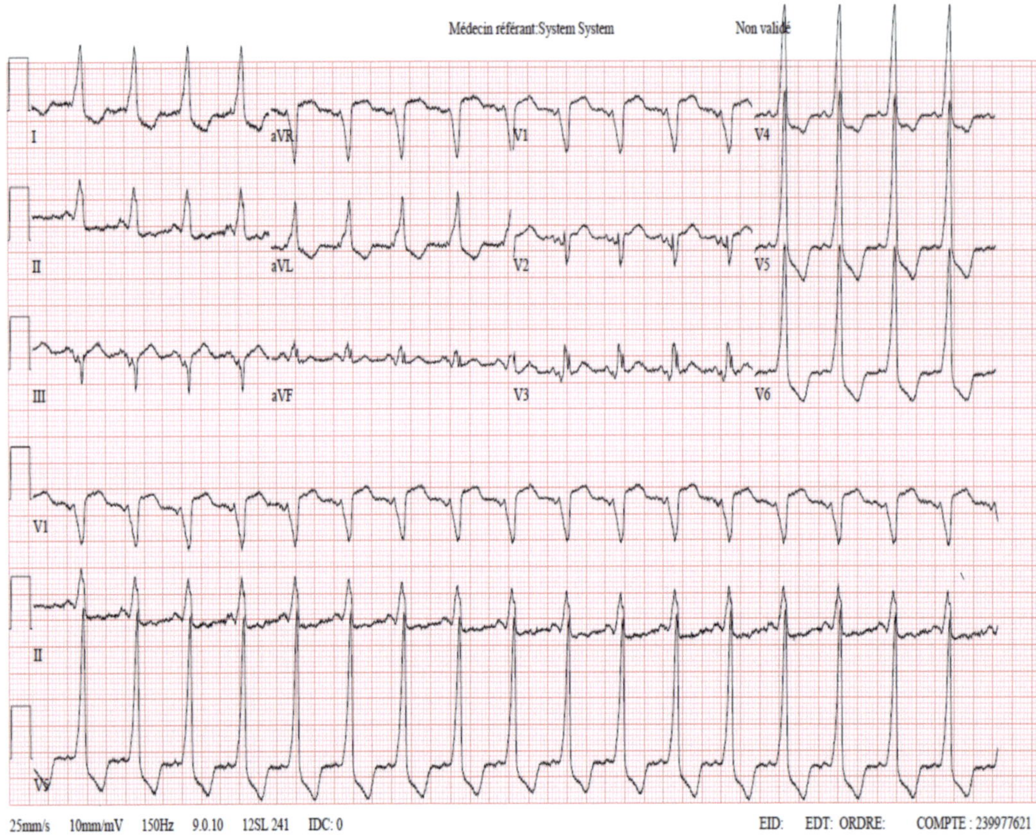

Fig. 1 Twelve-lead ECG recorded at admittance to the Cardiology Department

Applying the Brugada algorithm [2] to the tachycardia from Fig. 1, it can be seen that: 1. There is no absence of an RS complex in the precordial leads (otherwise said, there are rS complexes in leads V1 to V3); we therefore move to the second step of the algorithm: 2. This step analyzes the absence of an R to S interval > 100 ms in any precordial lead. This is actually the case (Fig. 3). Therefore, according to the Brugada algorithm, the tachycardia is ventricular in nature.

The Vereckei algorithm [3] for the differential diagnosis of wide QRS complex tachycardias also suggests VT as the correct answer. The first step of the algorithm looks for A–V dissociation, which is not seen on the ECG from Fig. 1, since the P–QRS relationship is 1:1. The second step of the algorithm looks for an initial predominant R wave in lead aVR, which, again, is not the case (Fig. 4).

The third step "QRS morphology unlike BBB or fascicular block" does not suggest SVT with RBBB, based on the morphological characteristics presented above (QRS transition in lead V3). This takes us to the fourth step of the algorithm: the vi/vt index. This index compares the amplitude of the first 40 ms of a QRS complex to the amplitude of the last 40 ms of the QRS complex in a lead where the QRS has both an R and an S wave. In the present case, this is illustrated in Fig. 5.

Even though both the Brugada and Vereckei algorithms suggest ventricular tachycardia as the right answer, it should be remembered that both algorithms are not accurate enough in distinguishing VT from pre-excitation syndromes.

However, the new Vereckei algorithm [4], demonstrated to perform better in distinguishing pre-excited atrial fibrillation/ventricular pre-excitation from VT, correctly identifies ventricular

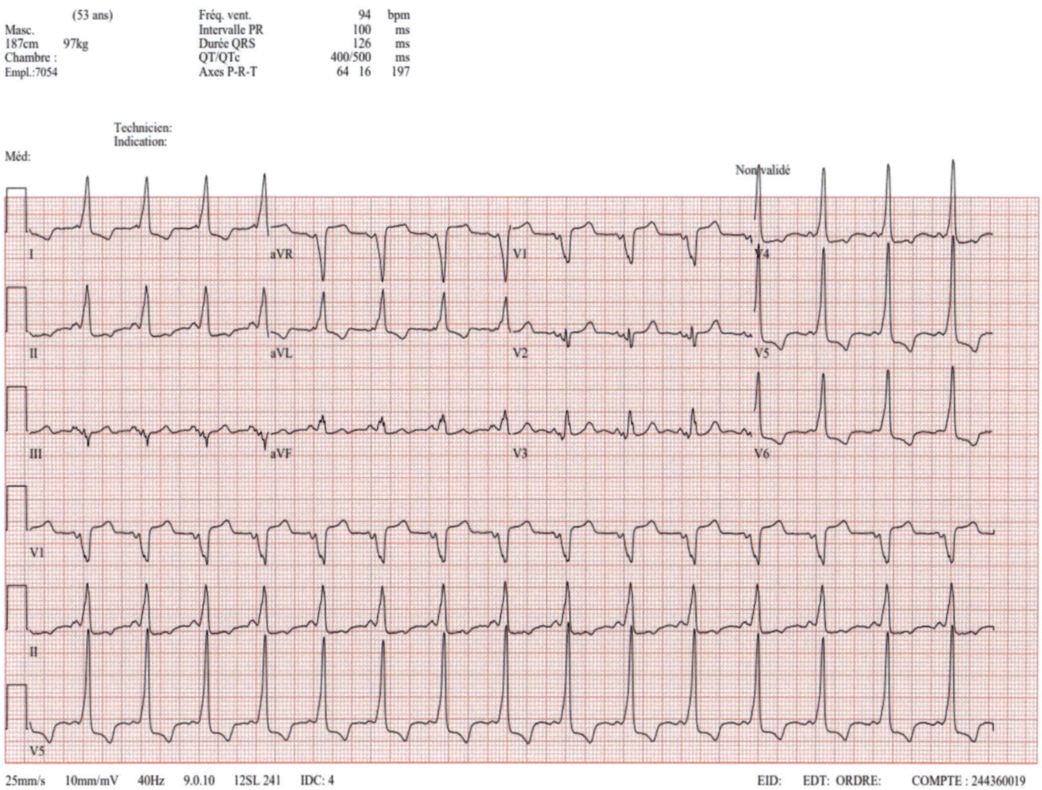

Fig. 2 Twelve-lead ECG recorded after the end of the episode of palpitations

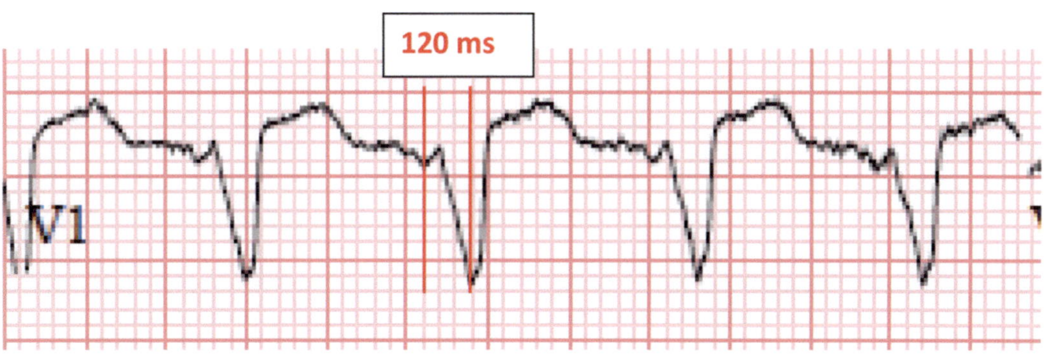

Fig. 3 Lead V6 from the tachycardia presented in Fig. 1, showing an R to S interval of 120 ms, argument in favor of ventricular tachycardia

pre-excitation in this case. The first step of this algorithm looks for the presence of atrioventricular dissociation. This is not the case, since P waves are present with a 1:1 P-to-QRS relationship. Step 2 of this algorithm "in lead aVR, positive onset of the QRS complex, and the area above the baseline of the QRS complex greater than the area below the baseline" is not in favor of VT (Fig. 6). The absence of this criterion takes us to step 3 of the algorithm.

Step 3 of the algorithm: "presence of a QR complex in one or more of the leads V2 to V6" is not in favor of ventricular tachycardia, since there are no QR complexes present (Fig. 7).

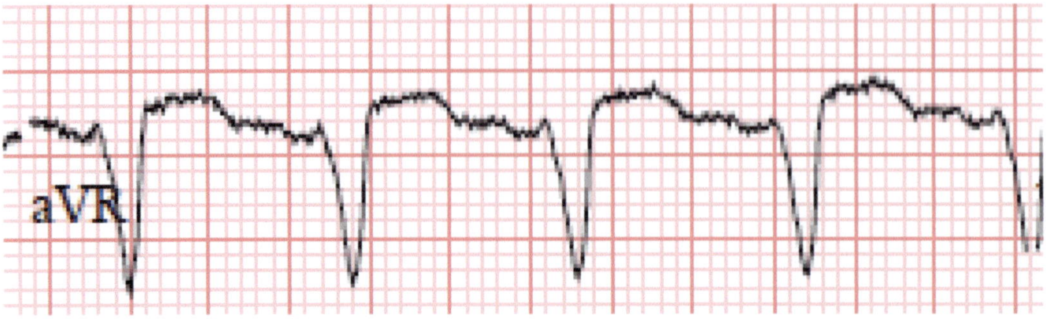

Fig. 4 Lead aVR from the tachycardia presented in Fig. 1, showing the absence of an initial positive tall R wave, criterion not in favor of ventricular tachycardia (but not excluding it either)

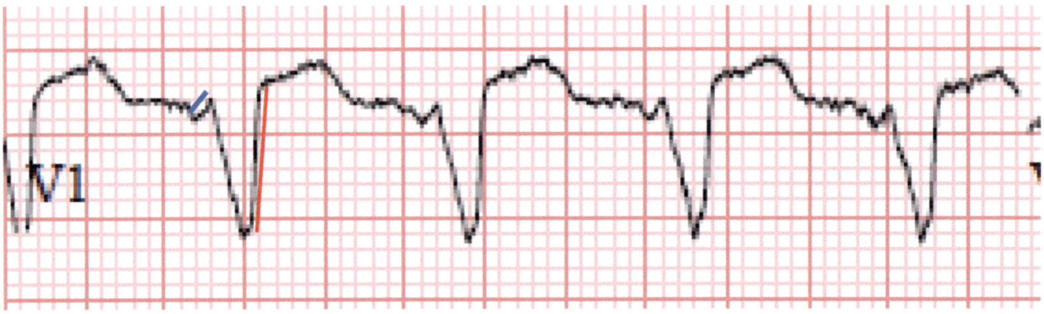

Fig. 5 The vi/vt index from the Vereckei algorithm in lead V6. The ratio of the initial 40 ms and the last 40 ms of the QRS complex is 1 mV vs 8 mV; therefore, 1/8 = 0.12, which is <1. This is in favor of ventricular tachycardia

Step 4 of this algorithm "predominantly negative QRS complexes in lead V4 to V6" is in favor of ventricular pre-excitation, since the QRS complexes in these leads are mostly positive (the absence of this criterion is in favor of ventricular pre-excitation).

Besides the new Vereckei algorithm, a simple comparison of ECG 1 and 2 provides the correct answer to the question. Analyzing the ECG from Fig. 2, it can be seen that the morphology of the QRS complex is identical to the one from the tachycardia in Fig. 1. On this ECG, P waves are clearly visible, with 1 P wave preceding each QRS complex, best seen in leads II, III, aVF, and V2–V5 (Fig. 8).

The PR interval is short (< 120 ms), and delta waves are present, arguments in favor of ventricular pre-excitation. The morphology of the P waves is compatible with a sinus node origin: positive P waves in leads II, III, and aVF, negative in lead aVR, and biphasic (positive–negative) in lead V1. This is therefore sinus rhythm (sinus tachycardia).

Going back to the ECG from Fig. 1, one can see that P waves with an identical morphology are present, also with a 1:1 P-to-QRS relationship. There is therefore sinus tachycardia with ventricular pre-excitation. An antidromic tachycardia with 1:1 ventriculo-atrial conduction would show negative P waves in leads II, III, and aVF, which is not the case. Therefore, answer d—"antidromic tachycardia using a right-sided bypass tract"—is not correct. For this reason, answer c—"Atypical aVNRT with LBBB"—is also incorrect, since during AVNRT, atria are depolarized in a caudal-to-cranial manner, implying the presence of negative P waves in the inferior leads on the 12-lead ECG.

The correct answer is e—"Sinus tachycardia with ventricular pre-excitation".

This case demonstrates that the existing algorithms are not perfect in differentiating between

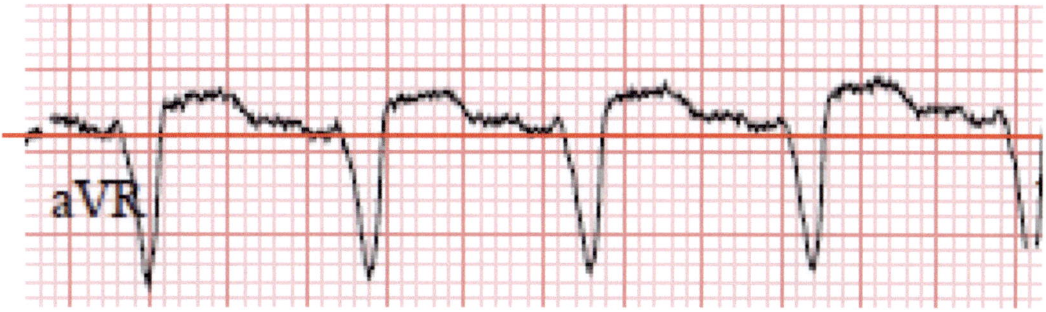

Fig. 6 Lead aVR from the tachycardia presented in Fig. 1, showing a small initial r wave but above the baseline of the QRS complex that is smaller than the area below the baseline, criterion not in favor of ventricular tachycardia (but not excluding it either)

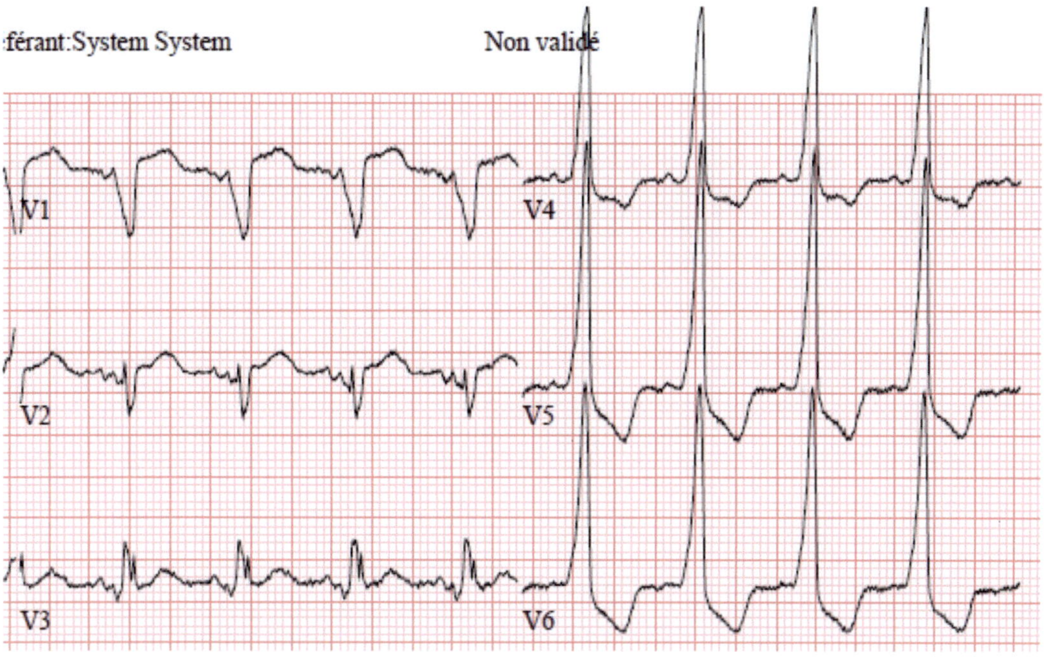

Fig. 7 Precordial leads from the ECG from Fig. 1, demonstrating the absence of "QR" complexes from V2 to V6, criterion not in favor of ventricular tachycardia (but not excluding it either)

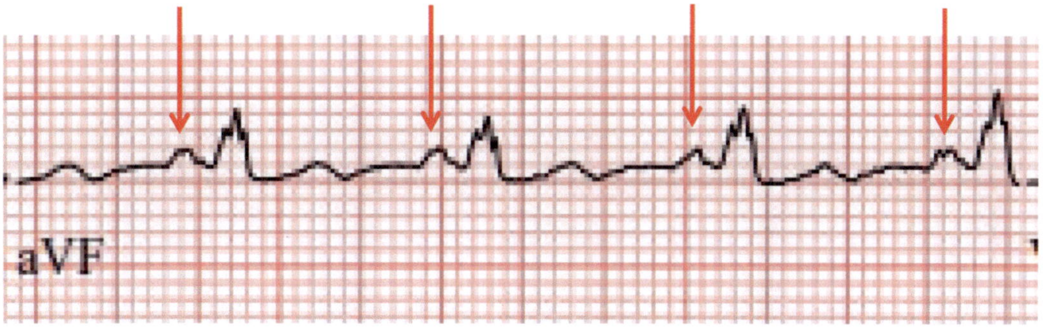

Fig. 8 Lead aVF from the tachycardia recorded in Fig. 2, showing the presence of P waves (red arrows) with a 1:1 P-to-QRS relationship

several etiologies of a wide QRS complex tachycardia and that evaluation of several ECGs of the same patients is sometimes needed and represents the best way to establish the correct diagnosis.

References

1. Surawicz B, Childers R, Deal BJ, Gettes LS, Bailey JJ, Gorgels A, et al. AHA/ACCF/HRS recommendations for the standardization and interpretation of the electrocardiogram: part III: intraventricular conduction disturbances: a scientific statement from the American Heart Association Electrocardiography and Arrhythmias Committee, Council on Clinical Cardiology; the American College of Cardiology Foundation; and the Heart Rhythm Society. Endorsed by the International Society for Computerized Electrocardiology. J Am Coll Cardiol. 2009;53(11):976–81.
2. Brugada P, Brugada J, Mont L, Smeets J, Andries EW. A new approach to the differential diagnosis of a regular tachycardia with a wide QRS complex. Circulation. 1991;83(5):1649–59.
3. Vereckei A, Duray G, Szenasi G, Altemose GT, Miller JM. Application of a new algorithm in the differential diagnosis of wide QRS complex tachycardia. Eur Heart J. 2007;28(5):589–600.
4. Vereckei A, Simon A, Szenasi G, Miller JM. The application of a new, modified algorithm for the differentiation of regular ventricular and pre-excited Tachycardias. Heart Lung Circ. 2023;32(6):719–25.

ECG 14

Crina Muresan

1 Case Presentation

A 64-year-old male patient with a history of severe aortic stenosis and COPD presents to the Emergency Department for an episode of constrictive chest pain, palpitations, and syncope. His lab work showed an important inflammatory syndrome (CRP = 180 mg/L), severe anemia (Hb = 6.9 g/dL), and hyperthyroidism (TSH = 0.01 IU/L). A 12-lead ECG was recorded at admittance to the Cardiology Department and is presented in Fig. 1.

Question: What is the nature of the tachycardia presented in Fig. 1?

(a) Ventricular tachycardia originating from the basal–septal left ventricle
(b) Atrial tachycardia with right bundle branch block
(c) Antidromic tachycardia using a left-sided by-pass tract
(d) Atrial fibrillation with right bundle branch block
(e) Fascicular ventricular tachycardia (re-entry in the left posterior fascicle)

Hint: A helping ECG is provided in Fig. 2.

C. Muresan (✉)
Department of Cardiology, Emile Muller Hospital, Mulhouse, France
e-mail: crina.muresan@ghrmsa.fr

Correct answer: b. Atrial tachycardia with right bundle branch block.

Explanation The ECG in Fig. 1 shows a regular wide QRS complex tachycardia with a heart rate of 164 bpm and RBBB morphology. The width of the QRS complex is 144 ms. The QRS axis is at +120°. The differential diagnosis of this wide QRS complex tachycardia with RBBB morphology includes: ventricular tachycardia (myocardial-related VT, bundle branch re-entry VT, and fascicular VT), supraventricular tachycardia (atrial fibrillation, atrial flutter, atrial tachycardia, AVNRT, and AVRT) with functional or pre-existing bundle branch block, and antidromic tachycardia (in pre-excitation syndromes).

The morphology of the right bundle branch block is that of a typical one: QRS duration >120 ms; there is an "RSR'" pattern in lead V1; there is an "RS" pattern in leads V5, V6, I, and aVL; and the duration of the S wave in leads I and V6 is >40 ms [1]. So, at this point of the analysis, the tachycardia may be an SVT with RBBB.

Applying the Brugada algorithm [2] to the tachycardia from Fig. 1, it can be seen that: 1. There is no absence of an RS complex in the precordial leads (otherwise said, there are RS complexes in leads V4 to V6). 2. There is no R to S interval > 100 ms in any precordial lead (see

L. Muresan (ed.), *ECG Interpretation of Wide QRS Complex Tachycardia*,
https://doi.org/10.1007/978-3-031-97030-6_15

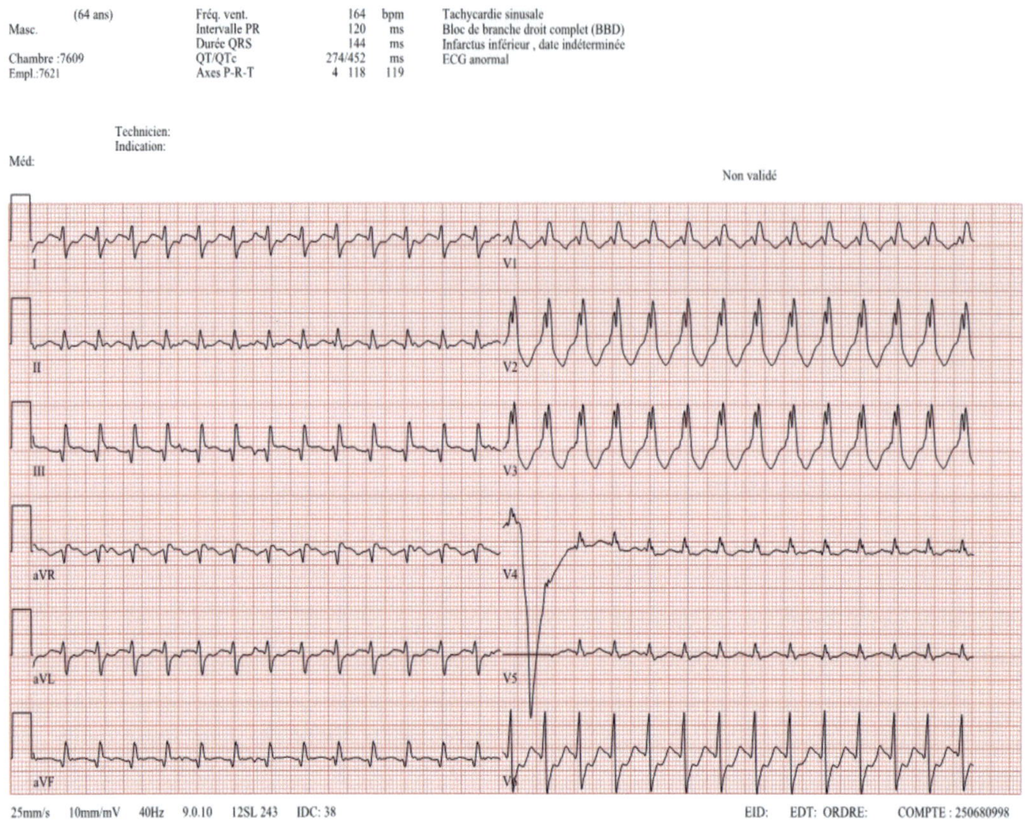

Fig. 1 ECG recorded at admittance to the Emergency Department

Fig. 3). 3. There is no AV dissociation visible (actually, there are no P waves visible). Therefore, we need to move to the fourth step of the algorithm and analyze the morphology of the QRS complexes during tachycardia.

For a RBBB morphology wide QRS complex tachycardia, an argument in favor of VT would be the presence of a taller left peak of the QRS complex in lead V1 (the rabbit ear sign) or for biphasic RS or QR complexes, which is not the case (the aspect is RSR', with the amplitude of the first R wave being smaller than the amplitude of the R' wave). Next, in lead V6, an argument in favor of VT would be the presence of an "rS" complex (a ratio of R/S <1), which is not the case either (Fig. 3). Therefore, we have no argument in favor of VT and, according to this algorithm, the tachycardia can therefore be classified as SVT with RBBB.

The Vereckei algorithm [3] for the differential diagnosis of wide QRS complex tachycardias also suggests SVT with RBBB as the correct answer. The first step of the algorithm looks for A–V dissociation, which is not seen on the present ECG. The second step of the algorithm looks for an initial predominant R wave in lead aVR, which, again, is not the case. The third step "QRS morphology unlike BBB or fascicular block" is in fact in favor of SVT with typical BBB.

The ECG in Fig. 2 shows sinus tachycardia with a heart rate of 109 bpm and right bundle branch block. P waves are visible best in leads I, II, and aVF (Fig. 4). The morphology of the QRS is identical to the one from Fig. 1 during tachycardia. This suggests that the tachycardia from Fig. 1 is a supraventricular tachycardia with RBBB. Therefore, answer a—"Ventricular tachycardia originating from the basal–septal left ventricle"—and answer e—"Fascicular ventricular tachycardia (reentry in the left posterior fascicle)"—are not correct.

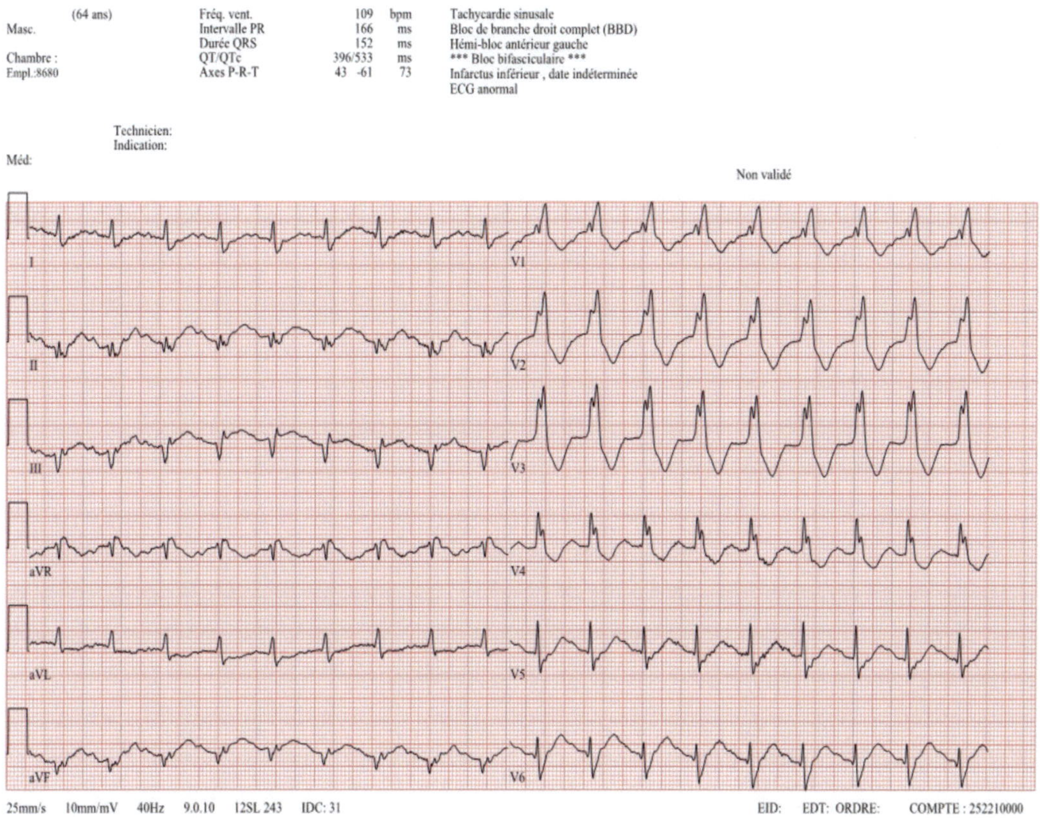

Fig. 2 Twelve-lead ECG recorded 1 h after the first ECG

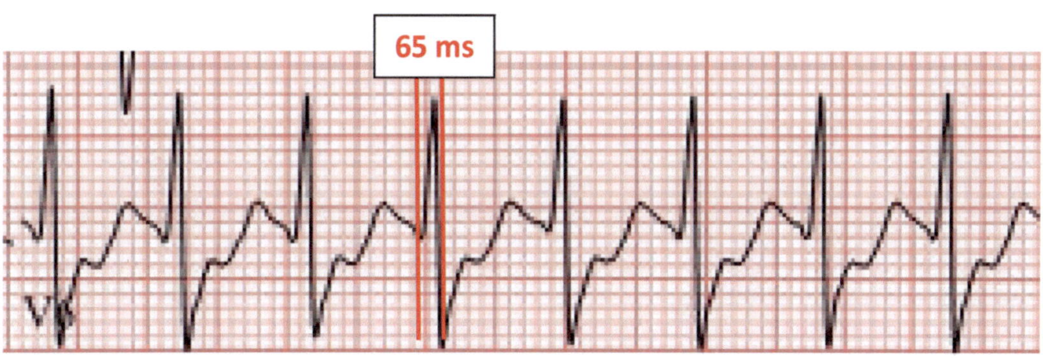

Fig. 3 Lead V6 from the ECG presented in Fig. 1, showing the presence of an RS interval of 65 ms, not in favor of ventricular tachycardia (but not excluding it either)

Answer d is also not correct since atrial fibrillation would have an irregular rhythm. Answer c—"Antidromic tachycardia using a left-sided by-pass tract"—is not correct either, since there is no ventricular pre-excitation, as can be seen from the ECGs in Figs. 2 and 5.

An ECG of the patient is presented after the correction of anemia and antibiotic treatment. Sinus bradycardia with RBBB is present, confirming that the tachycardia from Fig. 1 is actually supraventricular tachycardia with RBBB (Fig. 5). The reason for which P waves are not visible during tachycardia in Fig. 1 is that they are actually superposed on the preceding T wave. This tendency is better observed in Figs. 2 and 4, where the heart rate is slower (109 bpm vs 164 bpm in

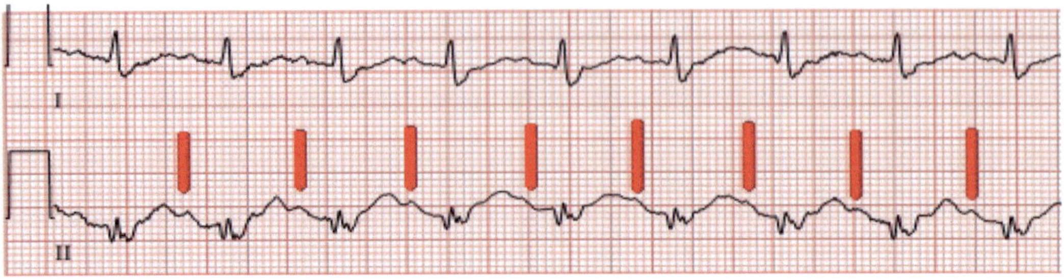

Fig. 4 Sinus rhythm evidenced by the presence of a sinus P wave before each QRS complex

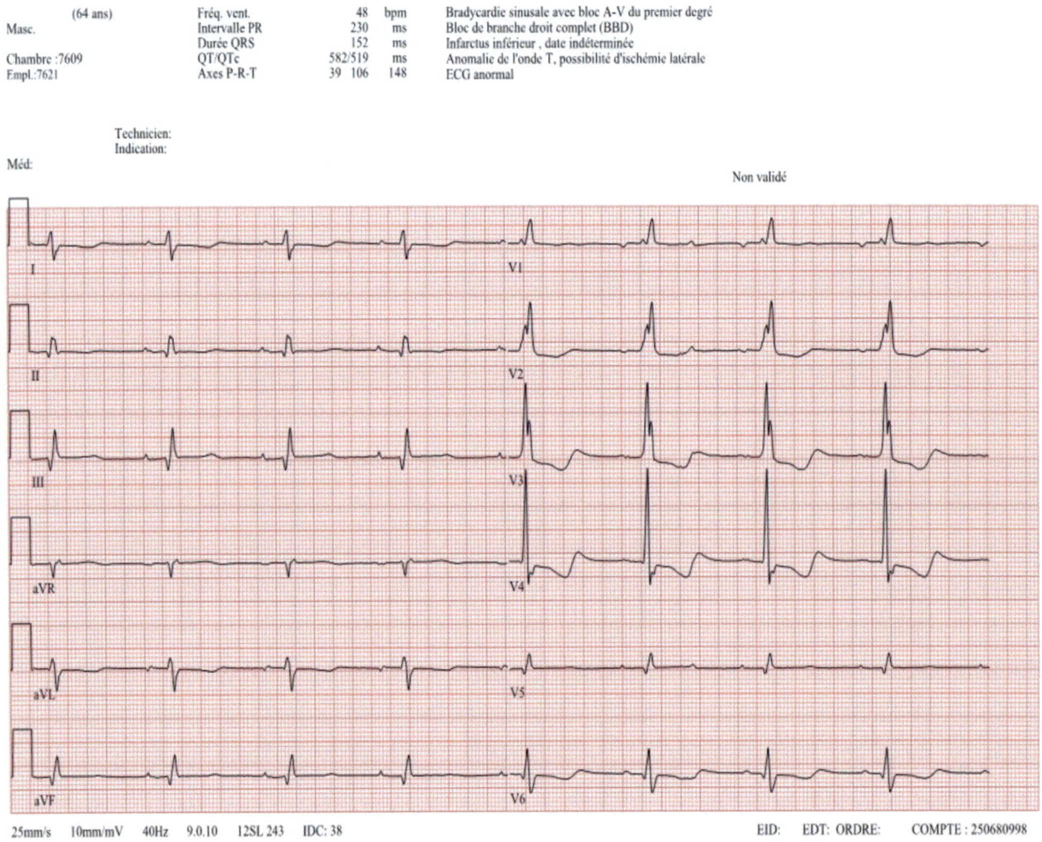

Fig. 5 Twelve-lead ECG showing sinus rhythm with a heart rate of 48 bpm and complete right bundle branch block

Fig. 1), showing P waves at the end of preceding T waves.

References

1. Wellens HJ, Bar FW, Lie KI. The value of the electrocardiogram in the differential diagnosis of a tachycardia with a widened QRS complex. Am J Med. 1978;64(1):27–33.
2. Brugada P, Brugada J, Mont L, Smeets J, Andries EW. A new approach to the differential diagnosis of a regular tachycardia with a wide QRS complex. Circulation. 1991;83(5):1649–59.
3. Vereckei A, Duray G, Szenasi G, Altemose GT, Miller JM. Application of a new algorithm in the differential diagnosis of wide QRS complex tachycardia. Eur Heart J. 2007;28(5):589–600.

ECG 15

Raphael Martins

1 Case Presentation

A 79-year-old male patient with a history of remote inferolateral myocardial infarction (1993), with ischemic cardiomyopathy with moderate left ventricular dysfunction (LVEF of 40–45%), typical counter-clockwise atrial flutter treated with RF ablation (2021), gastric ulcer, and lung carcinoma, presents an episode of palpitations during his hospitalization in the Cardiology Department where he had been admitted 2 days prior for an episode of constrictive chest pain. A 12-lead ECG was recorded during palpitations and is presented in Fig. 1. His coronary angiography demonstrated severe proximal LAD stenosis, severe proximal CX stenosis, and diffuse atheroma of the right coronary artery.

Question: What is the rhythm presented in Fig. 1?

(a) Sinus rhythm with ventricular bigemini
(b) Sinus rhythm with supraventricular bigemini with permanent RBBB
(c) Atrial fibrillation with ventricular bigemini
(d) Atrial fibrillation and bidirectional ventricular tachycardia
(e) Sinus rhythm and bidirectional ventricular tachycardia

Hint: A helping ECG is provided in Fig. 2

Correct answer: e. Sinus rhythm and bidirectional ventricular tachycardia

Explanation The ECG in Fig. 1 shows a regularly irregular rhythm with a heart rate of 121 bpm. There are two types of QRS complexes, both having an RBBB morphology, alternating between each other (to facilitate explanation, the first QRS morphology on the ECG is labeled "morphology A" and the second morphology on the ECG "morphology B") (Fig. 3).

The width of the QRS complex is 144 ms for morphology A and 140 ms for morphology B, as measured in lead V1. There is a left axis deviation for morphology A (QRS axis at −60°) and extreme (north-west) axis deviation (−170°) for morphology B. Neither of the two QRS morphologies corresponds to the typical right bundle branch block morphology [1], since the R/S ratio is <1 in lead V6. For morphology B, the R/S ratio is <1, already starting from lead V2, which is completely atypical for an RBBB. They are, therefore, ventricular in nature. Thus, answer b—"Sinus rhythm with supraventricular bigemini with permanent RBBB"—can be excluded. Another argument for the ventricular nature of

R. Martins (✉)
Department of Cardiology, CHU Rennes, Rennes, France
e-mail: raphael.martins@chu-rennes.fr

L. Muresan (ed.), *ECG Interpretation of Wide QRS Complex Tachycardia*,
https://doi.org/10.1007/978-3-031-97030-6_16

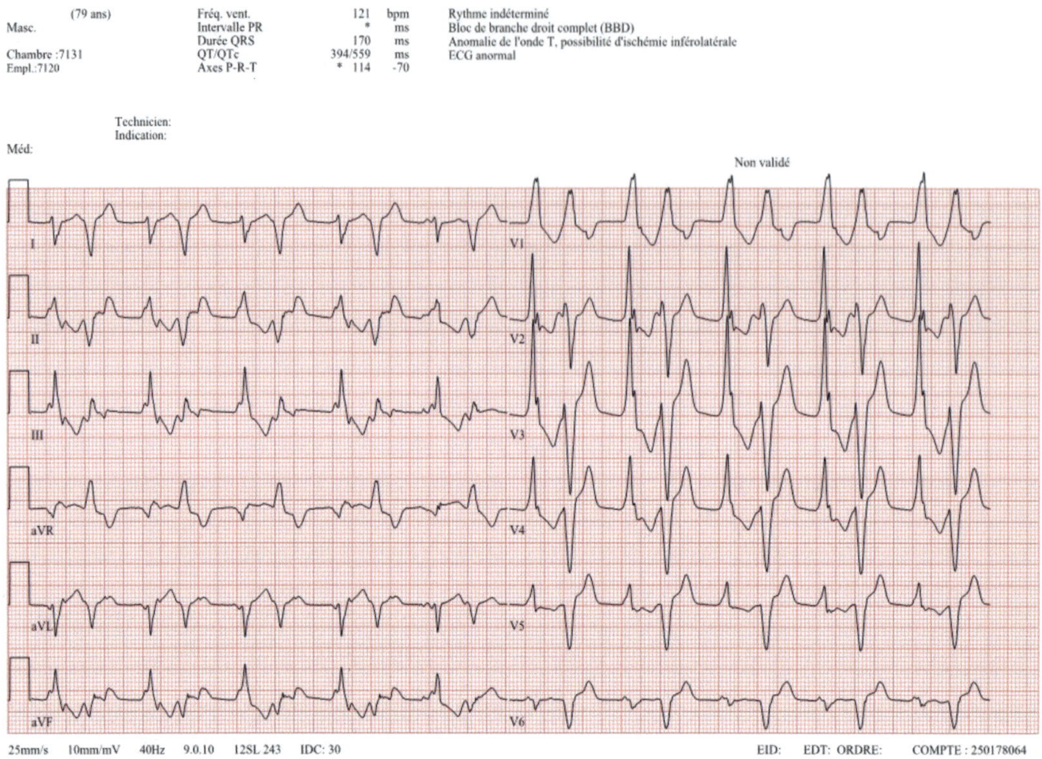

Fig. 1 ECG recorded at admittance to the Emergency Department

this rhythm is the presence of a fusion beat (ninth QRS complex recorded in the limb leads).

There is indeed an alternation between two QRS morphologies, and sinus rhythm with ventricular bigemini could theoretically be the case. In order to characterize the atrial rhythm, one needs to look for P waves. This is not obvious because at a first glance, there are none clearly visible. However, at a closer inspection, a P wave can be seen preceding every other QRS complex (best seen in leads III and aVL, as indicated by the vertical red lines in Fig. 4). The morphology of this P wave is compatible with a sinus origin (positive P wave in leads I, aVL, II, III, and aVF). Nevertheless, the PR interval is too short for these P waves to be transmitted to the ventricles, and, as said above, the morphology of the QRS complex is not evocative of a supraventricular rhythm with a functional RBBB. Therefore, these P waves are not conducted to the ventricles, and answer a—"Sinus rhythm with ventricular bigemini"—is not correct. Since P waves are present, answers c—"Atrial fibrillation with ventricular bigemini"—and d—"Atrial fibrillation and bidirectional ventricular tachycardia"—are not correct either.

A second type of P wave can also be seen, superposed on the T wave of the "B-type" QRS complexes. These are close to the QRS complex, and therefore, they can be retrograde P waves. A possible explanation for their presence is that these represent retrograde activation of the atria, and these P waves do not reset the sinus node (perhaps being blocked in the sino-atrial junction); therefore, the sinus node is not refractory and can initiate a sinus impulse. An alternative hypothesis is that sinus tachycardia is present, and these retrograde P waves depolarize the sinus node, which recovers rapidly and initiates a sinus P wave. Whatever the case, these retrograde P waves are another argument for the ventricular nature of the preceding QRS complexes. The cor-

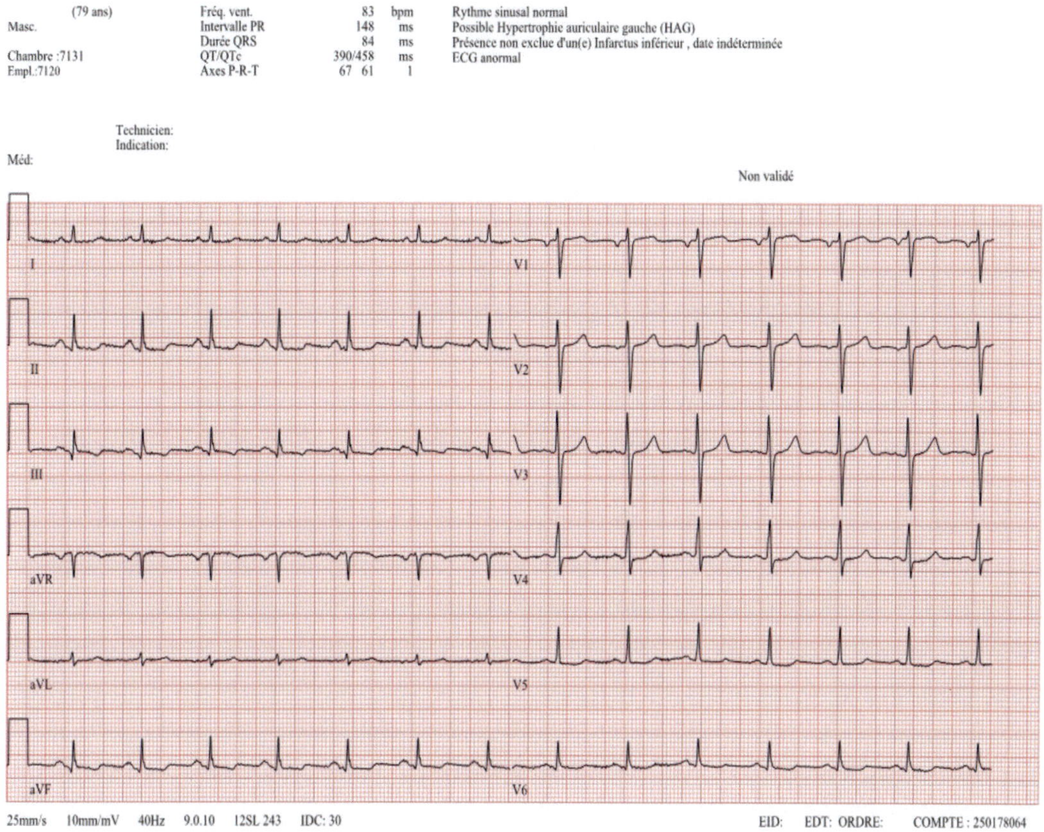

Fig. 2 Twelve-lead ECG recorded 10 min after the first ECG

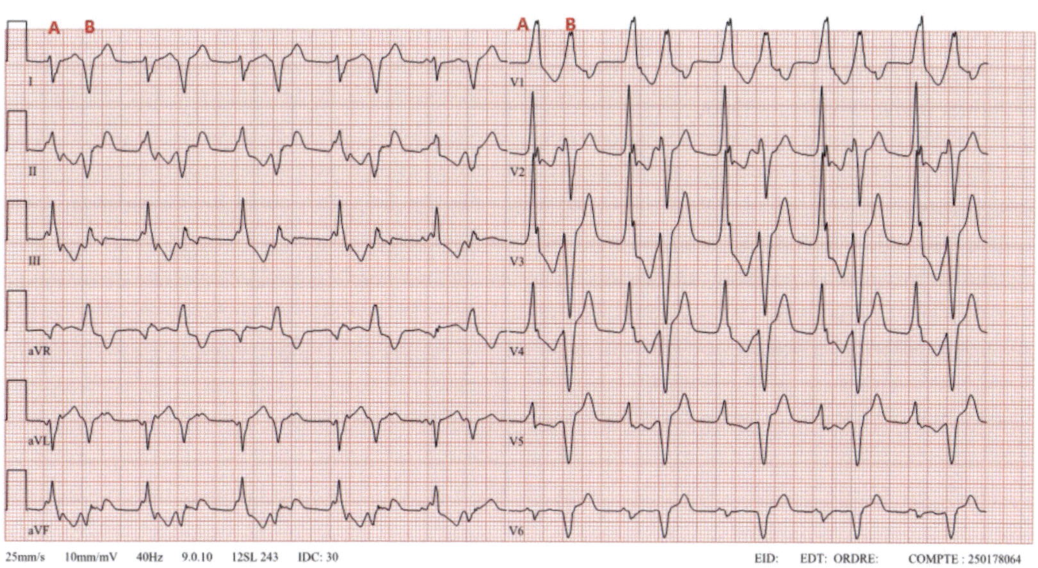

Fig. 3 Annotation of the two alternating QRS morphologies from Fig. 1: A and B

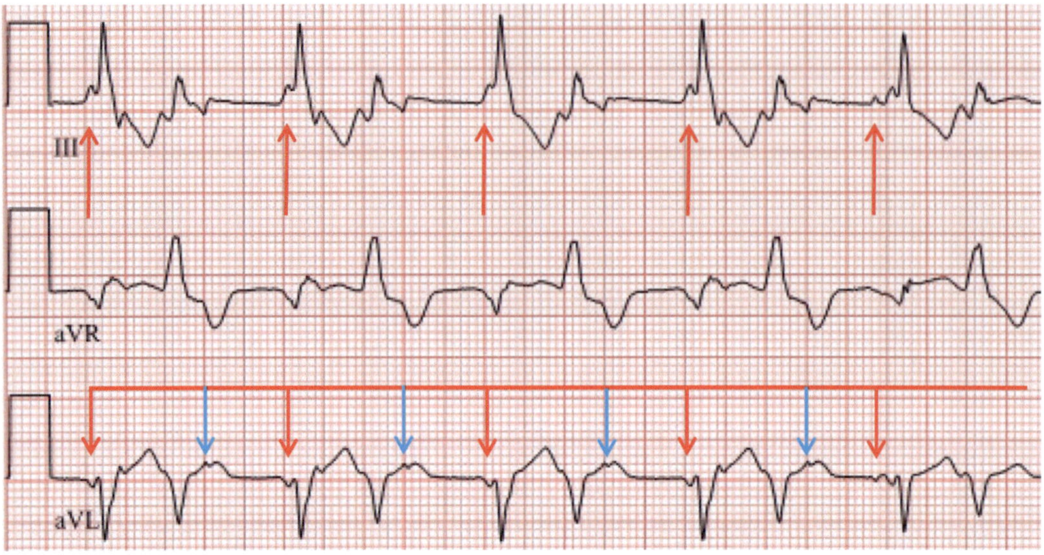

Fig. 4 Leads III, avR, and aVL from the tachycardia presented in Fig. 1. The red vertical lines identify the presence of a P wave preceding every second QRS complex. The last P wave of the five P waves indicated by the red arrows is better seen, being positive in lead aVL. The vertical blue arrows indicate the presence of other P waves, superposed on the preceding T wave, after every second QRS complex, possibly being retrogradely conducted. Both atrial rhythms are regular

rect answer is therefore e—"Sinus rhythm and bidirectional ventricular tachycardia".

The ECG in Fig. 2 shows sinus rhythm with a heart rate of 83 bpm, QRS axis at +60°, absence of ventricular hypertrophy, and absence of ischemia. There is no ventricular pre-excitation present and no atrial fibrillation.

Bidirectional ventricular tachycardia is a special and rare type of ventricular tachycardia that was first described in the context of digoxin intoxication [2, 3].

The mechanism underlying bidirectional ventricular tachycardia is not fully understood but appears to be related either to triggered activity (after depolarization), abnormal automaticity, or re-entry. Treatment of this arrhythmia should address the underlying cause. Antiarrhythmic drugs can also be useful.

References

1. Surawicz B, Childers R, Deal BJ, Gettes LS, Bailey JJ, Gorgels A, et al. AHA/ACCF/HRS recommendations for the standardization and interpretation of the electrocardiogram: part III: intraventricular conduction disturbances: a scientific statement from the American Heart Association Electrocardiography and Arrhythmias Committee, Council on Clinical Cardiology; the American College of Cardiology Foundation; and the Heart Rhythm Society. Endorsed by the International Society for Computerized Electrocardiology. J Am Coll Cardiol. 2009;53(11):976–81.
2. Almarzuqi A, Kimber S, Quadros K, Senaratne J. Bidirectional ventricular tachycardia: challenges and solutions. Vasc Health Risk Manag. 2022;18:397–406.
3. Kummer JL, Nair R, Krishnan SC. Images in cardiovascular medicine. Bidirectional ventricular tachycardia caused by digitalis toxicity. Circulation. 2006;113(7):e156–7.

ECG 16

Jacques Levy

1 Case Presentation

A 70-year-old male patient with a history of persistent atrial fibrillation, asthma, amiodarone-induced hyperthyroidism, severe obstructive sleep apnea, and severe obesity (BMI of 49.38 kg/m^2) presents to the Emergency Department for dyspnea at mild physical effort, asthenia, and fatigue that had progressively worsened during the past 4 weeks. His ECG ad admittance is presented in Fig. 1. Transthoracic echocardiography showed an LVEF of 48–50%, a nondilated left ventricle, moderate LA dilation (surface of 30 cm^2), and mild pulmonary hypertension (sPAP of 45 mmHg). Since atrial fibrillation was considered at least partially responsive for the patient's symptoms, chemical cardioversion was attempted with 300 mg of Flecainide orally. Twenty four hours after the administration of Flecainide, the patient presented an episode of palpitations and pre-syncope. A 12-lead ECG was recorded and is presented in Figs. 2 and 3.

Question: What is the nature of the tachycardia presented in Fig. 2?

(a) Monomorphic ventricular tachycardia
(b) Atrial flutter with 1:1 atrioventricular conduction and left bundle branch block
(c) Antidromic tachycardia using a right-sided bypass tract
(d) Atrial tachycardia with left bundle branch block
(e) Antidromic tachycardia using a right-sided bypass tract

Hint: Look at the QRS duration during atrial fibrillation in Figs. 1 and 3.

Correct answer: a. Monomorphic ventricular tachycardia

Explanation: The ECG in Fig. 1 shows a regular wide QRS complex tachycardia with a heart rate of 183 bpm with LBBB morphology. The width of the QRS complex is 180 ms. The QRS axis is at +40°. The differential diagnosis of this wide QRS complex tachycardia with LBBB morphology includes: ventricular tachycardia (myocardial-related VT and bundle branch re-entry VT), supraventricular tachycardia (atrial fibrillation, atrial flutter, atrial tachycardia, AVNRT, and AVRT) with functional or pre-existing bundle branch block, and antidromic tachycardia (in pre-excitation syndromes).

At a first glance, the morphology of the left bundle branch block of the QRS complex during tachycardia from Fig. 2 suggests that it might be

J. Levy (✉)
Department of Cardiology, Emile Muller Hospital, Mulhouse, France
e-mail: LEVYJ@ghrmsa.fr

L. Muresan (ed.), *ECG Interpretation of Wide QRS Complex Tachycardia*,
https://doi.org/10.1007/978-3-031-97030-6_17

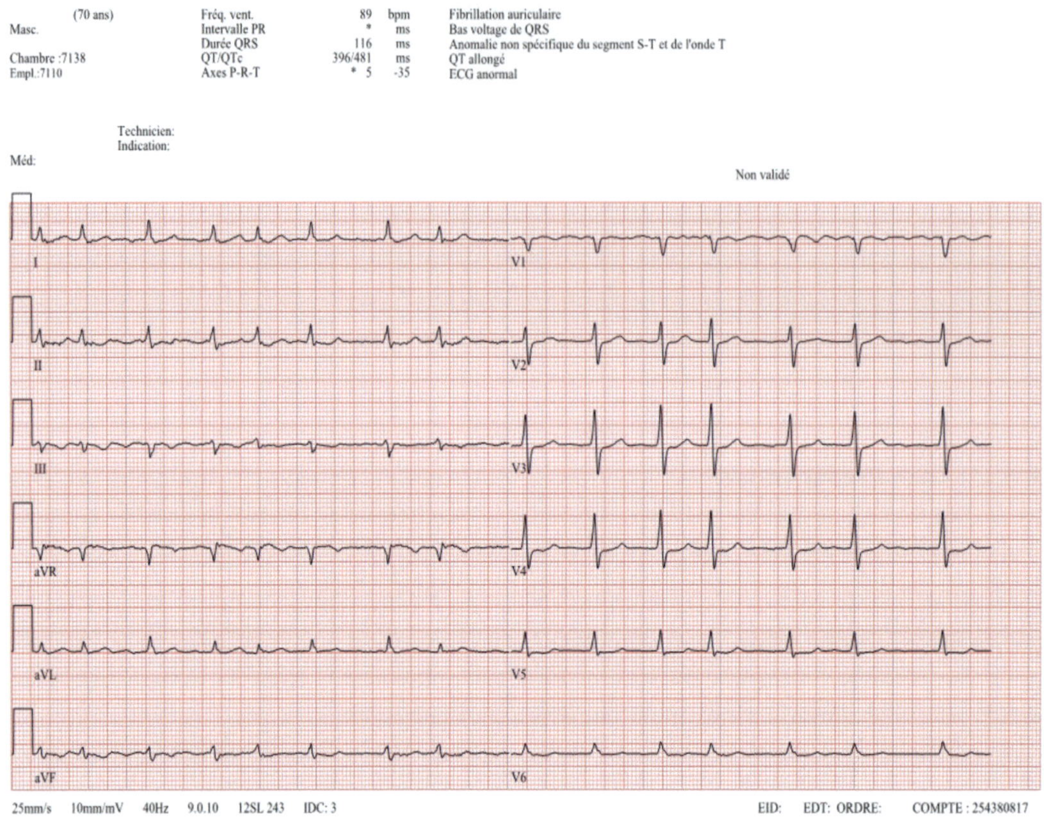

Fig. 1 Twelve-lead ECG recorded at admittance to the Cardiology Department

a typical one: QRS duration >120 ms; absence of q waves in leads V5 and V6; monomorphic R wave (usually notched) in leads I, V5, and V6; and ST segment and T wave modification opposite to the major deflection of the QRS complex: ST segment elevation with positive T waves in leads V1–V3 [1]. So, at this point of the analysis, we cannot say whether this is VT or SVT with BBB. Antidromic tachycardia is unlikely (even though not impossible) given the absence of pre-excitation on the ECG from Fig. 1.

In order to differentiate between VT and SVT with BBB, one needs to better analyze the morphology of the QRS complex, and for that, it is important to correctly delineate the beginning and the end of the QRS complex (Fig. 4). Once this has been done, one can analyze the morphological criteria according to the existing definitions/algorithms.

Applying the Brugada algorithm [2] to the tachycardia from Fig. 2, it can be seen that: (1) There is no absence of an RS complex in the precordial leads (otherwise said, there are rS complexes in leads V4); we therefore move to the second step of the algorithm: (2) This step analyzes the absence of an R-to-S interval >100 ms in any precordial lead. If we take a closer look at the single precordial lead where an "RS" complex is present, lead V4, and measure the RS interval, we can see that it is of 140 ms, and this criterion suggests VT (see Figs. 5 and 6).

Unlike the Brugada algorithm, the Vereckei algorithm [3] for the differential diagnosis of wide QRS complex tachycardias suggests SVT and LBBB as the correct answer. The first step of the algorithm looks for A–V dissociation, which is not seen on the present ECG. The second step of the algorithm looks for an initial predominant R wave in lead aVR, which, again, is not the case (Fig. 7). The third step "QRS morphology unlike BBB or fascicular block" is in fact in favor of

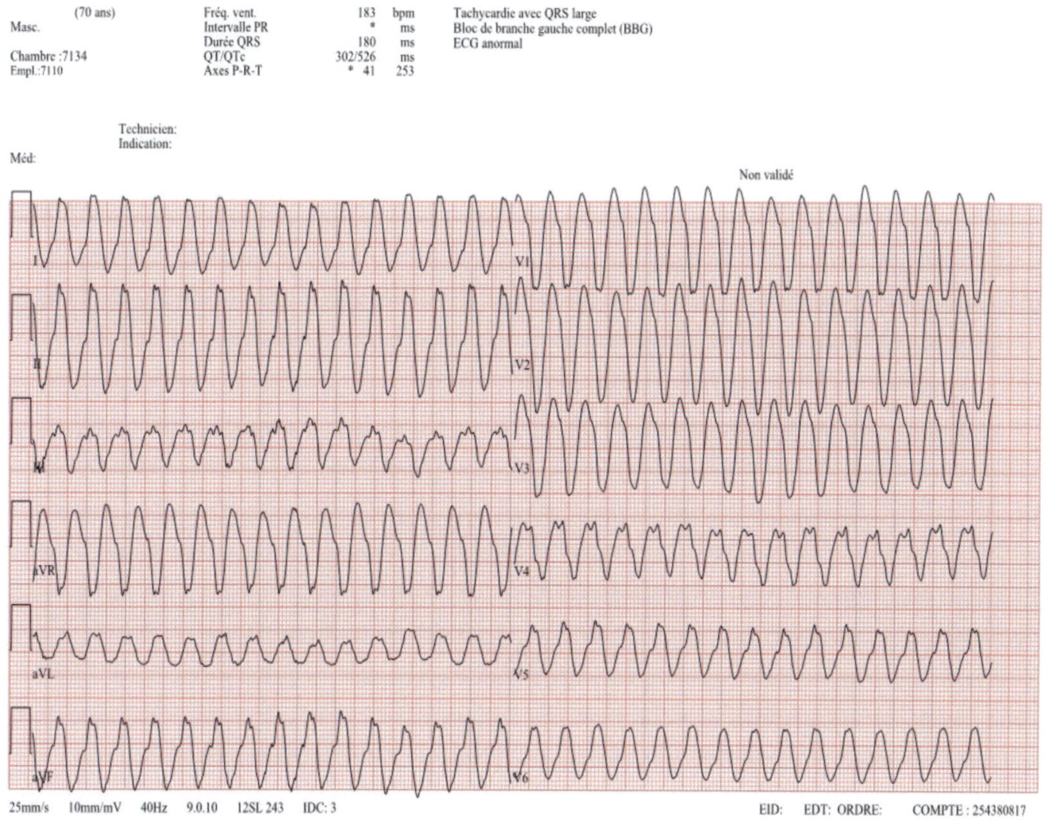

Fig. 2 Twelve-lead ECG recorded after the administration of Flecainide

SVT with typical LBBB based on the morphological criteria explained above [1].

Like the Brugada algorithm, the Basel algorithm [4] is also in favor of ventricular tachycardia as the right answer. According to this algorithm, a positive diagnosis of VT is established if at least two out of three criteria are present: (1) Structural heart disease (history of myocardial infarction, congestive heart failure (LVEF <35%) and the presence of an ICD and CRT), which the patient does not have. (2) The time to first peak in lead II >40 ms (Fig. 8). (3) The time to first peak in lead aVR >40 ms (Fig. 9) [4].

Other arguments in favor of ventricular tachycardia are: (1) For an LBBB QRS morphology, a QRS duration of over 160 ms [5]. (2) A duration of >60 ms from the onset of the QRS to the nadir of the S wave in lead V1 (see Fig. 6) [6].

The duration of the QRS complex before the administration of Flecainide (Fig. 1) is 116 ms, compared to 130 ms in Fig. 3. A widening of the QRS complex with 15–20% in patients taking Flecainide is an argument in favor of an increased risk of developing malignant ventricular arrhythmias [7, 8].

Therefore, the correct diagnosis is monomorphic ventricular tachycardia.

The wide QRS complex tachycardia terminated spontaneously. Flecainide was interrupted, and electrical cardioversion of atrial fibrillation was performed. No VT occurrence was observed during the rest of the patient's stay in hospital.

The present case illustrates the fact that sometimes there is discordance between the different existing algorithms for the differential diagnosis of ventricular tachycardia and that several elements need to be taken into account to establish the correct diagnosis.

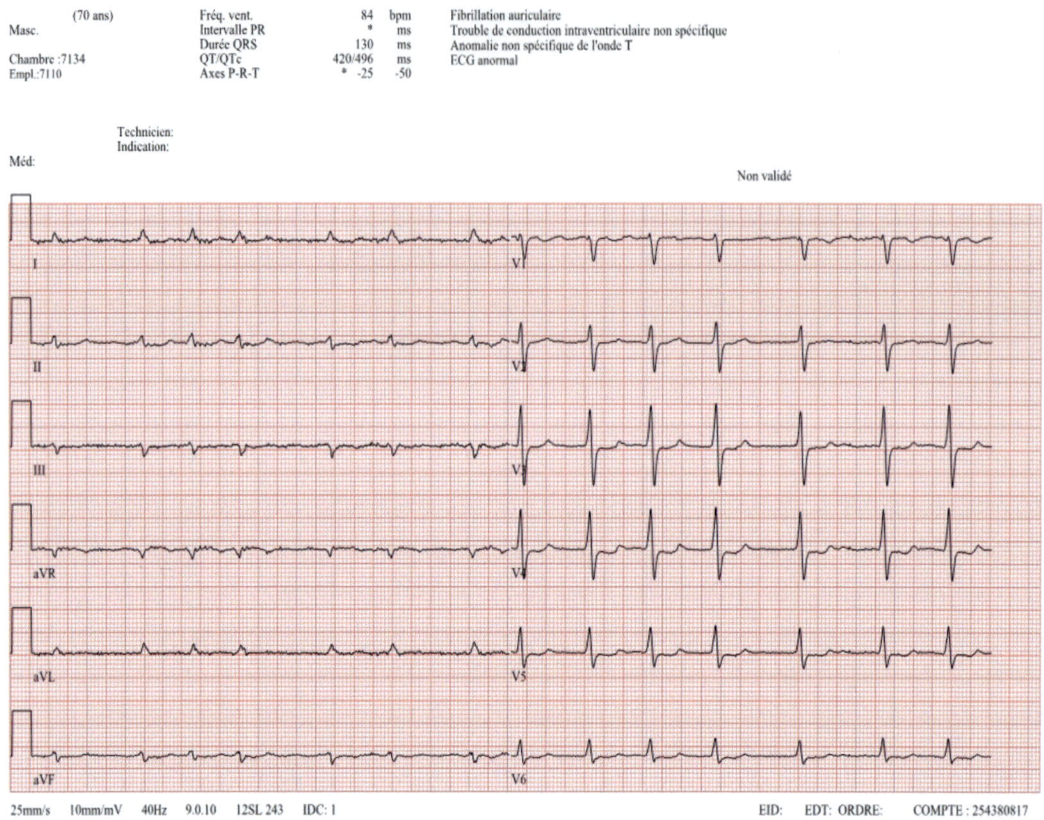

Fig. 3 ECG recorded after termination of the tachycardia

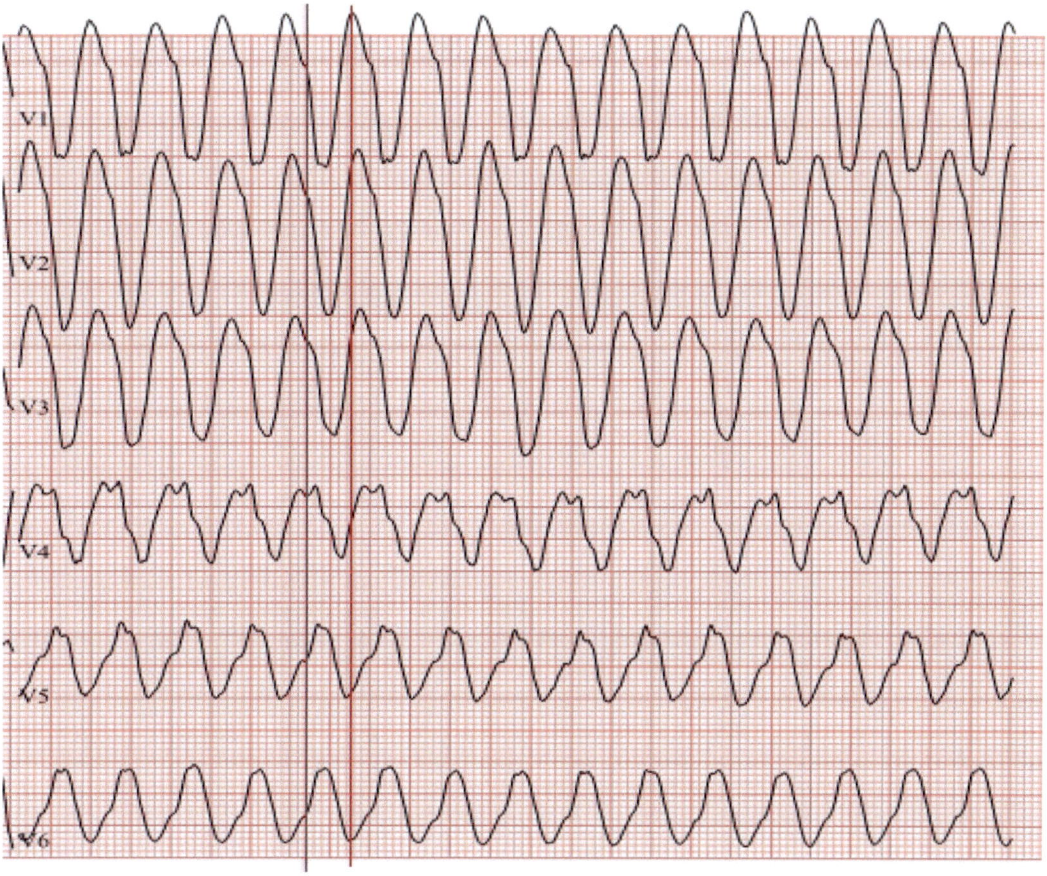

Fig. 4 Delineation of the QRS complex in the precordial leads during tachycardia

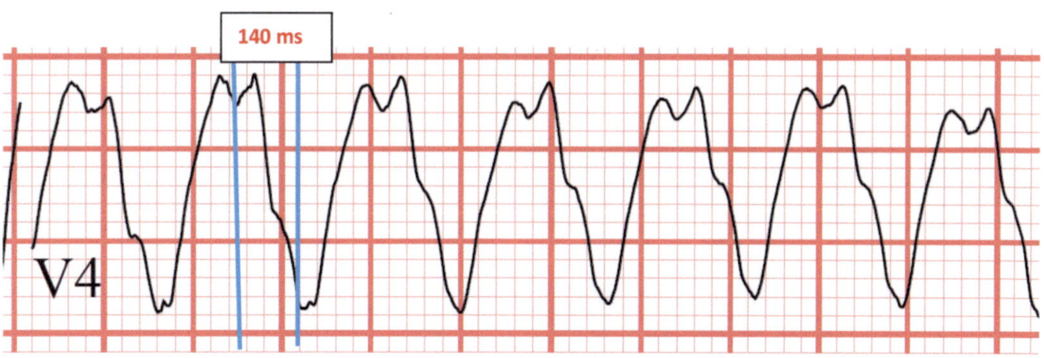

Fig. 5 Detailed analysis of the QRS morphology in lead V4 during the wide QRS complex tachycardia. The RS interval measures 140 ms, criterion in favor of ventricular tachycardia

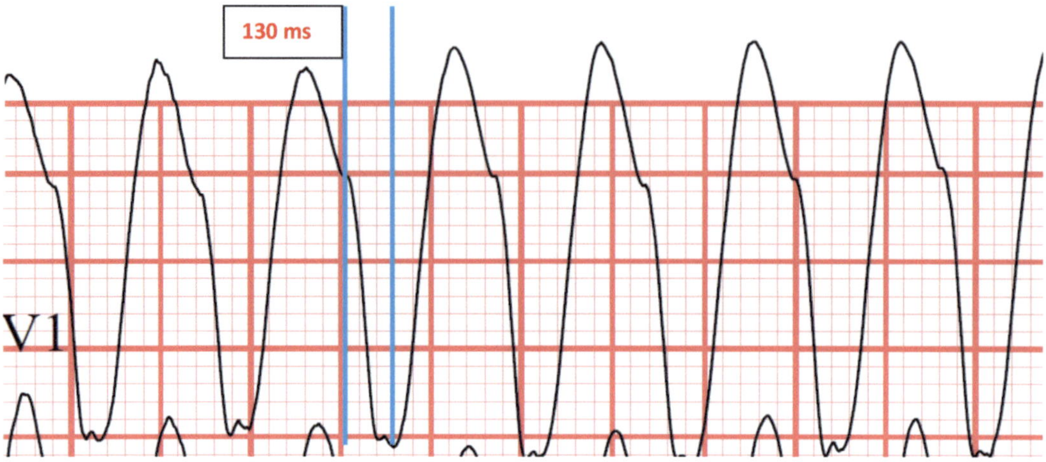

Fig. 6 Detailed analysis of the QRS morphology in lead V1 during the wide QRS complex tachycardia. The RS interval measures 130 ms, criterion in favor of ventricular tachycardia

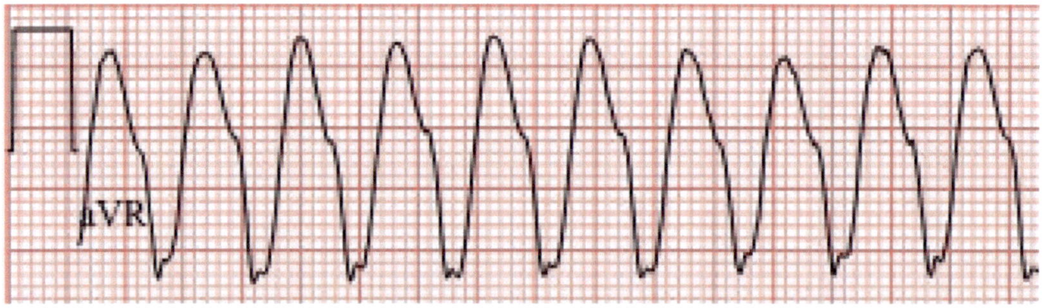

Fig. 7 Lead aVR from the ECG from Fig. 1 recorded during the wide QRS complex tachycardia. The QRS morphology is "QS" not "R", criterion not in favor of ventricular tachycardia (but not excluding it either)

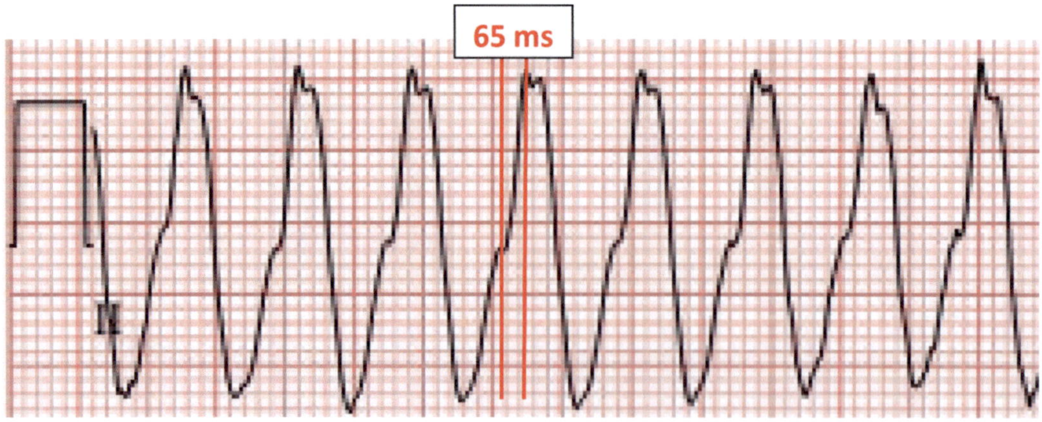

Fig. 8 Lead II from the ECG from Fig. 1 showing the time to first peak of 65 ms, criterion in favor of ventricular tachycardia

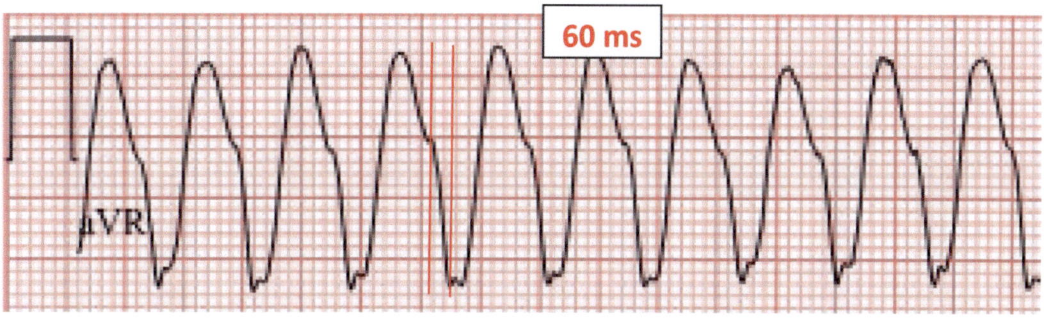

Fig. 9 Lead aVR from the ECG from Fig. 1 showing the time to first peak of 60 ms, criterion in favor of ventricular tachycardia

References

1. Surawicz B, Childers R, Deal BJ, Gettes LS, Bailey JJ, Gorgels A, et al. AHA/ACCF/HRS recommendations for the standardization and interpretation of the electrocardiogram: part III: intraventricular conduction disturbances: a scientific statement from the American Heart Association Electrocardiography and Arrhythmias Committee, Council on Clinical Cardiology; the American College of Cardiology Foundation; and the Heart Rhythm Society. Endorsed by the International Society for Computerized Electrocardiology. J Am Coll Cardiol. 2009;53(11):976–81.
2. Brugada P, Brugada J, Mont L, Smeets J, Andries EW. A new approach to the differential diagnosis of a regular tachycardia with a wide QRS complex. Circulation. 1991;83(5):1649–59.
3. Vereckei A, Duray G, Szenasi G, Altemose GT, Miller JM. Application of a new algorithm in the differential diagnosis of wide QRS complex tachycardia. Eur Heart J. 2007;28(5):589–600.
4. Moccetti F, Yadava M, Latifi Y, Strebel I, Pavlovic N, Knecht S, et al. Simplified integrated clinical and electrocardiographic algorithm for differentiation of wide QRS complex tachycardia: the basel algorithm. JACC Clin Electrophysiol. 2022;8(7):831–9.
5. Eckardt L, Breithardt G, Kirchhof P. Approach to wide complex tachycardias in patients without structural heart disease. Heart. 2006;92(5):704–11.
6. Kindwall KE, Brown J, Josephson ME. Electrocardiographic criteria for ventricular tachycardia in wide complex left bundle branch block morphology tachycardias. Am J Cardiol. 1988;61(15):1279–83.
7. Falk RH. Flecainide-induced ventricular tachycardia and fibrillation in patients treated for atrial fibrillation. Ann Intern Med. 1989;111(2):107–11.
8. Razavi M. Safe and effective pharmacologic management of arrhythmias. Tex Heart Inst J. 2005;32(2):209–11.

ECG 17

Charline Daval

1 Case Presentation

A 74-year-old male patient with a history of non-ischemic cardiomyopathy with severe LV systolic dysfunction (LVEF of 35%), implanted with a CRT-D device for the primary prevention of sudden cardiac death, device extraction due to an episode of device-related infective endocarditis, persistent symptomatic typical atrial flutter treated with catheter ablation (2021), and paroxysmal atrial fibrillation presents to the Emergency Department for an episode of decompensated heart failure. His ECG at admittance is presented in Fig. 1.

Question: What is the nature of the tachycardia presented in Fig. 1?

(a) Sinus tachycardia with left bundle branch block
(b) Ventricular tachycardia originating from the peri-tricuspid region
(c) Ventricular tachycardia originating from the inferoseptal LV
(d) Atrial tachycardia with left bundle branch block
(e) Atrial fibrillation with left bundle branch block

C. Daval (✉)
Department of Cardiology, Emile Muller Hospital, Mulhouse, France
e-mail: charline.daval@ghrmsa.fr

Hint: A second ECG recorded after the administration of 5 mg of bisoprolol orally is presented in Fig. 2.

Correct answer: e. Atrial fibrillation with left bundle branch block

Explanation: The ECG in Fig. 1 shows an irregular wide QRS complex tachycardia with a heart rate of 105 bpm and LBBB morphology. The width of the QRS complex is 196 ms. The QRS axis is at −60°. The differential diagnosis of this irregular wide QRS complex tachycardia with LBBB morphology includes: ventricular tachycardia (myocardial-related VT and bundle branch re-entry VT) and supraventricular tachycardia (atrial fibrillation, atrial flutter, atrial tachycardia, and AVNRT) with functional or pre-existing bundle branch block. Antidromic tachycardia (in pre-excitation syndromes) is generally regular and is less likely present in this case.

The morphology of the left bundle branch block of the QRS complex during tachycardia from Fig. 1 suggests that it might be a typical one: the QRS duration is >120 ms; there is a monomorphic R wave in leads I, aVL, and V6; and there is ST segment and T wave modifications opposite to the major deflection of the QRS complex: ST segment elevation with positive T waves in leads V1–V5 [1]. However, there are

L. Muresan (ed.), *ECG Interpretation of Wide QRS Complex Tachycardia*,
https://doi.org/10.1007/978-3-031-97030-6_18

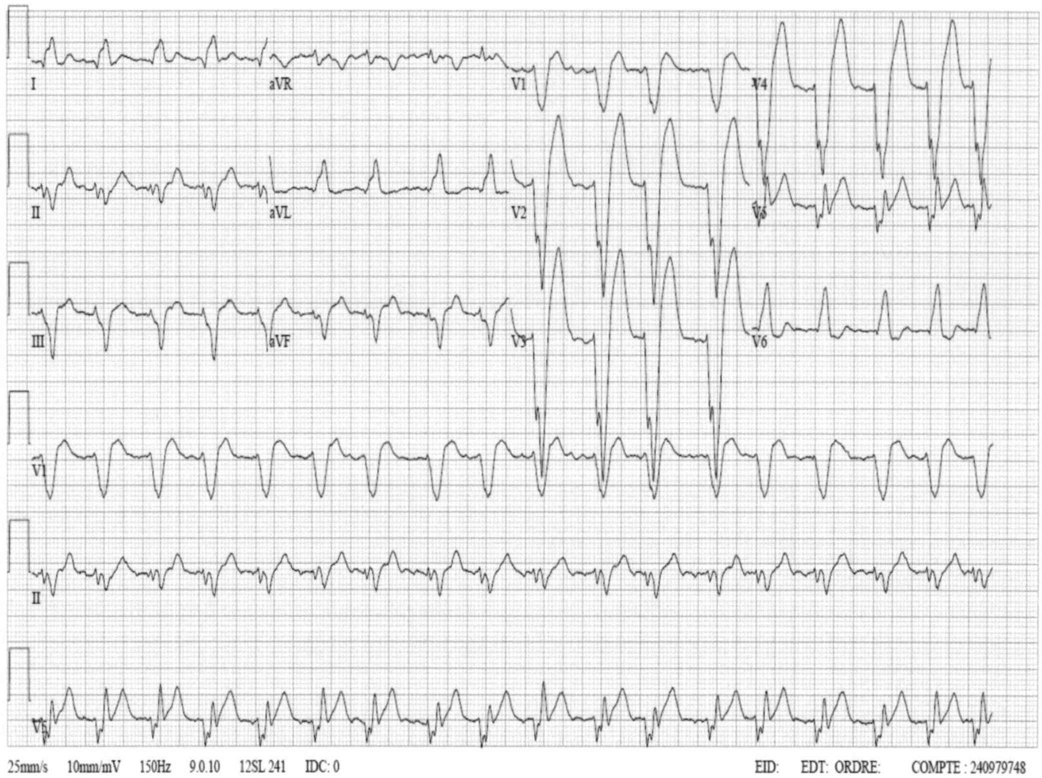

Fig. 1 Twelve-lead ECG recorded at admittance to the Cardiology Department

small q waves present in leads I, aVL, and V6, which are not in favor of a typical left bundle branch block. So, at this point of the analysis, we cannot say whether this is VT or SVT with LBBB.

Applying the Brugada algorithm [2] to the tachycardia from Fig. 1, it can be seen that: (1) There is no absence of an RS complex in the precordial leads (otherwise said, there are rS complexes in leads V2–V4); we therefore move to the second step of the algorithm: (2) This step analyzes the absence of an R-to-S interval >100 ms in any precordial lead, which is actually the case (Fig. 3).

Other arguments from the Brugada algorithm in favor of ventricular tachycardia are: for a wide QRS complex tachycardia with LBBB morphology, such as the present case, the presence of an "r wave" >0.04 s in lead V1 or V2 is not the case in the ECG presented in Fig. 1. The presence of a notched S wave in lead V1 or V2 is actually the case (see Fig. 4). And the presence of a delayed S nadir >0.06 s in lead V1 or V2 is also the case [3] (see Fig. 3).

The Vereckei algorithm [4] for the differential diagnosis of wide QRS complex tachycardias also suggests VT as the correct answer. The first step of the algorithm looks for A–V dissociation. If we analyze the atrial activity, we can see that the atrial rhythm is actually atrial fibrillation (Fig. 5). So, we cannot say if there is A–V dissociation. We, therefore, need to move to step 2 of the algorithm.

The second step of the algorithm looks for an initial predominant R wave in lead aVR, which, again, is not the case. The third step "QRS morphology unlike BBB or fascicular block" does not suggest SVT with BBB, given the presence of q waves in leads I, aVL, and V6, which is atypical for an LBBB [1]. The fourth step of the algorithm analyzes the vi/vt index. This index compares the amplitude of the first 40 ms of a QRS complex to

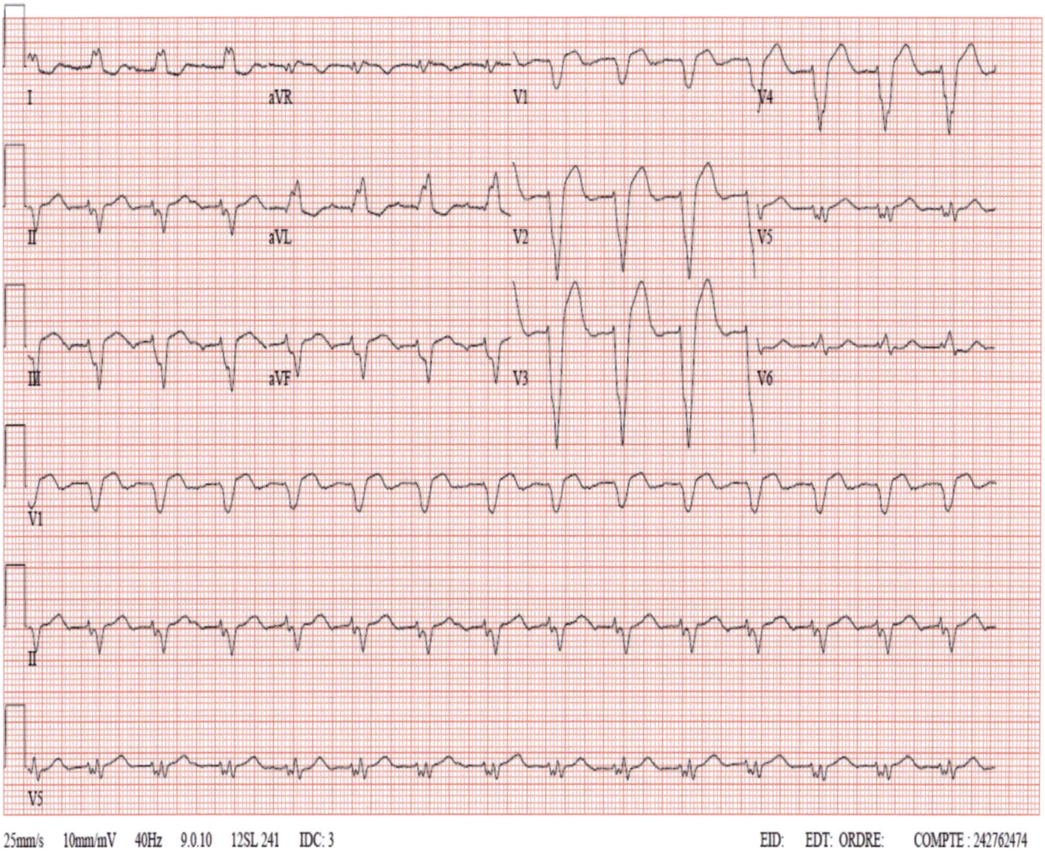

Fig. 2 ECG after administration of bisoprolol 5 mg orally

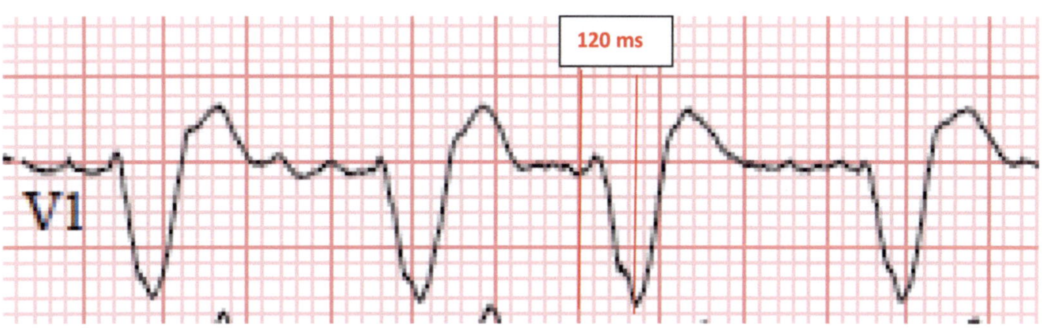

Fig. 3 Lead V1 from the tachycardia presented in Fig. 1 showing an R-to-S interval of 120 ms, argument in favor of ventricular tachycardia

the amplitude of the last 40 ms of the QRS complex in a lead where the QRS has both an R and an S wave. In the present case, this is illustrated in Fig. 6.

Another argument in favor of ventricular tachycardia for an LBBB QRS morphology would be a QRS duration of over 160 ms [5], which is also the case.

Based on these arguments, the diagnosis of ventricular tachcyardia would normally be retained. However, the ECG in Fig. 2 shows that the morphology of the QRS is basically the same

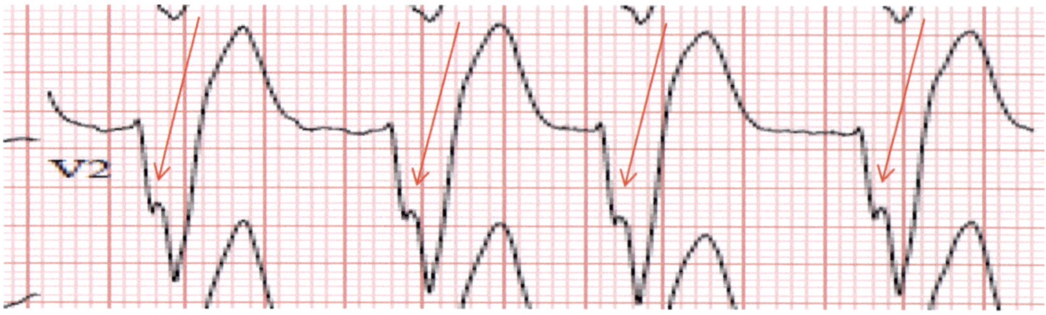

Fig. 4 The QRS complex presents a notch on the descending part of the S wave (Josephson's sign), criterion in favor of ventricular tachycardia

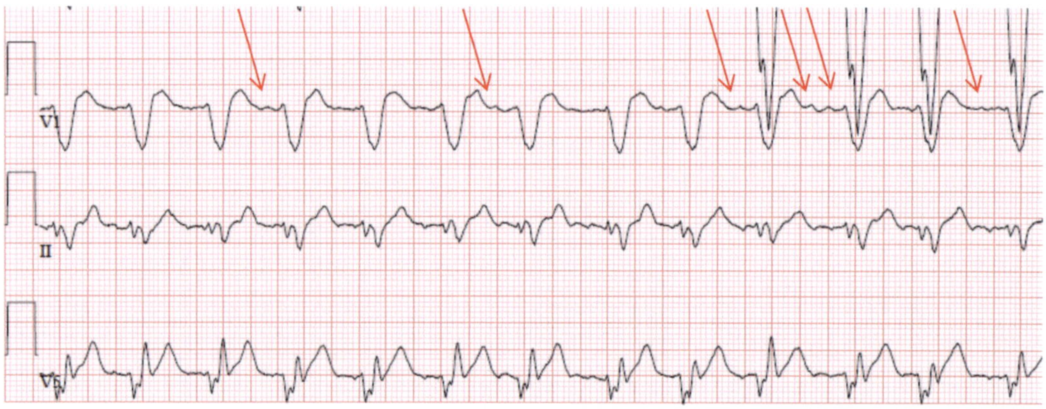

Fig. 5 Leads V1, II, and V5 demonstrating atrial fibrillation (red arrows point to the different morphologies of the f waves)

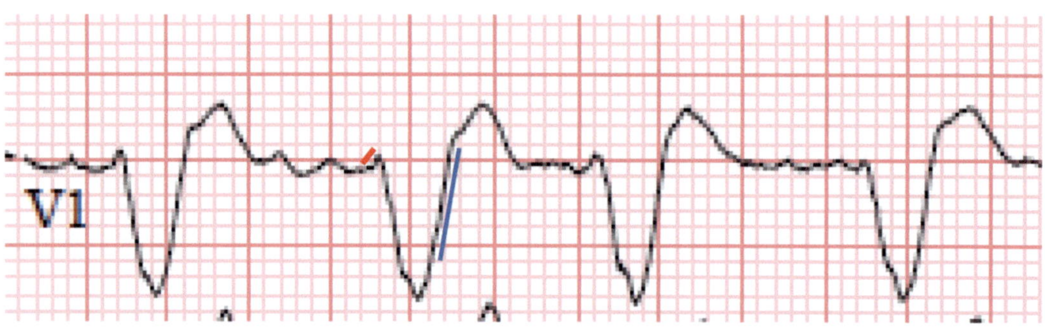

Fig. 6 The vi/vt index from the Vereckei algorithm in lead V1. The ratio of the initial 40 ms and the last 40 ms of the QRS complex is: 1 mV vs 7 mV; therefore, 1/7 = 0.14, which is <1. This is in favor of ventricular tachycardia

with the one from Fig. 1. This is actually sinus rhythm with LBBB (P waves are best seen at the end of the T waves, being positive in lead I and aVL, with a rate of 88 bpm).

This case demonstrates that the existing algorithms are not perfect in differentiating between several etiologies of a wide QRS complex tachycardia and that the evaluation of several ECGs of the same patients is sometimes needed and represents the best way to establish the correct diagnosis.

References

1. Surawicz B, Childers R, Deal BJ, Gettes LS, Bailey JJ, Gorgels A, et al. AHA/ACCF/HRS recommendations for the standardization and interpretation of the electrocardiogram: part III: intraventricular conduction disturbances: a scientific statement from the American Heart Association Electrocardiography and Arrhythmias Committee, Council on Clinical Cardiology; the American College of Cardiology Foundation; and the Heart Rhythm Society. Endorsed by the International Society for Computerized Electrocardiology. J Am Coll Cardiol. 2009;53(11):976–81.
2. Brugada P, Brugada J, Mont L, Smeets J, Andries EW. A new approach to the differential diagnosis of a regular tachycardia with a wide QRS complex. Circulation. 1991;83(5):1649–59.
3. Kindwall KE, Brown J, Josephson ME. Electrocardiographic criteria for ventricular tachycardia in wide complex left bundle branch block morphology tachycardias. Am J Cardiol. 1988;61(15):1279–83.
4. Vereckei A, Duray G, Szenasi G, Altemose GT, Miller JM. Application of a new algorithm in the differential diagnosis of wide QRS complex tachycardia. Eur Heart J. 2007;28(5):589–600.
5. Eckardt L, Breithardt G, Kirchhof P. Approach to wide complex tachycardias in patients without structural heart disease. Heart. 2006;92(5):704–11.

ECG 18

Serban Schiau

1 Case Presentation

A 77-year-old male patient with a history of ischemic cardiomyopathy with moderate systolic dysfunction (LVEF of 40%), remote anterior myocardial infarction at the age of 70, severe aortic stenosis treated with a TAVI procedure at the age of 76, and paroxysmal atrial fibrillation presents to the Emergency Department for signs and symptoms of congestive heart failure (dyspnea on exertion during a mild physical effort). His ECG at admittance is presented in Fig. 1.

Question: What is the nature of the tachycardia presented in Fig. 1?

(a) Sinus tachycardia with right bundle branch block
(b) Ventricular tachycardia originating from the inferoseptal LV wall
(c) Fascicular ventricular tachycardia (re-entry in the anterior fascicle)
(d) Fascicular ventricular tachycardia (re-entry in the posterior fascicle)
(e) Atrial fibrillation with right bundle branch block

Hint: A second ECG recorded after the administration of 300 mg of iv amiodarone is presented in Fig. 2.

Correct answer: e. Atrial fibrillation with right bundle branch block

Explanation: The ECG in Fig. 1 shows an irregular wide QRS complex tachycardia with a heart rate of 160 bpm and RBBB morphology. The width of the QRS complex is 125 ms. There is extreme (north-west) axis deviation. The differential diagnosis of this irregular wide QRS complex tachycardia with RBBB morphology includes: ventricular tachycardia (myocardial-related VT, bundle branch re-entry VT, and fascicular VT) and supraventricular tachycardia (atrial fibrillation, atrial flutter, atrial tachycardia, AVNRT, and AVRT) with functional or pre-existing bundle branch block. Antidromic tachycardia (in pre-excitation syndromes) is generally regular and is less likely present in this case.

The morphology of the right bundle branch block is that of a typical one: QRS duration >120 ms, an "RSR'" pattern in lead V1, an "RS" pattern in leads I, aVL, V5, and V6, and a duration of the S wave of >40 ms in lead V6 [1].

Applying the Brugada algorithm [2] to the tachycardia from Fig. 1, it can be seen that: (1) There is no absence of an RS complex in the

S. Schiau (✉)
Department of Cardiology, "Emile Muller" Hospital, Mulhouse, France
e-mail: serban.schiau@ghrmsa.fr

L. Muresan (ed.), *ECG Interpretation of Wide QRS Complex Tachycardia*,
https://doi.org/10.1007/978-3-031-97030-6_19

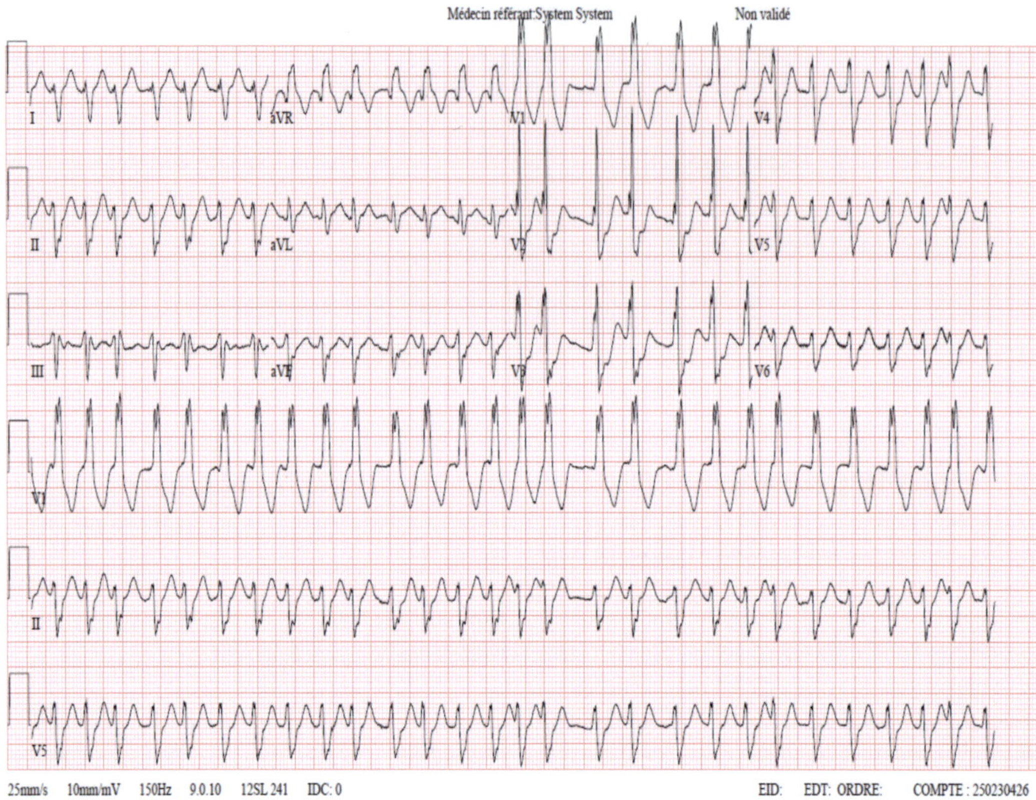

Fig. 1 Twelve-lead ECG recorded at admittance to the Cardiology Department

precordial leads (otherwise said, there are RS complexes in leads V2–V6). (2) There is no R-to-S interval >100 ms in any precordial lead (Fig. 3). (3) There is no AV dissociation visible (actually there are no P waves visible). Therefore, we need to move to the fourth step of the algorithm and analyze the morphology of the QRS complexes during tachycardia.

For an RBBB morphology wide QRS complex tachycardia, an argument in favor of VT would be the presence of a taller left peak of the QRS complex in lead V1 (the rabbit ear sign) or for biphasic RS or QR complexes, which is not the case (the aspect is RSR', with the amplitude of the first R wave being smaller than the amplitude of the R' wave) (Fig. 4).

Next, in lead V6, an argument in favor of VT would be the presence of an "rS" complex (a ratio of R/S <1), which is actually the case either (Fig. 5). Therefore, we have one argument in favor of VT. Another argument in favor of ventricular tachycardia is the "extreme north-west" axis deviation.

The Vereckei algorithm [3] for the differential diagnosis of wide QRS complex tachycardias suggests SVT with RBBB as the correct answer. The first step of the algorithm looks for A–V dissociation, which is not seen on the present ECG. The second step of the algorithm looks for an initial predominant R wave in lead aVR, which, again, is not the case (Fig. 6).

The third step "QRS morphology unlike BBB or fascicular block" is in fact in favor of SVT (atrial fibrillation) with typical BBB: the presence of an irregular rhythm, with no visible P waves and a large QRS complex with typical RBBB morphology.

Like the Vereckei algorithm, the Basel algorithm [4] is also in favor of supraventricular tachycardia with RBBB as the right answer. According to this algorithm, a positive diagnosis of VT is established if at least two out of three

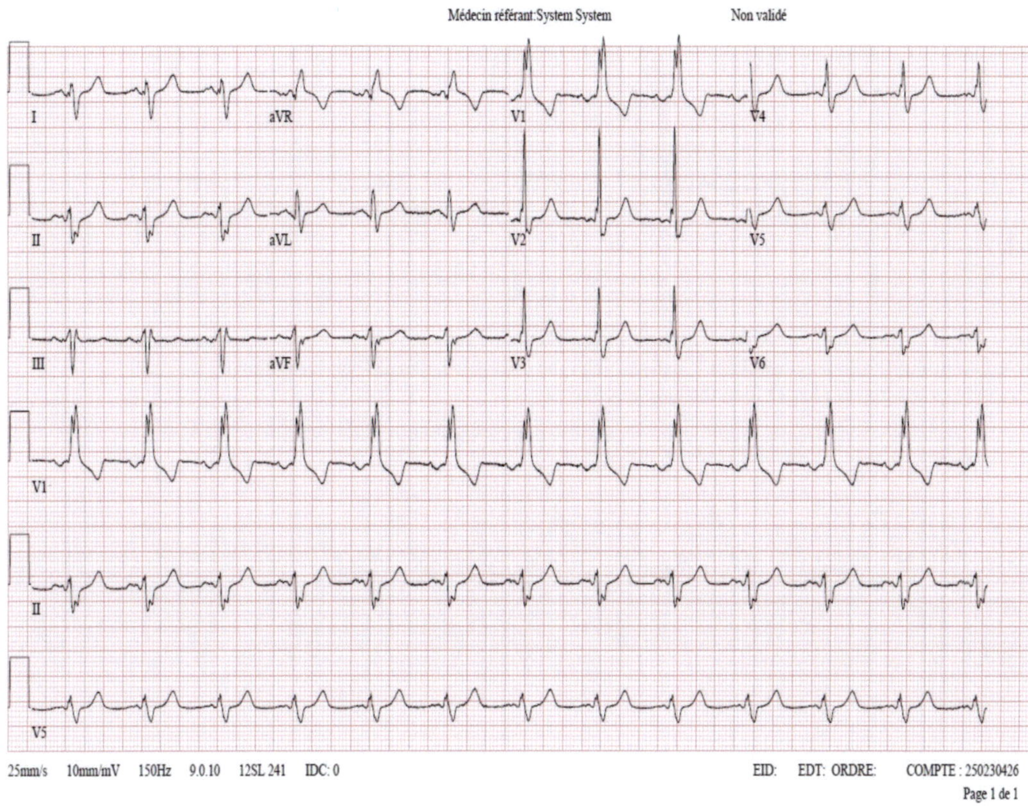

Fig. 2 ECG after administration of 300 mg of iv amiodarone

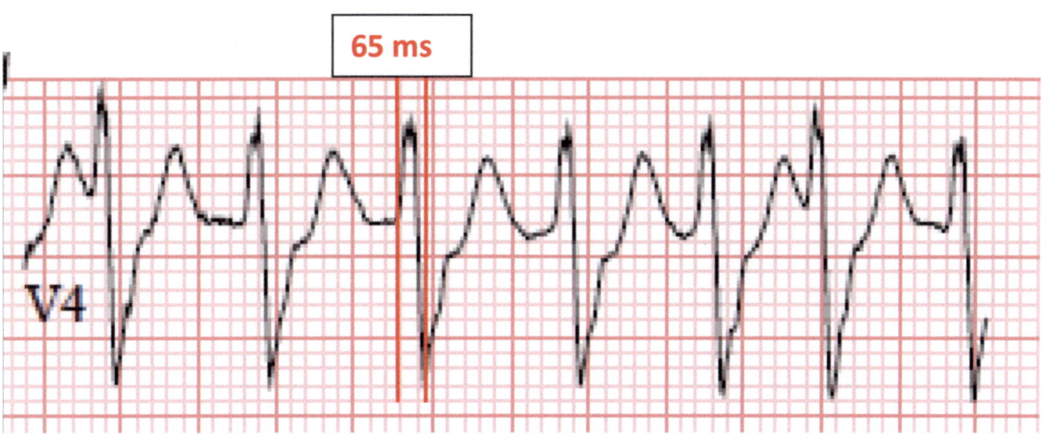

Fig. 3 Lead V4 from the wide QRS complex tachycardia presented in Fig. 1 showing an R-to-S interval of 65 ms (<100 ms), argument not favoring the diagnosis of ventricular tachycardia (but not excluding it either)

criteria are present: (1) Structural heart disease (history of myocardial infarction, congestive heart failure (LVEF <35%), the presence of an ICD and CRT), which the patient has (remote myocardial infarction). (2) The time to first peak in lead II >40 ms (Fig. 7), which is not the case. (3) The time to first peak in lead aVR >40 ms (Fig. 8), which is also not the case [4]. Therefore,

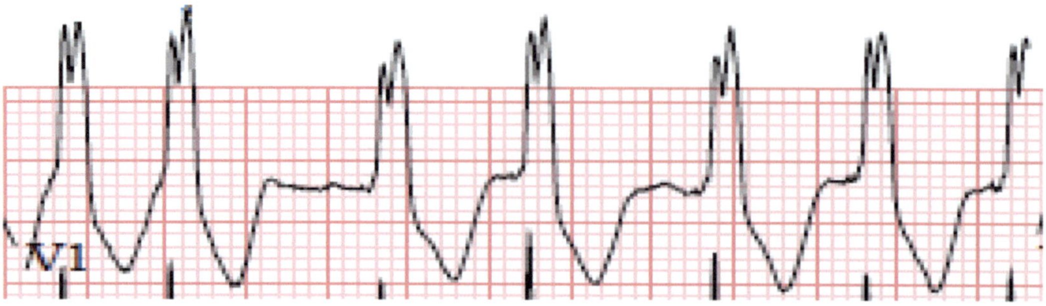

Fig. 4 Lead V1 from the wide QRS complex tachycardia presented in Fig. 1 showing an "RSR'" pattern, with the amplitude of the R wave lesser than the amplitude of the R' wave, argument not favoring the diagnosis of ventricular tachycardia (but not excluding it either)

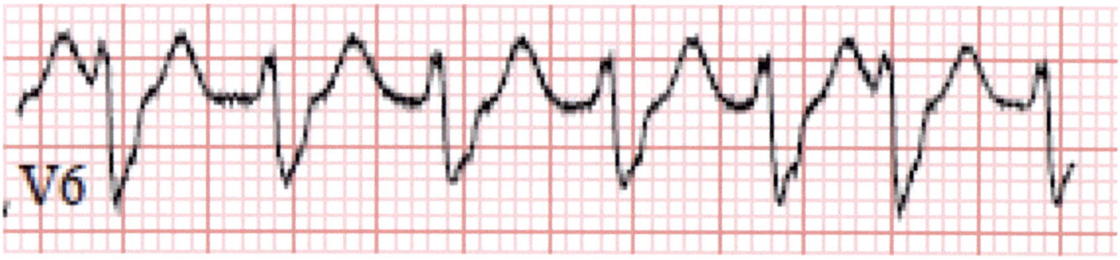

Fig. 5 Lead V6 from the wide QRS complex tachycardia presented in Fig. 1 showing an R-to-S ratio of <1, argument in favor of ventricular tachycardia.

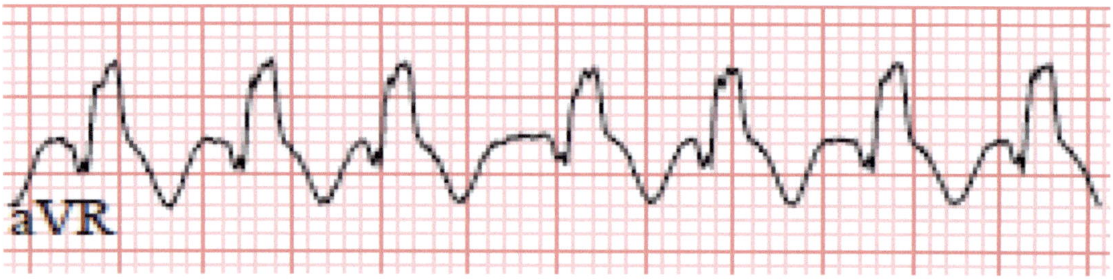

Fig. 6 Lead aVR from the wide QRS complex tachycardia presented in Fig. 1 showing the "rSR'" pattern, or the absence of an initial tall R wave, argument not favoring the diagnosis of ventricular tachycardia (but not excluding it either)

according to the Basel algorithm, there is only one criterion in favor of VT, and the diagnosis of VT cannot be established.

The ECG from Fig. 2, recorded after the administration of 300 mg of iv amiodarone, shows the presence of sinus rhythm with a heart rate of 73 bpm, with extreme (north-west) axis deviation and with typical RBBB morphology. The morphology of the QRS is identical to the one from the ECG presented in Fig. 1, recorded during the wide QRS complex tachycardia. This is a very strong argument for the tachycardia from Fig. 1 being SVT with RBBB.

Therefore, the correct answer is: b. Atrial fibrillation with right bundle branch block". This case demonstrates that sometimes different algorithms point to different diagnosis and that in case of doubt, several arguments need to be con-

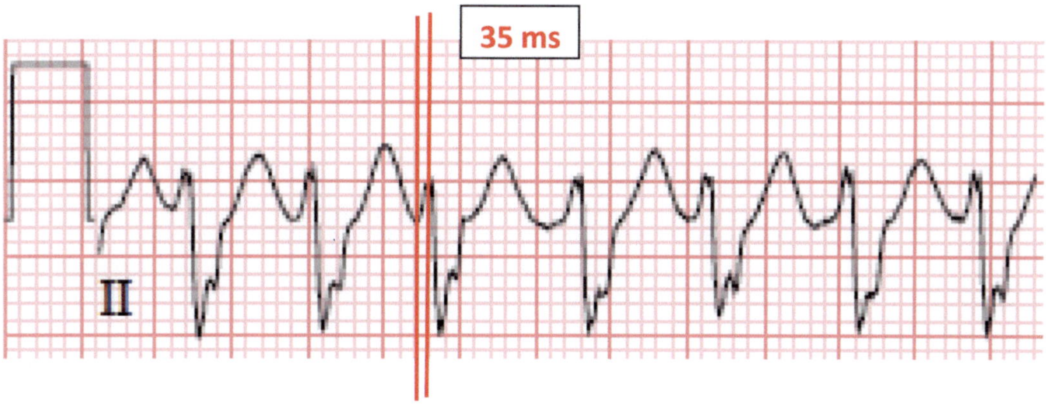

Fig. 7 Lead II from the ECG from Fig. 1 showing the time to first peak of 35 ms, criterion not in favor of ventricular tachycardia

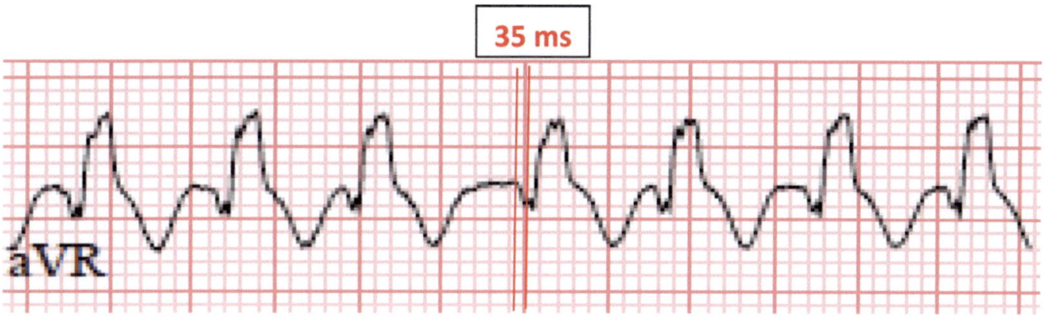

Fig. 8 Lead aVR from the ECG from Fig. 1 showing the time to first peak of 35 ms, criterion not in favor of ventricular tachycardia

sidered in order to reach the correct diagnosis; relying on a single diagnostic criterion risks to establish a wrong conclusion.

The patient was scheduled for a catheter ablation procedure of his atrial fibrillation.

References

1. Wellens HJ, Bar FW, Lie KI. The value of the electrocardiogram in the differential diagnosis of a tachycardia with a widened QRS complex. Am J Med. 1978;64(1):27–33.
2. Brugada P, Brugada J, Mont L, Smeets J, Andries EW. A new approach to the differential diagnosis of a regular tachycardia with a wide QRS complex. Circulation. 1991;83(5):1649–59.
3. Vereckei A, Duray G, Szenasi G, Altemose GT, Miller JM. Application of a new algorithm in the differential diagnosis of wide QRS complex tachycardia. Eur Heart J. 2007;28(5):589–600.
4. Moccetti F, Yadava M, Latifi Y, Strebel I, Pavlovic N, Knecht S, et al. Simplified integrated clinical and electrocardiographic algorithm for differentiation of wide QRS complex tachycardia: the basel algorithm. JACC Clin Electrophysiol. 2022;8(7):831–9.

ECG 19

Lucien Diene

1 Case Presentation

A 58-year-old male patient with a history of coronary artery disease, remote anterior myocardial infarction (2009) treated with PTCA + stent implantation at the level of the proximal LAD coronary artery, and with ischemic cardiomyopathy with severe LV systolic dysfunction (LVEF of 31%) is admitted to the Cardiology Department due to an episode of palpitations with sudden onset and regular rhythm, accompanied by presyncope and chest pain, that had started 15 min before arriving at the Emergency Department. His ECG recorded at admittance to the Cardiology Department is presented in Fig. 1.

Question: What is the nature of the rhythm presented in Fig. 1?

(a) Ventricular tachycardia originating from the inferior lateral LV wall
(b) Ventricular tachycardia originating from the anterior lateral LV wall
(c) Ventricular tachycardia originating from the anterior septal LV wall
(d) Antidromic tachycardia using a left-sided bypass tract
(e) AVNRT with right bundle branch block

L. Diene (✉)
Department of Cardiology, Clinique Le Noirmont, Le Noirmont, Switzerland

Hint: A second ECG recorded several minutes later is presented in Fig. 2.

Correct answer: b. Ventricular tachycardia originating from the anterior lateral LV wall

Explanation: The ECG in Fig. 1 shows a regular wide QRS complex tachycardia with a heart rate of 170 bpm and RBBB morphology. The width of the QRS complex is 176 ms. The QRS axis is at +160°. The differential diagnosis of this regular wide QRS complex tachycardia with RBBB morphology includes: ventricular tachycardia (myocardial-related VT, bundle branch reentry VT, and fascicular tachycardia), supraventricular tachycardia (atrial flutter, atrial tachycardia, AVNRT, and AVRT) with functional or pre-existing bundle branch block, and antidromic tachycardia (in pre-excitation syndromes).

The morphology of the right bundle branch block of the QRS complex during tachycardia from Fig. 1 is not that of a typical one [1]: the QRS duration is indeed >120 ms, and the QRS has an "RSR'" morphology in lead V1. However, the QRS complex has a "QS" morphology in V4–V6; there are deep "Q" waves in leads V2 and V3, elements which are not in favor of a typical right bundle branch block. This makes SVT with RBBB highly unlikely.

L. Muresan (ed.), *ECG Interpretation of Wide QRS Complex Tachycardia*,
https://doi.org/10.1007/978-3-031-97030-6_20

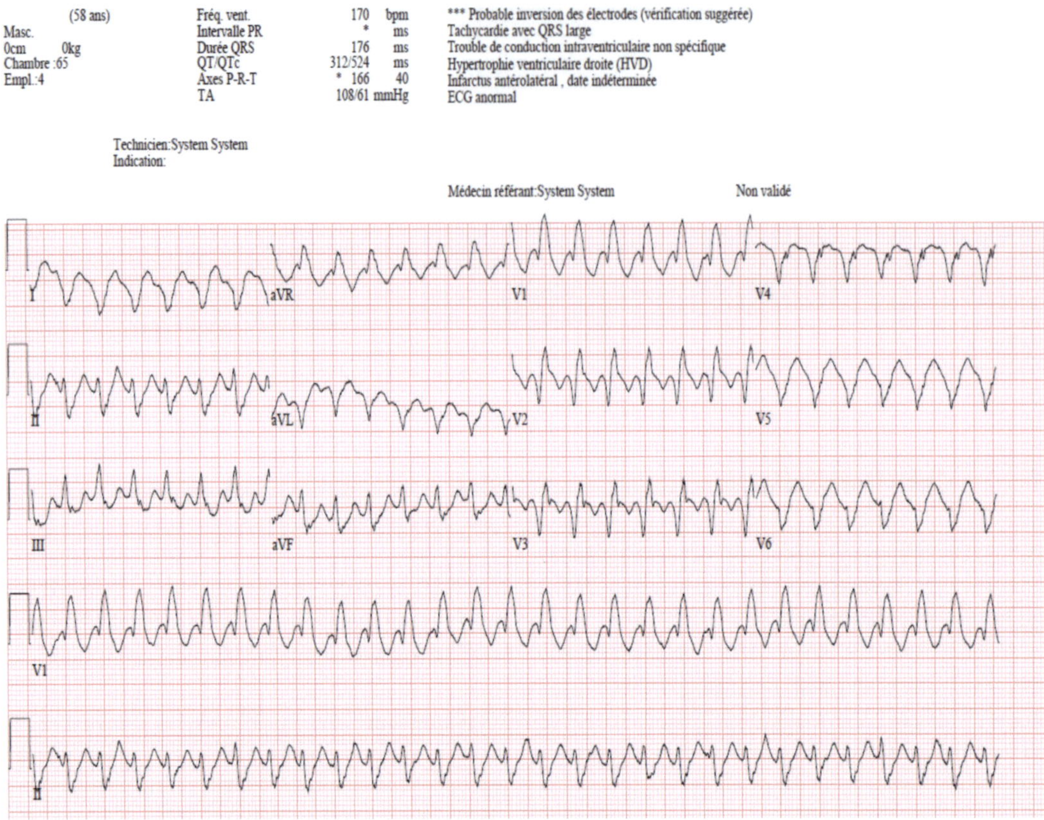

Fig. 1 Twelve-lead ECG recorded at admittance to the Cardiology Department

The ECG from Fig. 2 shows sinus rhythm with a heart rate of 58 bpm, QRS axis at +25°, absence of LV hypertrophy, with anteroseptal necrosis (QS aspect in leads V1–V3), biphasic T waves in V2 and V3, negative T waves in leads V4–V6, DI, and aVL, compatible with ischemia of the anterior LV wall; there are no signs of ventricular pre-excitation (no short PR interval and no delta waves). This makes antidromic tachycardia unlikely.

Applying the Brugada algorithm [2] to the tachycardia from Fig. 2, it can be seen that there is absence of RS complexes in the precordial leads (Fig. 3). This is a strong argument in favor of ventricular tachycardia.

Other morphological criteria from the Brugada algorithm favoring the diagnosis of ventricular tachycardia are the presence of an R-to-S ratio <1 in lead V6 (there is actually no R wave in lead V6 but a QS pattern) (Fig. 3).

The Vereckei algorithm [3] for the differential diagnosis of wide QRS complex tachycardias also suggests VT as the correct answer. The first step of the algorithm looks for A–V dissociation, which is not seen on the present ECG. The second step of the algorithm looks for an initial predominant R wave in lead aVR, which is also not the case (Fig. 4).

The third step of the algorithm "QRS morphology unlike BBB or fascicular block" does not suggest SVT with RBBB, based on the arguments exposed above. Therefore, the diagnosis is that of ventricular tachycardia.

Other arguments in favor of ventricular tachycardia are: a QRS transition in the precordial leads in V4 for an RBBB morphology wide QRS complex tachycardia (Fig. 3) and a QRS duration >140 ms (QRS duration of 176 ms).

The diagnosis is therefore ventricular tachycardia. Its origin is at the level of the left ventricle

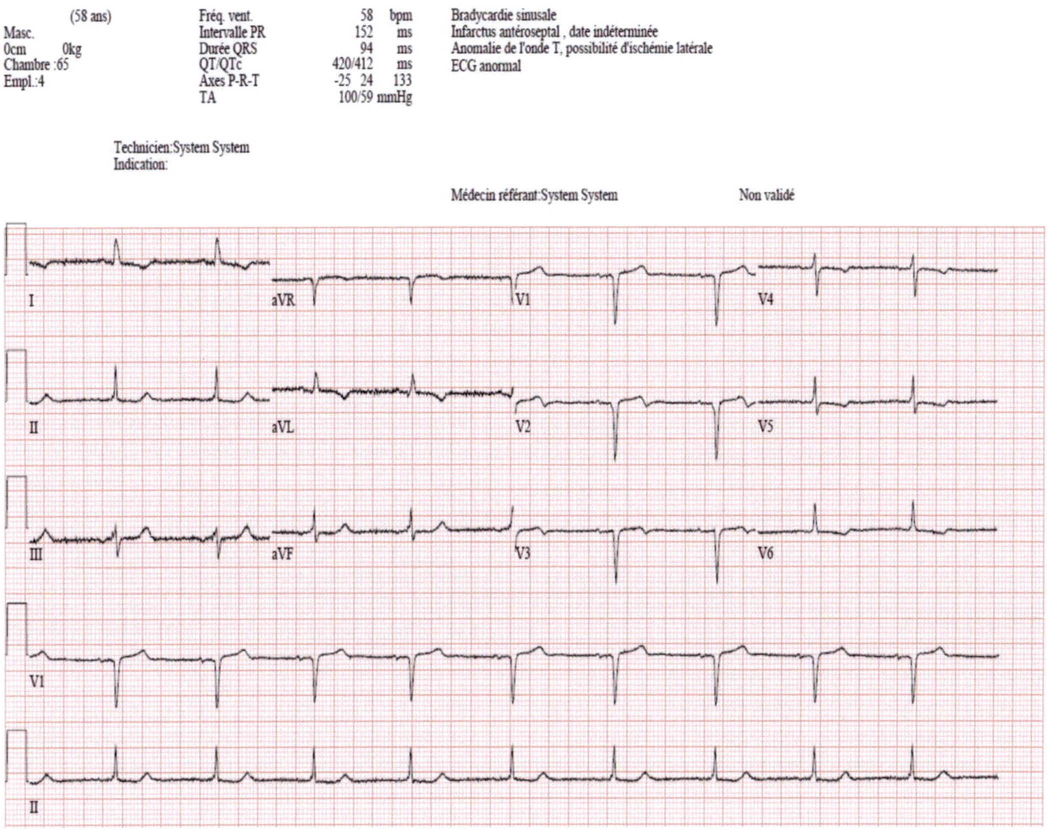

Fig. 2 Twelve-lead ECG recorded after the end of the episode of palpitations

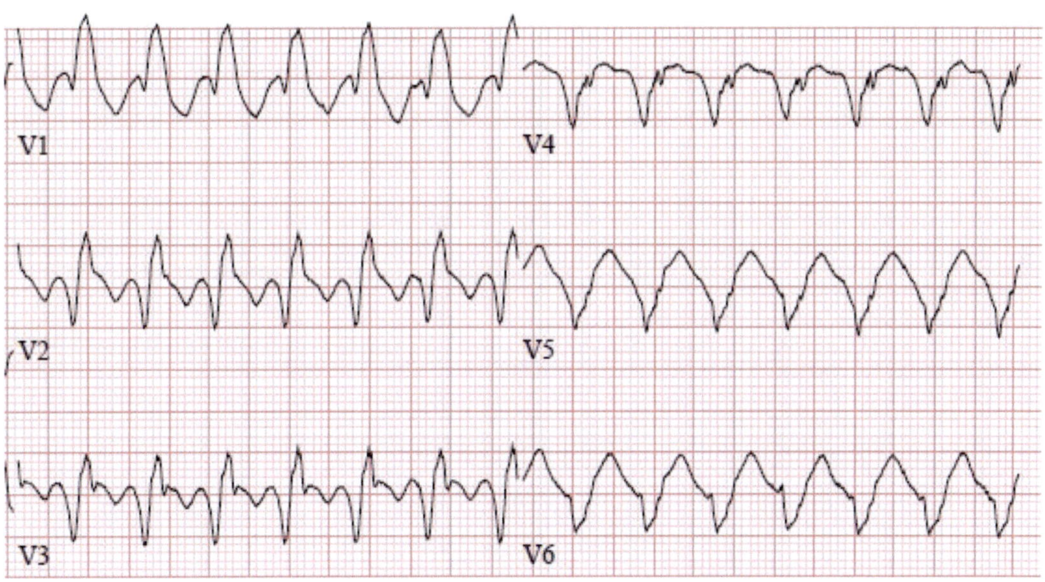

Fig. 3 Precordial leads in the wide QRS complex tachycardia presented in Fig. 1 showing the absence of RS complexes, a strong argument in favor of ventricular tachycardia

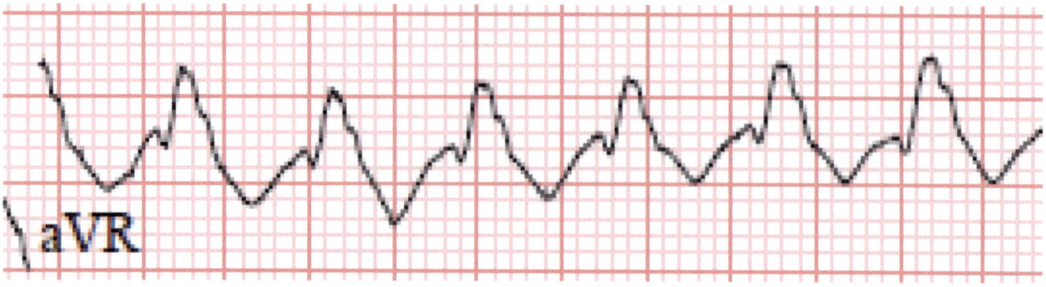

Fig. 4 Lead aVR from the tachycardia presented in Fig. 1, showing the absence of an initial tall R wave, argument not in favor of ventricular tachycardia (but not excluding it either)

(RBBB morphology), anterior wall (positive QRS complexes in leads III and aVF), and at the level of the lateral wall (negative QRS complex in leads I and aVL).

References

1. Surawicz B, Childers R, Deal BJ, Gettes LS, Bailey JJ, Gorgels A, et al. AHA/ACCF/HRS recommendations for the standardization and interpretation of the electrocardiogram: part III: intraventricular conduction disturbances: a scientific statement from the American Heart Association Electrocardiography and Arrhythmias Committee, Council on Clinical Cardiology; the American College of Cardiology Foundation; and the Heart Rhythm Society. Endorsed by the International Society for Computerized Electrocardiology. J Am Coll Cardiol. 2009;53(11):976–81.
2. Brugada P, Brugada J, Mont L, Smeets J, Andries EW. A new approach to the differential diagnosis of a regular tachycardia with a wide QRS complex. Circulation. 1991;83(5):1649–59.
3. Vereckei A, Duray G, Szenasi G, Altemose GT, Miller JM. Application of a new algorithm in the differential diagnosis of wide QRS complex tachycardia. Eur Heart J. 2007;28(5):589–600.

ECG 20

Gabriel Gusetu

1 Case Presentation

A 57-year-old male patient with a history of arterial hypertension and dyslipidemia is admitted to the Cardiology Department for three episodes of palpitations accompanied by dyspnea, anxiety, and lightheadedness that had occurred during the past 48 h prior to his presentation to the hospital. His ECG recorded during the third episode of palpitations by the Mobile Emergency Medical Team is presented in Fig. 1.

Question: What is the nature of the tachycardia presented in Fig. 1?

(a) Ventricular tachycardia originating from the inferior septal LV wall
(b) Ventricular tachycardia originating from the inferior septal RV wall
(c) Bundle branch re-entry ventricular tachycardia
(d) Antidromic tachycardia using a right-sided bypass tract
(e) AVNRT with left bundle branch block

Hint: A second ECG recorded several minutes later is presented in Fig. 2.

G. Gusetu (✉)
Department of Cardiology, Hôpital Emile Muller, Mulhouse, France

Correct answer: c. Bundle branch re-entry ventricular tachycardia

Explanation: The ECG in Fig. 1 shows a regular wide QRS complex tachycardia with a heart rate of 240 bpm and LBBB morphology. The width of the QRS complex is 160 ms. The QRS axis is at −150° (north-west axis deviation). The differential diagnosis of this regular wide QRS complex tachycardia with LBBB morphology includes: ventricular tachycardia (myocardial-related VT, bundle branch re-entry VT, and fascicular VT), supraventricular tachycardia (atrial fibrillation, atrial flutter, atrial tachycardia, AVNRT, and AVRT) with functional or preexisting bundle branch block, and antidromic tachycardia (in pre-excitation syndromes).

The ECG from Fig. 2 shows sinus rhythm with a heart rate of 81 bpm, QRS axis at 0°, absence of LV hypertrophy, ST segment depression in leads V5 and V6, complete RBBB (QRS duration of 140 ms), first degree AV block (PR = 240 ms), and prolonged QT and QTc interval (QTc = 511 ms).

The morphology of the left bundle branch block of the QRS complex during tachycardia from Fig. 1 suggests that it might be that of a typical one [1]: QRS duration >120 ms; absence of q waves in leads V5 and V6; monomorphic notched R wave in leads I and V6; and ST segment and T wave modification opposite to the

L. Muresan (ed.), *ECG Interpretation of Wide QRS Complex Tachycardia*,
https://doi.org/10.1007/978-3-031-97030-6_21

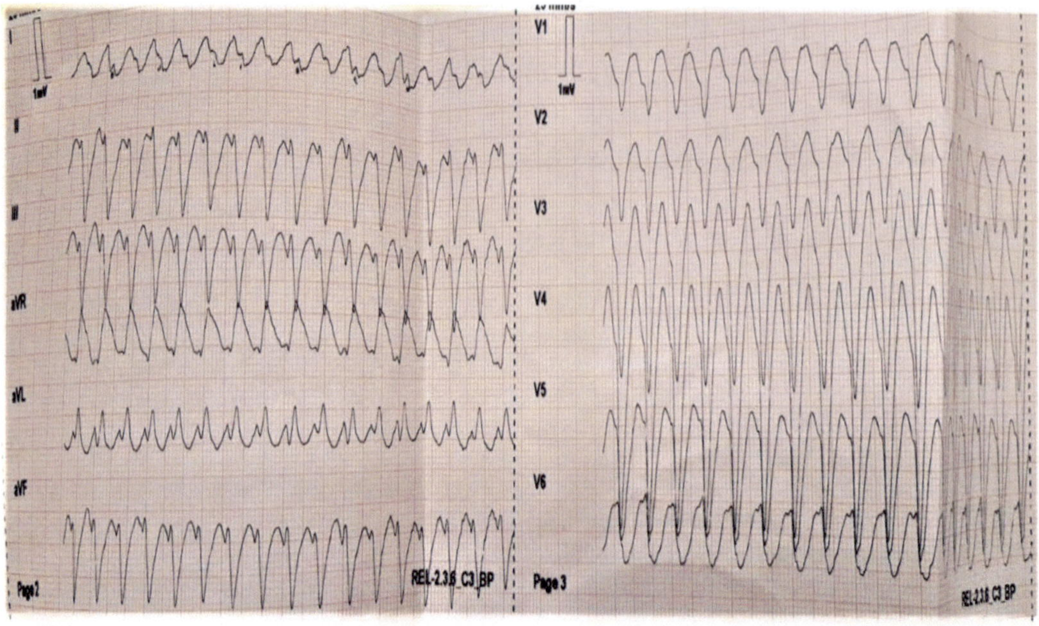

Fig. 1 Twelve-lead ECG recorded at admittance to the Cardiology Department

major deflection of the QRS complex: ST segment elevation with positive T waves in leads V1–V5. So, at this point of the analysis, we cannot say whether this is VT or SVT with LBBB. Antidromic tachycardia is unlikely (even though not impossible) given the absence of preexcitation on the ECG from Fig. 2, which shows AV conduction disorders (complete RBBB and first degree AV block).

Applying the Brugada algorithm [2] to the tachycardia from Fig. 2, it can be seen that there is no RS complex in the precordial leads (leads V1–V5 show a "QS" aspect and lead V6 a "unique R" morphology), which is an argument in favor of VT.

The Vereckei algorithm [3] for the differential diagnosis of wide QRS complex tachycardias also suggests VT as the correct answer. The first step of the algorithm looks for A–V dissociation, which is not seen on the present ECG. There might be P waves visible in the lead aVR but with a 1:1 V:A relationship (Fig. 3).

The second step of the algorithm looks for an initial predominant R wave in lead aVR, which is not the case (the aspect is "qR"; see Fig. 4).

The third step "QRS morphology unlike BBB or fascicular block" is not in favor of an SVT with LBBB, based on the arguments explained above. The fourth step of the algorithm analyzes the vi/vt index. This index compares the amplitude of the first 40 ms of a QRS complex to the amplitude of the last 40 ms of the QRS complex in a lead where the QRS has both an R and an S wave. In the present case, this is illustrated in Fig. 5.

Another argument in favor of ventricular tachycardia would be the extreme (north west) axis deviation.

Based on the abovementioned arguments, the tachycardia from Fig. 1 is VT.

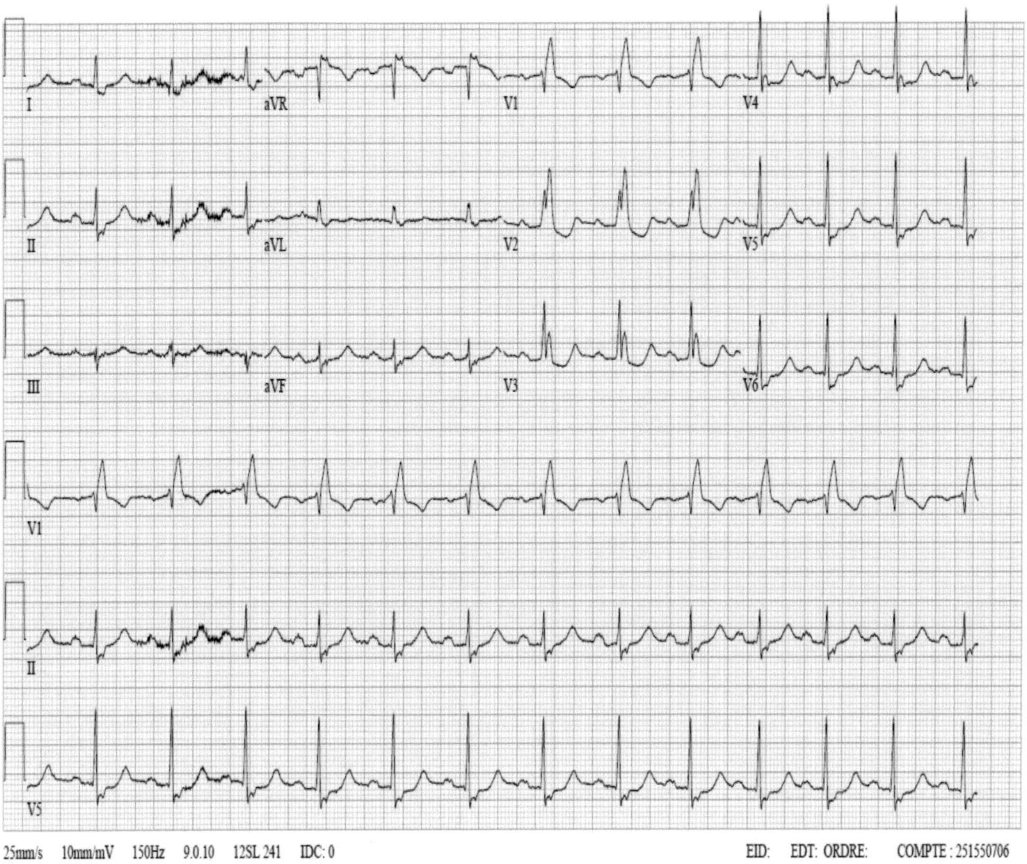

Fig. 2 Twelve-lead ECG recorded after the end of the episode of palpitations

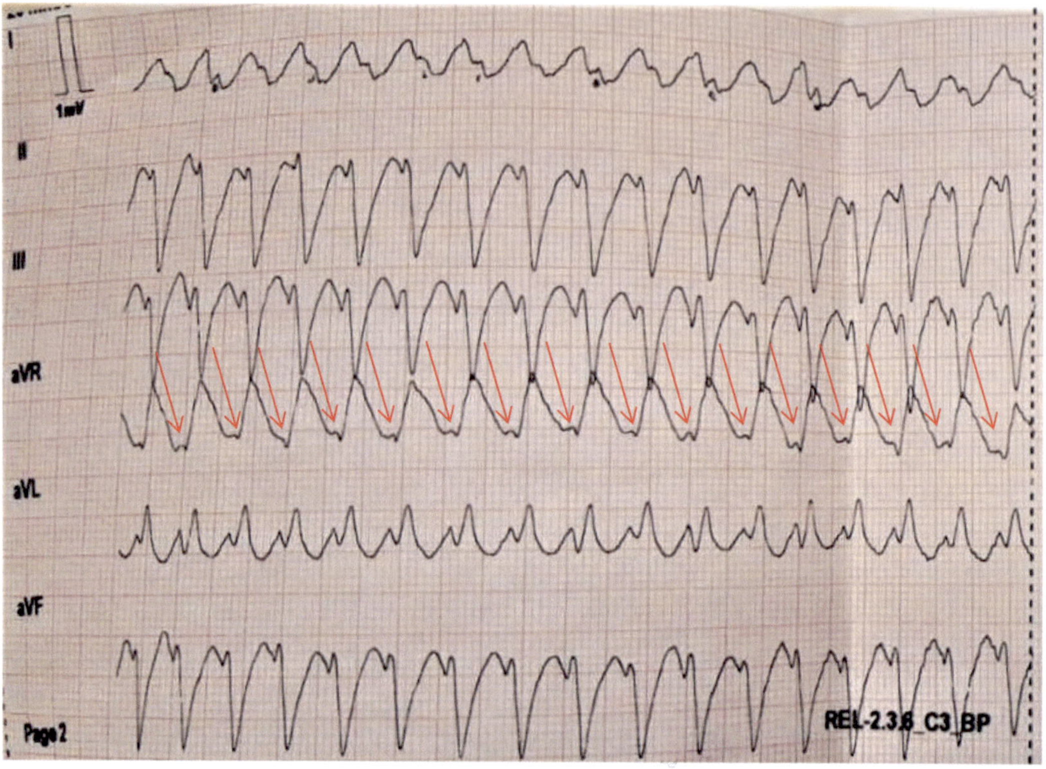

Fig. 3 Limb leads from the ECG in Fig. 1. Red arrows indicate possible P waves, with a 1:1 V:A conduction

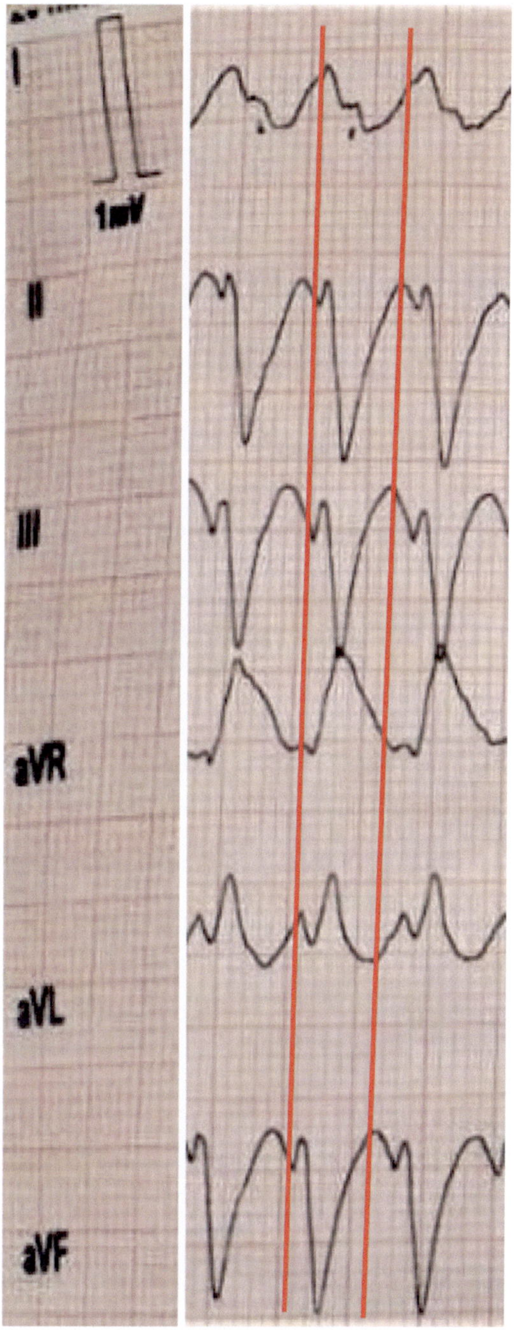

Fig. 4 Limb leads from the ECG in Fig. 1. The red vertical lines indicate the onset and the end of the QRS complex. This indicates a "qR" pattern in lead aVR

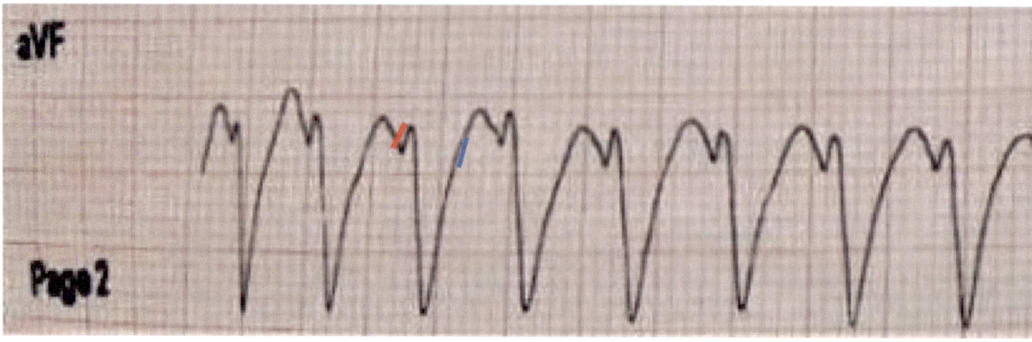

Fig. 5 The vi/vt index from the Vereckei algorithm in lead V1. The ratio of the initial 40 ms and the last 40 ms of the QRS complex is: 2 mV vs 2.5 mV; therefore, 2/2.5 = 0.8, which is <1. This is in favor of ventricular tachycardia

2 Additional Comments

The patient underwent an electrophysiological study. This confirmed the diagnosis of VT and elucidated its mechanism: bundle branch re-entry ventricular tachycardia. A schematic representation of the tachycardia circuit is presented in Fig. 6 and an ECG recorded during the electrophysiological study in Fig. 7.

Bundle branch re-entry ventricular tachycardia should be suspected in patients with a wide QRS complex tachcyardia who have conduction disorders on the ECG during sinus rhythm (prolonged PR interval, BBB) [4–8].

The fact that the patient had RBBB during sinus rhythm and LBBB during tachycardia shows that the right bundle is not completely incapable of conducting electical impulses during sinus rhythm, as shown in Fig. 7, right panel. The RBBB during sinus rhythm most likely shows different conduction velocities in the two branches, with hidden retrograde conduction from the left bundle into the right bundle, producing a functional block at this level (Fig. 8).

Treatment of bundle branch re-entry ventricular tachycardia is catheter ablation of one of the branches (usually the right bundle, which was also the choice for this patient).

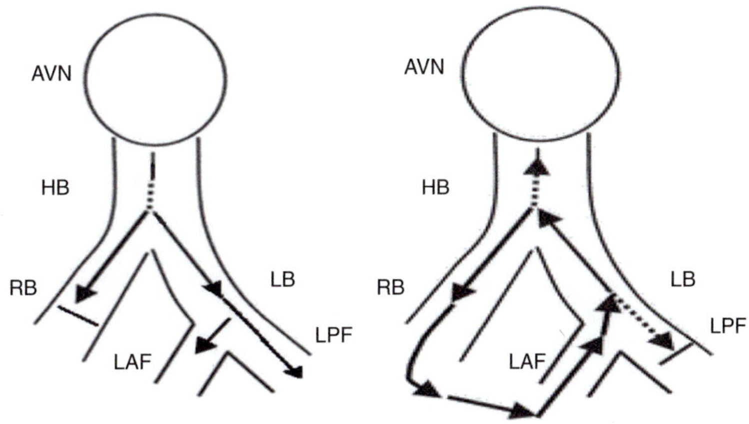

Fig. 6 *Left panel*: Diagram representing the depolarization of the LV during sinus rhythm in Fig. 2. *Right panel*: Diagram representing the depolarization of the LV during VT in Fig. 1. AVN atrioventricular node, HB His bundle, RB right bundle, LB left bundle, LAF left anterior fascicle, LPF left posterior fascicle

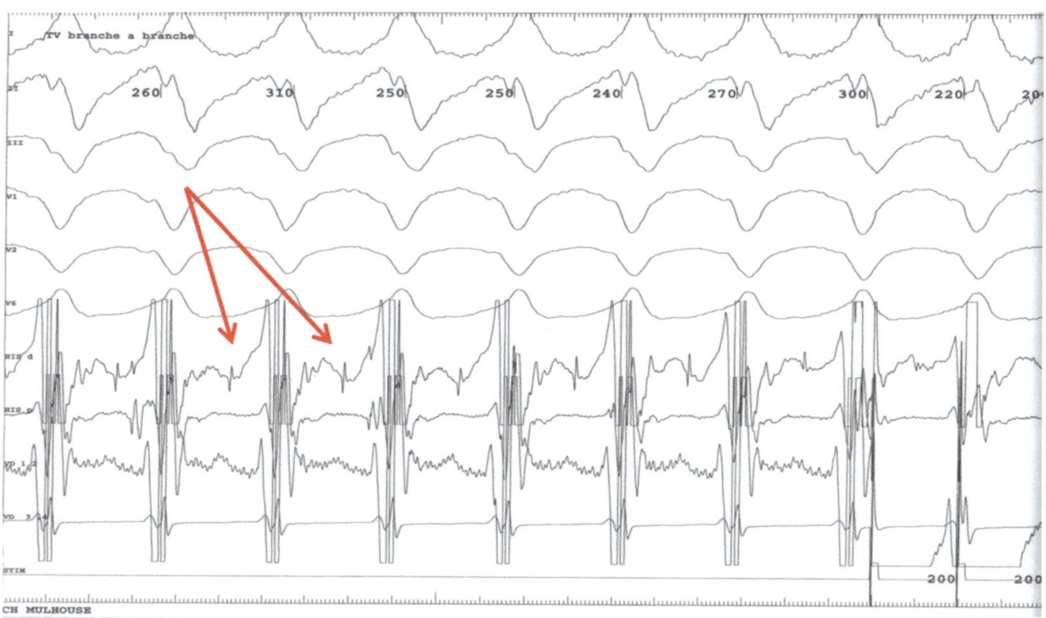

Fig. 7 ECG recorded during the wide QRS complex tachycardia showing surface leads I, II, III, V1, V2, V6, and intracavitary leads His d, His p, Vp 1, and Vp 2. The cycle length of the VT is 250 ms, identical to that of the clinical VT. It is worth noting that a His deflection precedes every QRS complex (red arrows), which is an argument in favor of bundle branch re-entry VT. His distal electrodes of the His catheter, His p proximal electrodes of the His catheter, Vp 1 distal electrodes of the RV catheter, Vp 2 proximal electrodes of the His catheter

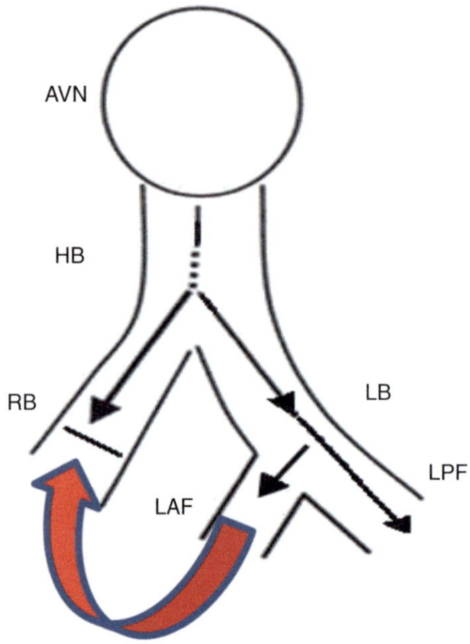

Fig. 8 Diagram representing the depolarization of the LV during sinus rhythm. The red curved arrow indicates the hidden retrograde conduction from the left bundle into the right bundle, explaining the presence of right bundle branch block during sinus rhythm but with possible anterior conduction during the bundle branch re-entry ventricular tachycardia. *AVN* atrioventricular node, HB His bundle, RB right bundle, LB left bundle, LAF left anterior fascicle, LPF left posterior fascicle

References

1. Surawicz B, Childers R, Deal BJ, Gettes LS, Bailey JJ, Gorgels A, et al. AHA/ACCF/HRS recommendations for the standardization and interpretation of the electrocardiogram: part III: intraventricular conduction disturbances: a scientific statement from the American Heart Association Electrocardiography and Arrhythmias Committee, Council on Clinical Cardiology; the American College of Cardiology Foundation; and the Heart Rhythm Society. Endorsed by the International Society for Computerized Electrocardiology. J Am Coll Cardiol. 2009;53(11):976–81.
2. Brugada P, Brugada J, Mont L, Smeets J, Andries EW. A new approach to the differential diagnosis of a regular tachycardia with a wide QRS complex. Circulation. 1991;83(5):1649–59.
3. Vereckei A, Duray G, Szenasi G, Altemose GT, Miller JM. Application of a new algorithm in the differential diagnosis of wide QRS complex tachycardia. Eur Heart J. 2007;28(5):589–600.
4. Blanck Z, Jazayeri M, Dhala A, Deshpande S, Sra J, Akhtar M. Bundle branch reentry: a mechanism of ventricular tachycardia in the absence of myocardial or valvular dysfunction. J Am Coll Cardiol. 1993;22(6):1718–22.
5. Lloyd EA, Zipes DP, Heger JJ, Prystowsky EN. Sustained ventricular tachycardia due to bundle branch reentry. Am Heart J. 1982;104(5 Pt 1):1095–7.
6. Mizusawa Y, Sakurada H, Nishizaki M, Ueda-Tatsumoto A, Fukamizu S, Hiraoka M. Characteristics of bundle branch reentrant ventricular tachycardia with a right bundle branch block configuration: feasibility of atrial pacing. Europace. 2009;11(9):1208–13.
7. Tchou P, Mehdirad AA. Bundle branch reentry ventricular tachycardia. Pacing Clin Electrophysiol. 1995;18(7):1427–37.
8. Touboul P, Kirkorian G, Atallah G, Moleur P. Bundle branch reentry: a possible mechanism of ventricular tachycardia. Circulation. 1983;67(3):674–80.

ECG 21

Gabriel Cismaru

1 Case Presentation

An 74-year-old male patient with a history of non-ischemic cardiomyopathy with severe LV systolic dysfunction (LVEF of 20%), nonsustained polymorphic ventricular tachycardia, amiodarone-induced hyperthyroidism, and chronic renal failure is admitted to the Cardiology Department for an episode of decompensated heart failure, presenting aggravated dyspnea on exertion and at rest, and peripheral edema that had occurred during the past 7 days prior to his presentation to the hospital. His ECG recorded at admittance to the Cardiology Department is presented in Fig. 1.

Question: What is the nature of the tachycardia presented in the ECG?

(a) Ventricular tachycardia originating from the inferior septal LV wall
(b) Ventricular tachycardia originating from the inferior septal RV wall
(c) Bundle branch re-entry ventricular tachycardia
(d) Antidromic tachycardia using a left-sided bypass tract
(e) Atrial flutter with 2:1 atrioventricular conduction, right bundle branch block, and left anterior fascicular block

Hint: A second ECG recorded after electrical cardioversion is presented in Fig. 2.

Correct answer: e. Atrial flutter with 2:1 atrioventricular conduction, right bundle branch block, and left anterior fascicular block

Explanation: The ECG in Fig. 1 shows a regular wide QRS complex tachycardia with a heart rate of 155 bpm and RBBB morphology. The width of the QRS complex is 155 ms. The QRS axis is at −75°. The differential diagnosis of this regular wide QRS complex tachycardia with RBBB morphology includes: ventricular tachycardia (myocardial-related VT and bundle branch re-entry VT), supraventricular tachycardia (atrial flutter, atrial tachycardia, AVNRT, and AVRT) with functional or pre-existing bundle branch block, and antidromic tachycardia (in pre-excitation syndromes).

The morphology of the left bundle branch block of the QRS complex during tachycardia from Fig. 1 is not that of a typical one [1]: the QRS duration is indeed >120 ms; there is an "rSR'" aspect in lead V1; there is a monomorphic R wave in leads I, aVL, and V6; and there is ST

G. Cismaru (✉)
Department of Cardiology, Rehabilitation Hospital, Cluj-Napoca, Romania

L. Muresan (ed.), *ECG Interpretation of Wide QRS Complex Tachycardia*,
https://doi.org/10.1007/978-3-031-97030-6_22

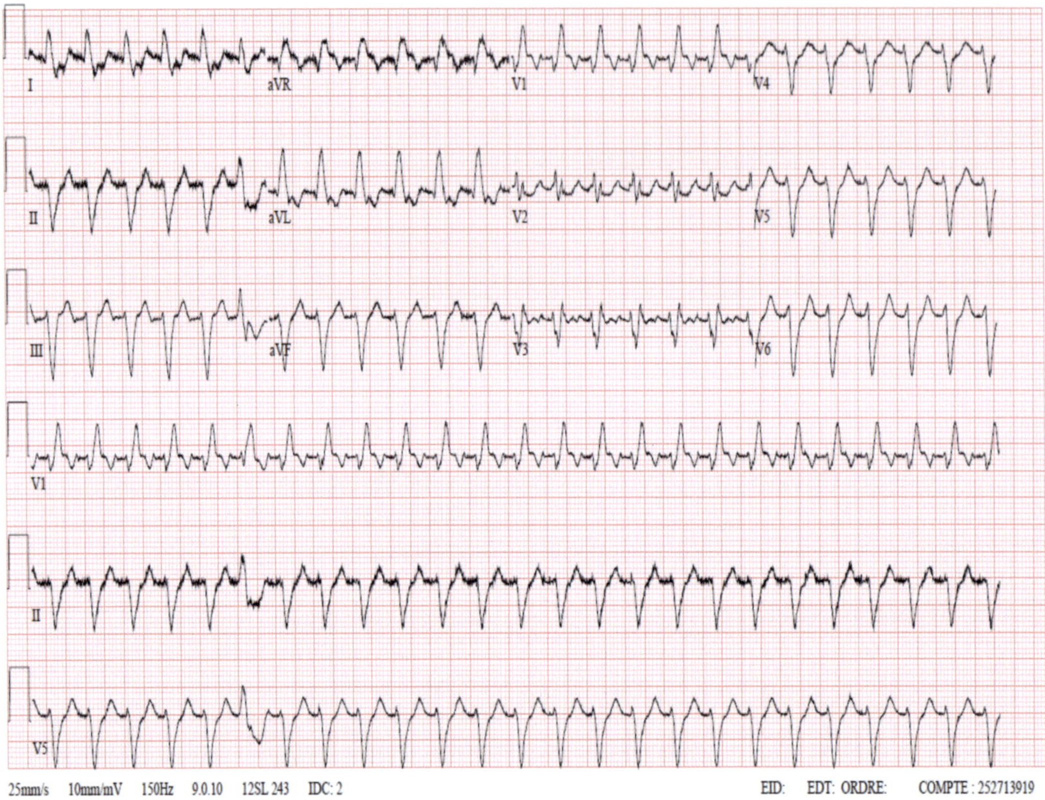

Fig. 1 Twelve-lead ECG recorded at admittance to the Cardiology Department

segment and T wave modifications opposite to the major deflection of the QRS complex; however, the R-to-S ratio in lead V6 is <1, which is not characteristic of a typical RBBB.

Applying the Brugada algorithm [2] to the tachycardia from Fig. 1, it can be seen that: (1) There is no absence of an RS complex in the precordial leads (otherwise said, there are rS complexes in leads V4–V6); we therefore move to the second step of the algorithm: (2) This step analyzes the absence of an R-to-S interval >100 ms in any precordial lead. This is not the case (Fig. 3).

Step 3 of the algorithm looks for A–V dissociation. There are no P waves visible; therefore, we need to move to step 4 of the algorithm.

For an RBBB morphology wide QRS complex tachycardia, an argument in favor of VT would be the presence of a taller left peak of the QRS complex in lead V1 (the rabbit ear sign) or for biphasic RS or QR complexes, which is not the case. Next, in lead V6, an argument in favor of VT would be the presence of an "rS" complex, which is actually the case (Fig. 4). This is therefore an argument in favor of VT. This can also be expressed as a ratio of R/S <1 in lead V6. So, according to the Brugada algorithm, the correct diagnosis is ventricular tachycardia.

The Vereckei algorithm [3] for the differential diagnosis of wide QRS complex tachycardias also suggests VT as the correct answer. The first step of the algorithm looks for A–V dissociation, which is not seen on the present ECG, since there are no visible P waves. The second step of the algorithm looks for an initial predominant R wave in lead aVR, which, again, is not the case (Fig. 5).

The third step "QRS morphology unlike BBB or fascicular block" does not suggest SVT with BBB, given the R-to-S ratio <1 in lead V6, which is atypical for an RBBB. The fourth step of the algorithm analyzes the vi/vt index. This index

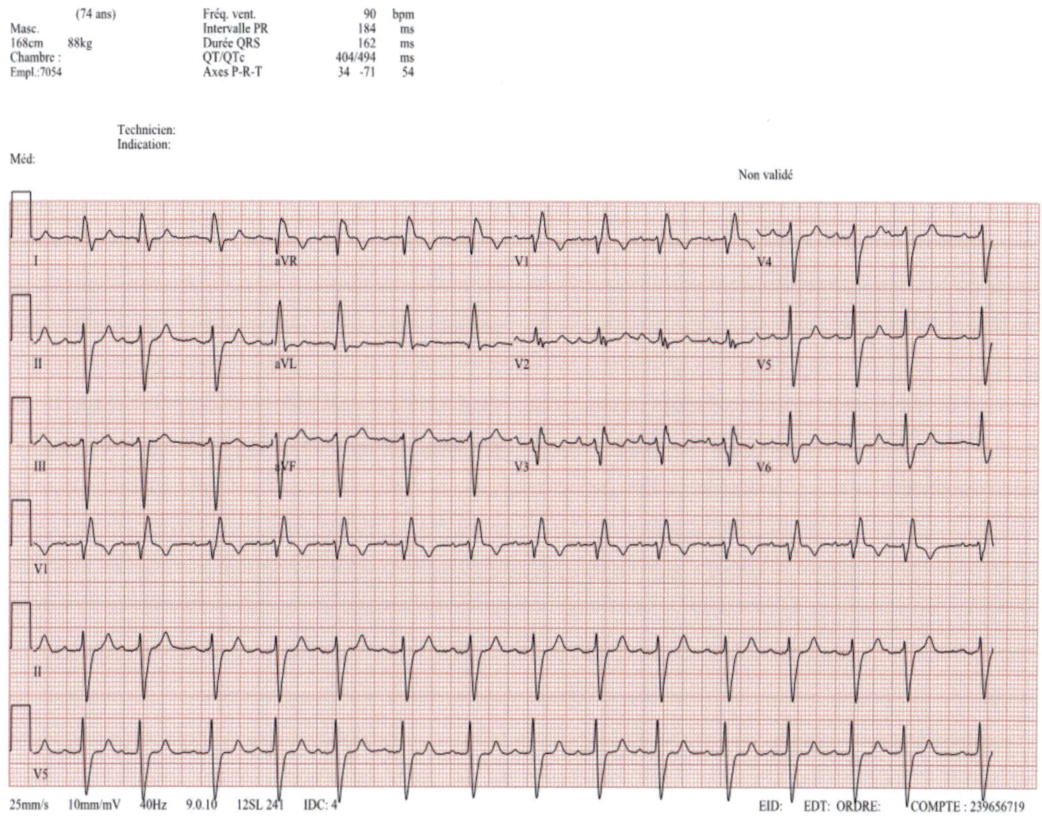

Fig. 2 Twelve-lead ECG recorded after the end of the episode of palpitations

Fig. 3 Lead V3 from the ECG presented in Fig. 1 showing an R-to-S interval of 70 ms, argument not in favor of ventricular tachycardia (but not excluding it either)

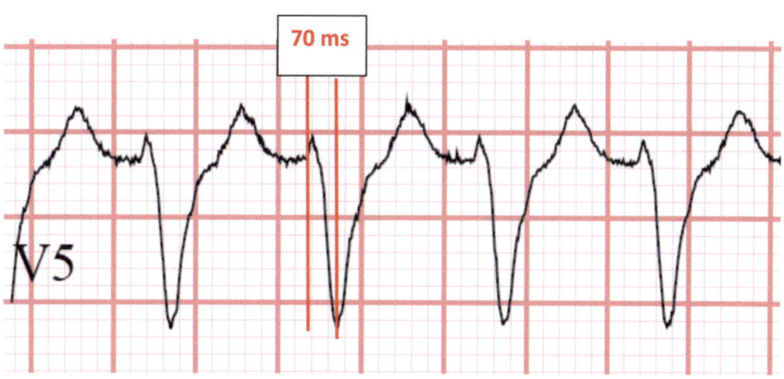

compares the amplitude of the first 40 ms of a QRS complex to the amplitude of the last 40 ms of the QRS complex in a lead where the QRS has both an R and as an S wave. In the present case, this is illustrated in Fig. 6.

Based on these arguments, the diagnosis of ventricular tachcyardia would normally be retained. However, the ECG in Fig. 2 recorded after electrical cardioversion shows sinus rhythm and the presece of QRS complexes that have the same morphology as the QRS complexes recroded in the ECG from Fig. 1. This is a very strong argument in favor of a supraventricular origin of the tachycardia from Fig. 1, with pre-existing

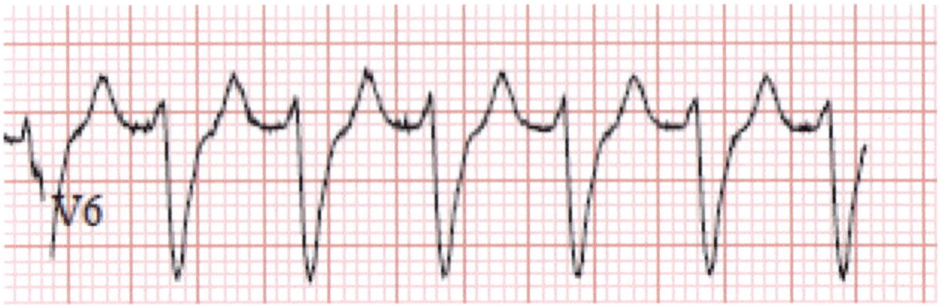

Fig. 4 Lead V6 from the ECG presented in Fig. 1, showing an R-to-S ratio of <1. This is in favor of ventricular tachycardia

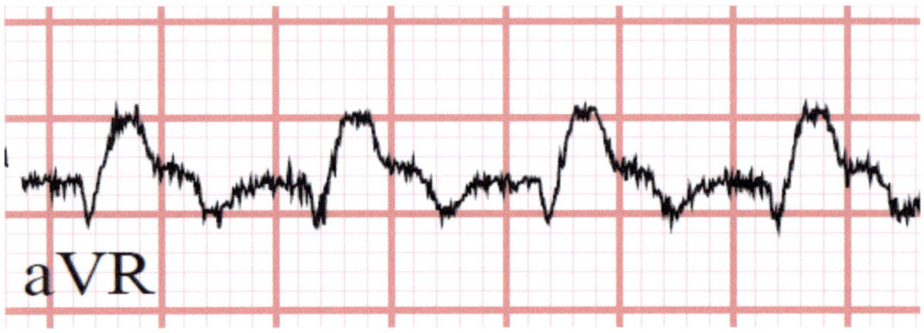

Fig. 5 Lead aVR from the ECG presented in Fig. 1, showing the absence of a tall initial R wave, argument not in favor of ventricular tachycardia (but not excluding it either)

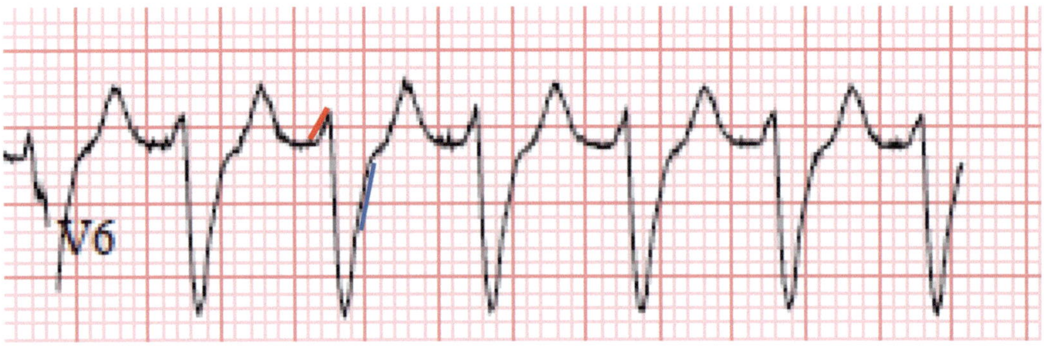

Fig. 6 The vi/vt index from the Vereckei algorithm in lead V6. The ratio of the initial 40 ms (red line) and the last 40 ms of the QRS complex (blue line) is: 3 mV vs 5 mV; therefore, 3/5 = 0.6, which is <1. This is in favor of ventricular tachycardia

RBBB. A close analysis of lead V1 identifies F waves (flutter) with a 2:1 atrioventricular conduction, compatible with atrial flutter (Fig. 7).

The patient underwent an electrophysiological study during which an atypical atrial flutter with 2:1 atrioventricular conduction and a heart rate of 155 bpm was induced. This was subsequently treated with catheter ablation, and the patient converted to sinus rhythm. The ECG recorded after the procedure is presented in Fig. 8.

This case demonstrates that the existing algorithms are not perfect in differentiating between several etiologies of a wide QRS complex tachycardia, especially in the presence of RBBB and LAFB, and that evaluation of several ECGs of the same patient (especially during sinus rhythm) is sometimes needed and represents the best way to establish the correct diagnosis.

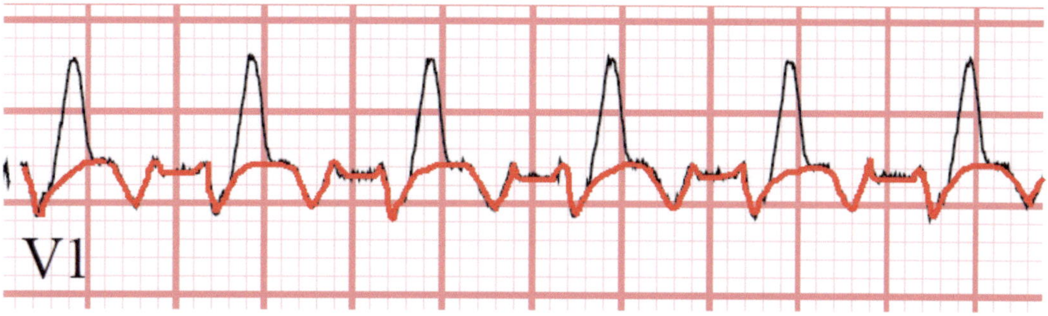

Fig. 7 Lead V1 from the ECG from Fig. 1 demonstrating atrial flutter with 2:1 atrioventricular conduction (in red, the atrial flutter F waves).

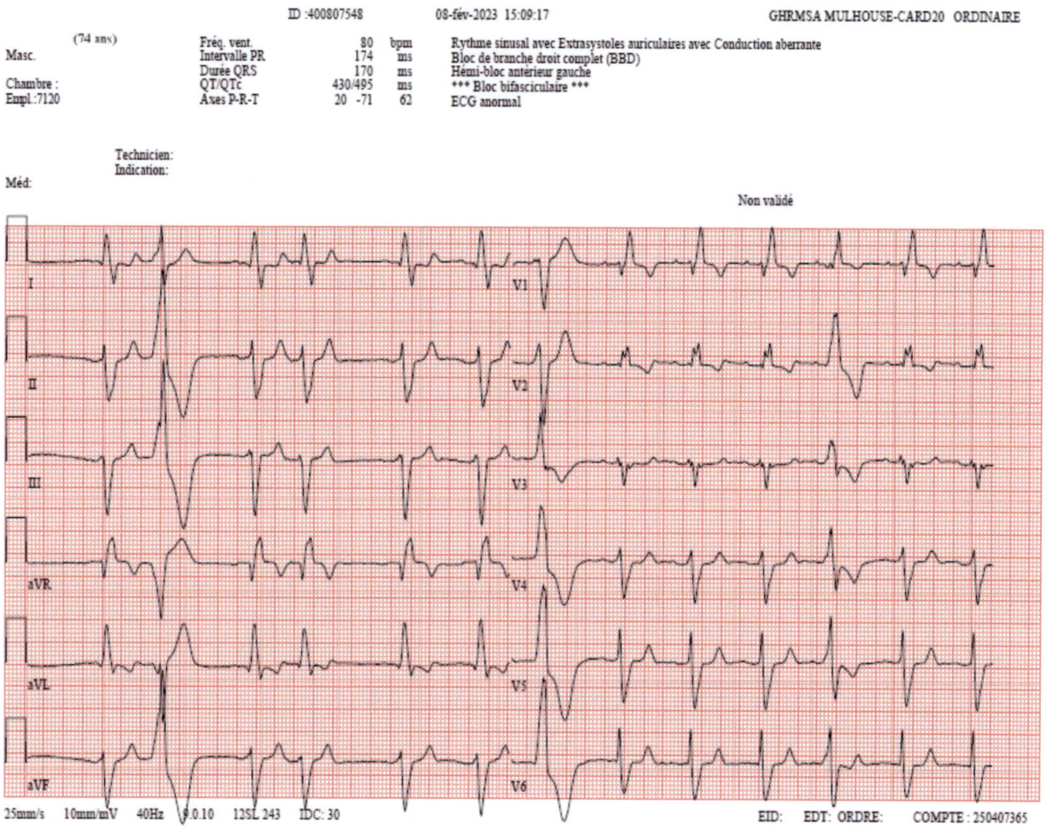

Fig. 8 ECG recorded after catheter ablation of atrial flutter

References

1. Surawicz B, Childers R, Deal BJ, Gettes LS, Bailey JJ, Gorgels A, et al. AHA/ACCF/HRS recommendations for the standardization and interpretation of the electrocardiogram: part III: intraventricular conduction disturbances: a scientific statement from the American Heart Association Electrocardiography and Arrhythmias Committee, Council on Clinical Cardiology; the American College of Cardiology Foundation; and the Heart Rhythm Society. Endorsed by the International Society for Computerized Electrocardiology. J Am Coll Cardiol. 2009;53(11):976–81.

2. Brugada P, Brugada J, Mont L, Smeets J, Andries EW. A new approach to the differential diagnosis of a regular tachycardia with a wide QRS complex. Circulation. 1991;83(5):1649–59.
3. Vereckei A, Duray G, Szenasi G, Altemose GT, Miller JM. Application of a new algorithm in the differential diagnosis of wide QRS complex tachycardia. Eur Heart J. 2007;28(5):589–600.

ECG 22

Radu Rosu

1 Case Presentation

A 71-year-old male patient with a history of arterial hypertension, diabetes mellitus, dyslipidemia, COPD, pulmonary embolism, tachycardia–bradycardia syndrome treated with a dual-chamber pacemaker, and antiarrhythmic treatment (beta-blockers) is admitted to the Cardiology Department for an episode of decompensated heart failure. The patient presented aggravated dyspnea on exertion, paroxysmal nocturnal dyspnea, and important peripheral edema, which had progressively worsened during the previous 3–4 weeks. His ECG recorded at admittance to the Cardiology Department is presented in Fig. 1. The pacemaker was programmed in DDD mode, with a lower rate interval of 60 bpm and an upper tracking rate of 120 bpm.

Question: What is the nature of the tachycardia presented in Fig. 1?

(a) Ventricular tachycardia originating from the inferior RV wall
(b) Atrial flutter with paced QRS complexes
(c) Sinus tachycardia with paced QRS complexes
(d) Pacemaker-mediated tachycardia
(e) Runaway pacemaker

Hint: A second ECG recorded after reprogramming the pacemaker in VVI mode at 60 bpm is presented in Fig. 2.

Correct answer: b. Atrial flutter with paced QRS complexes

Explanation: The ECG in Fig. 1 shows a regular wide QRS complex tachycardia with a heart rate of 120 bpm and LBBB morphology. The width of the QRS complex is 170 ms. The QRS axis is at −85°. Each of the QRS complexes is preceded by a pacing spike. Therefore, these are all paced QRS complexes. Hence, despite the LBBB morphology of the QRS, answer a—"Ventricular tachycardia originating from the inferior RV wall"—is not correct.

Runaway pacemaker is a rare pacemaker dysfunction characterized by fast and erratic spikes delivered at very high rates, which can induce ventricular fibrillation. This is obviously not the case; therefore, answer e—"Runaway pacemaker"—is not correct.

A careful analysis of the atrial rhythm from the ECG in Fig. 1 is not able to clearly identify P waves. However, analysis of the second ECG, after reprogramming the pacemaker in VVI mode at 60 bpm (Fig. 2) clearly shows typical atrial flutter with variable atrioventricular conduction.

R. Rosu (✉)
Department of Cardiology, Rehabilitation Hospital, Cluj-Napoca, Romania

L. Muresan (ed.), *ECG Interpretation of Wide QRS Complex Tachycardia*,
https://doi.org/10.1007/978-3-031-97030-6_23

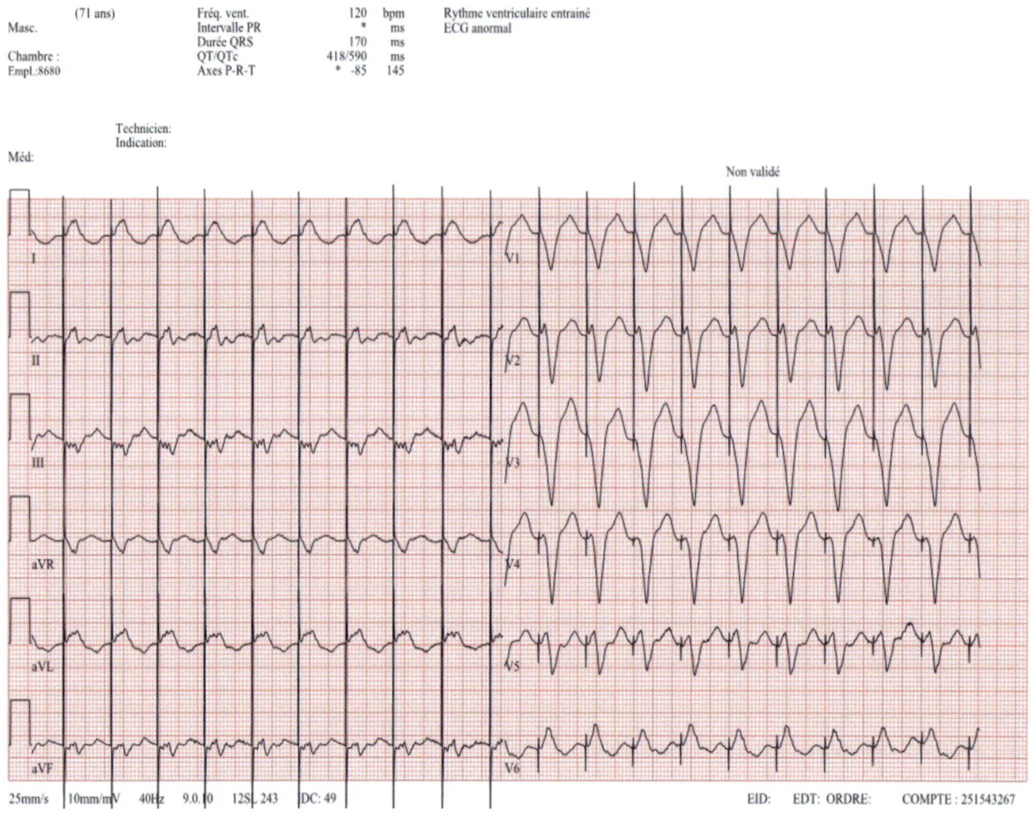

Fig. 1 Twelve-lead ECG recorded at admittance to the Cardiology Department

Therefore, the atrial rhythm on the ECG from Fig. 1 is also atrial flutter. Answer c—"Sinus tachycardia with paced QRS complexes"—is therefore incorrect.

The pacemaker paces the right ventricle with a heart rate of 120 bpm. This is the maximal tracking rate. There are two flutter waves for one paced QRS complex; hence, there is a 2:1 atrioventricular conduction. The explanation for this phenomenon is that in DDD mode, the pacemaker detects a first spontaneous flutter (F) wave, and as a result, an AV interval is initiated, after which pacing of the right ventricle occurs in the absence of spontaneous ventricular activity (for the programmed sensed AV interval). The second F wave falls into the PVARP (postventricular atrial refractory period) and does not initiate an AV interval. There is no ventricular pacing spike and no QRS complex initiated for this F wave. Then, the sequence is repeated [1].

Answer c—"Pacemaker-mediated tachycardia"—is not correct, since this requires retrograde conduction to be present (via the AV node) with depolarization of the atria (with a resulting P wave), which is detected by the (dual chamber) pacemaker, which paces the ventricle to maintain A–V synchrony. Since the patient is in atrial flutter, this answer cannot be correct.

The patient underwent radiofrequency ablation of the atrial flutter with conversion to sinus rhythm (Fig. 3).

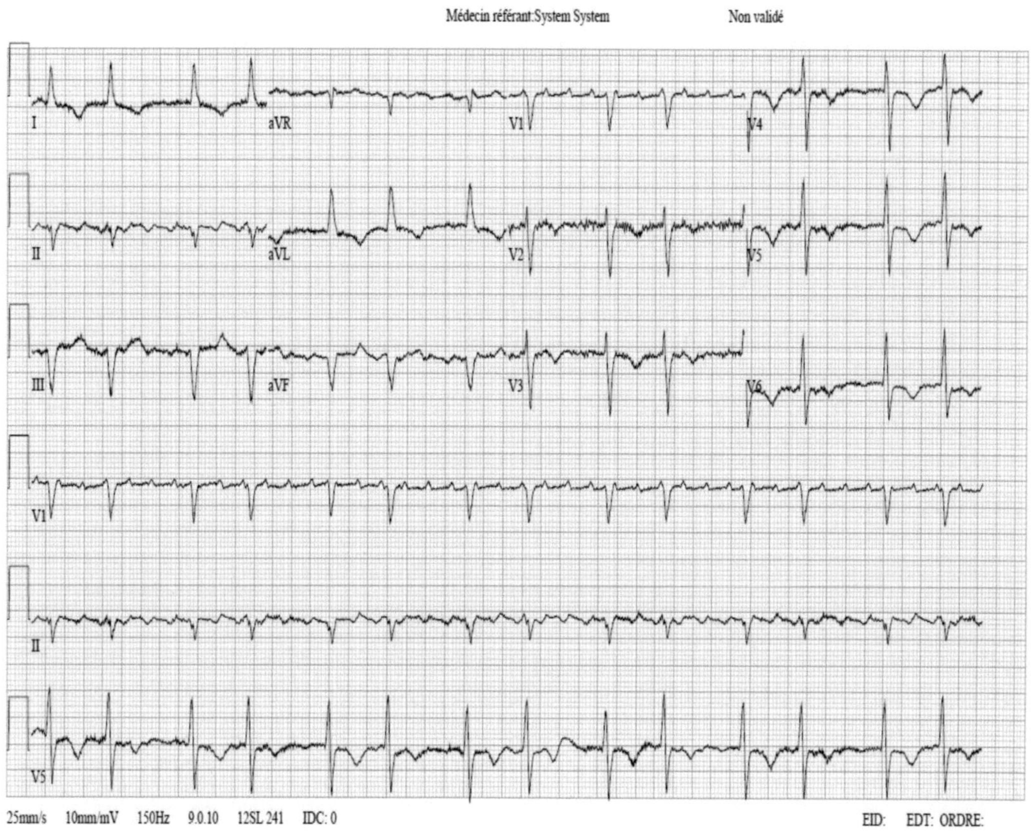

Fig. 2 Twelve-lead ECG recorded after reprogramming the pacemaker in VVI mode at 60 bpm

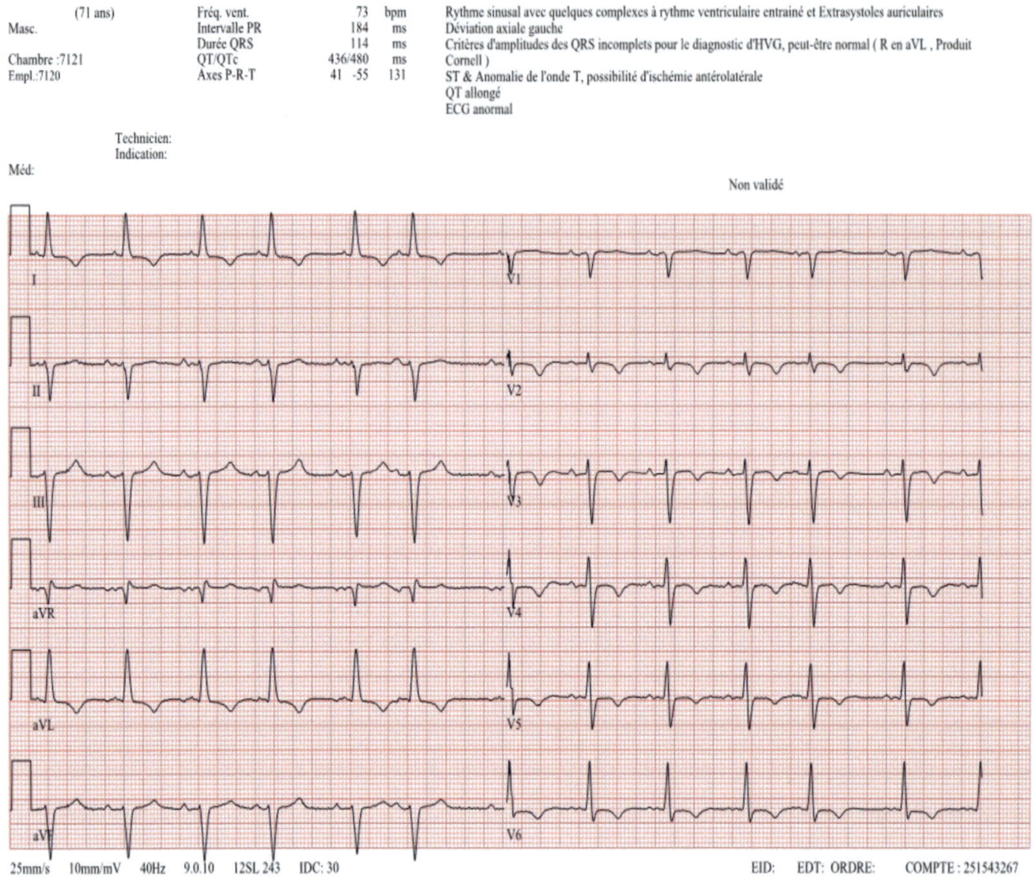

Fig. 3 Twelve-lead ECG recorded after catheter ablation of atrial flutter showing sinus rhythm with spontaneous atrioventricular conduction (pacemaker programmed in DDD at 60–120 bpm)

Reference

1. Greenspon AJ, Greenberg RM, Frankl WS. Tracking of atrial flutter during DDD pacing: another form of pacemaker-mediated tachycardia. Pacing Clin Electrophysiol. 1984;7(6 Pt 1):955–60.

ECG 23

Mihai Puiu

1 Case Presentation

A 76-year-old male patient with a history of ischemic cardiomyopathy with severe LV systolic dysfunction (LV EF of 20%), remote myocardial infarction, and severe coronary artery disease (chronic total occlusion of the right coronary artery, severe stenosis of the proximal circumflex artery, first marginal artery, and of the left anterior descending coronary artery, treated with PCI and stent implantation: two stents in the proximal LAD coronary artery) is admitted to the Cardiology Department for pre-syncope and palpitations accompanied by dyspnea, anxiety, and chest pain. His ECG recorded in the Cardiology Department is presented in Fig. 1.

Question: What is the nature of the tachycardia presented in the ECG in Fig. 1?

(a) Ventricular tachycardia originating from the left ventricular outflow tract
(b) Ventricular tachycardia originating from the right ventricular outflow tract
(c) Ventricular tachycardia originating from the inferior lateral LV wall
(d) Antidromic tachycardia using a right-sided bypass tract
(e) Atrial flutter with left bundle branch block and 1:1 AV conduction

Hint: A second ECG recorded after electrical cardioversion is presented in Fig. 2.

Correct answer: a. Ventricular tachycardia originating from the left ventricular outflow tract

Explanation: The ECG in Fig. 1 shows a regular wide QRS complex tachycardia with a heart rate of 199 bpm and LBBB morphology. The width of the QRS complex is 122 ms. The QRS axis is at +110°. The differential diagnosis of this regular wide QRS complex tachycardia with LBBB morphology includes: ventricular tachycardia (myocardial-related VT, bundle branch reentry VT, and fascicular VT), supraventricular tachycardia (atrial fibrillation, atrial flutter, atrial tachycardia, AVNRT, and AVRT) with functional or pre-existing bundle branch block, and antidromic tachycardia (in pre-excitation syndromes).

The ECG from Fig. 2 shows sinus rhythm with a heart rate of 85 bpm, QRS axis at +70°, absence of LV hypertrophy, ST segment depression in leads V4–V6, DII, DIII, and aVF, and ST segment elevation in lead aVR and V1 in favor of possible ongoing ischemia in the left main coronary artery or severe three-vessel disease. There

M. Puiu (✉)
Department of Cardiology, Rehabilitation Hospital, Cluj-Napoca, Romania

L. Muresan (ed.), *ECG Interpretation of Wide QRS Complex Tachycardia*,
https://doi.org/10.1007/978-3-031-97030-6_24

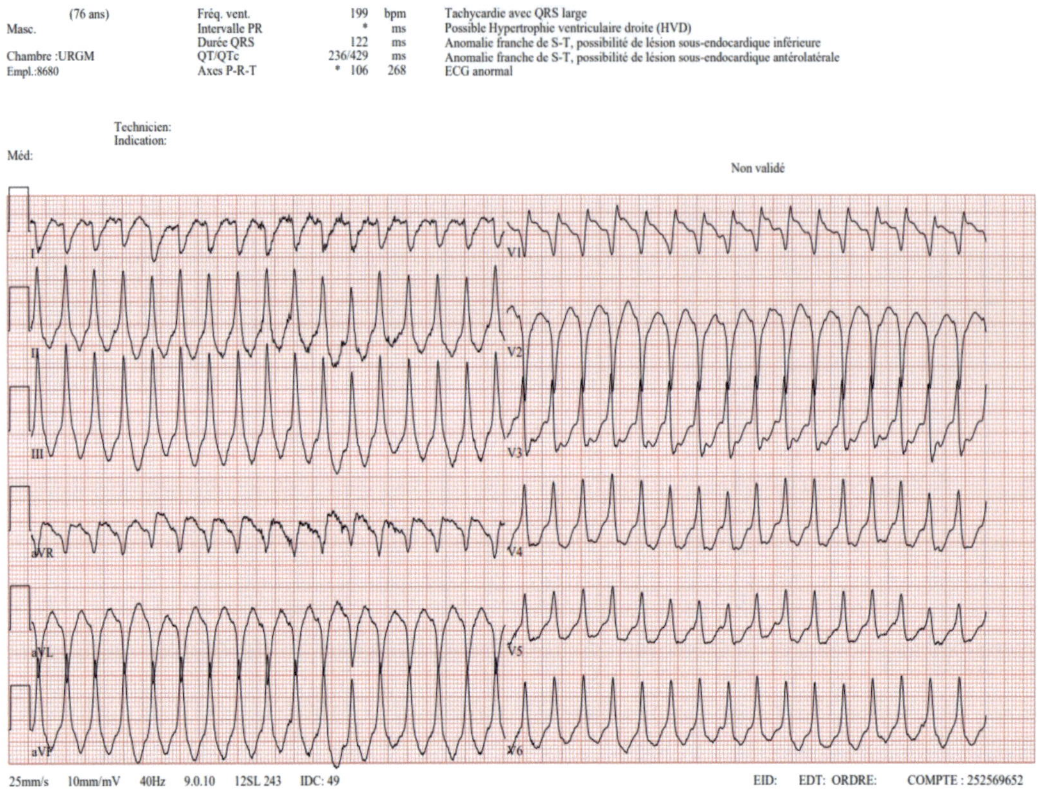

Fig. 1 Twelve-lead ECG recorded at admittance to the Cardiology Department

are no signs of ventricular pre-excitation (no delta waves and no short PR interval), so the likelihood of the tachycardia from Fig. 1 to be antidromic tachycardia is quite low.

The morphology of the left bundle branch block of the QRS complex during tachycardia from Fig. 1 is not that of a typical one [1]: the QRS complex is mostly negative (has a deep Q wave) in lead V1, and the QRS width is >120 ms; however, there is a "Qr" aspect in lead V1; the transition in precordial leads takes places in lead V3, and there is an "rS" aspect in leads I and aVL, which are not characteristic of a typical LBBB. This makes SVT with LBBB unlikely.

Applying the Brugada algorithm [2] to the tachycardia from Fig. 1, it can be seen that: (1) There is no absence of an RS complex in the precordial leads (otherwise said, there are "rS" complexes in lead V3); we therefore move to the second step of the algorithm: (2) This step analyzes the absence of an R to S interval >100 ms in any precordial lead. This is not the case (Fig. 3).

Step 3 of the algorithm looks for A–V dissociation. If we analyze the atrial activity, we can see that there are P waves visible after each QRS complex, best visible in leads V3 and V5 (Fig. 4). So, there is a 1:1 P to QRS relationship. We therefore need to move to step 4 of the algorithm.

For a wide QRS complex tachycardia with LBBB, an argument in favor of VT is the presence of an "r wave" >0.04 s in lead V1 or V2, which is actually the case in the ECG presented in Fig. 1 [3] (Fig. 5). Therefore, according to the Brugada algorithm, the tachycardia presented in Fig. 1 is ventricular tachycardia.

The Vereckei algorithm [4] for the differential diagnosis of wide QRS complex tachycardias also suggests VT as the correct answer. The first step of the algorithm looks for A–V dissociation, which is not seen on the present ECG. The sec-

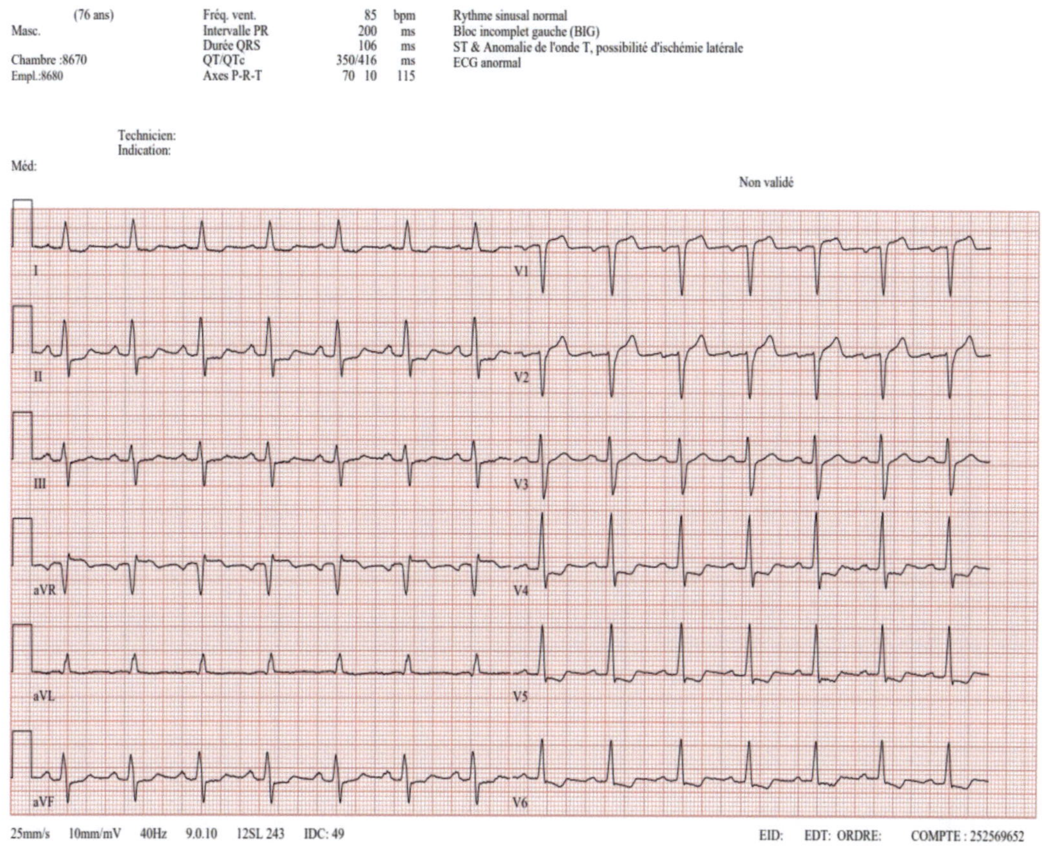

Fig. 2 Twelve-lead ECG recorded after the end of the episode of palpitations

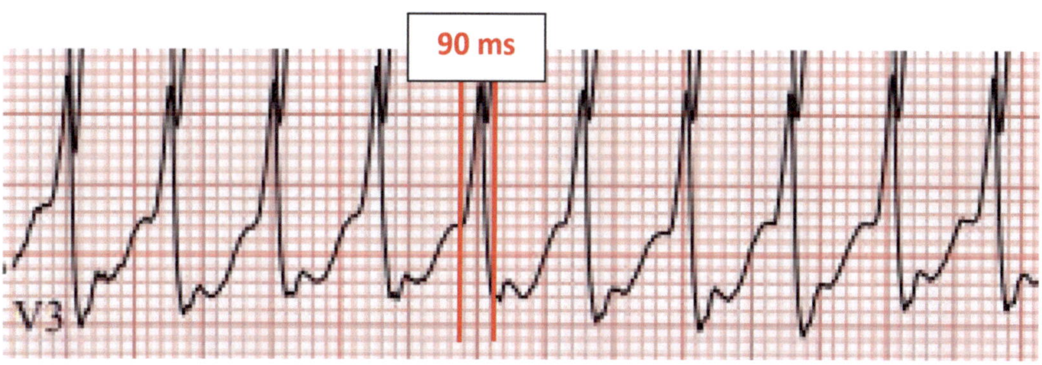

Fig. 3 Lead V3 from the tachycardia from Fig. 1 showing an RS interval of 90 ms, argument not in favor of ventricular tachycardia (but not excluding it either)

ond step of the algorithm looks for an initial predominant R wave in lead aVR, which, again, is not the case (Fig. 6). The third step "QRS morphology unlike BBB or fascicular block" does not suggest SVT with BBB, given the presence of a "Qr" aspect in lead V1; the transition in precordial leads takes places in lead V3, and an "rS" aspect in lead DI and aVL. Therefore, according to this algorithm, the tachycardia is ventricular in nature.

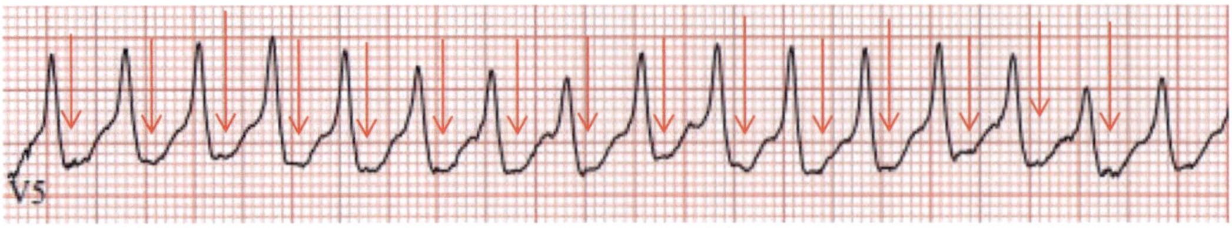

Fig. 4 Lead V5 demonstrating V:A conduction with one P wave visible after each QRS complex (red arrows point to the P waves)

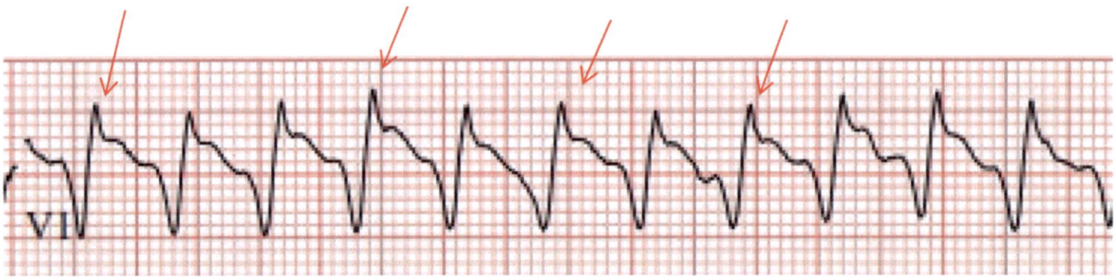

Fig. 5 For a LBBB wide QRS complex tachycardia, presence of an "R" wave >0.04 s in lead V (red arrows) 1 is a criterion in favor of ventricular tachycardia

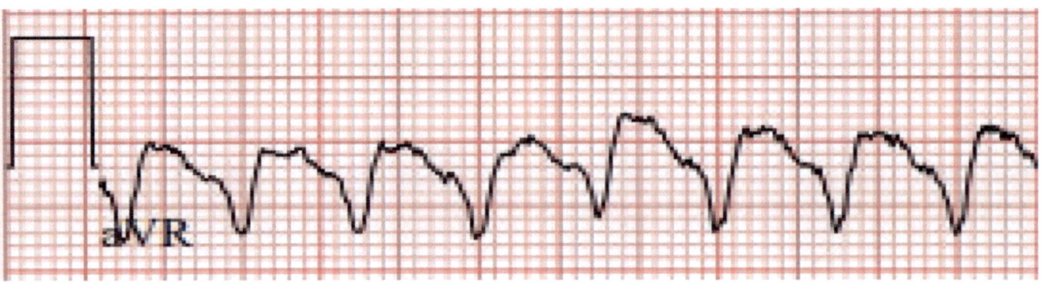

Fig. 6 Lead aVR from the tachycardia presented in Fig. 1, showing the presence of a "QS" pattern, not in favor of ventricular tachycardia (but not excluding it either)

The Basel algorithm [5] is also in favor of ventricular tachycardia as the right answer. According to this algorithm, a positive diagnosis of VT is established if at least two out of three criteria are present: (1) Structural heart disease (history of myocardial infarction, congestive heart failure (LVEF <35%), and the presence of an ICD and CRT), which the patient has. (2) The time to first peak in lead II >40 ms (Fig. 7), which is also the case. (3) The time to first peak in lead aVR >40 ms (Fig. 8), which is also the case [5]. Therefore, according to the Basel algorithm, the diagnosis of VT can be established.

Based on these arguments, the diagnosis of ventricular tachcyardia was established.

The morphology of the VT is in favor of an outflow tract origin, given the LBBB morphology and inferior axis [6–8]. The presence of a deep S wave in lead I and an abrupt transition from V2 to V3 are in favor of an LVOT origin [9–11].

The patient underwent an electrophysiological study which confirmed the diagnosis of ventriculr tachycardia and a catheter ablation procedure.

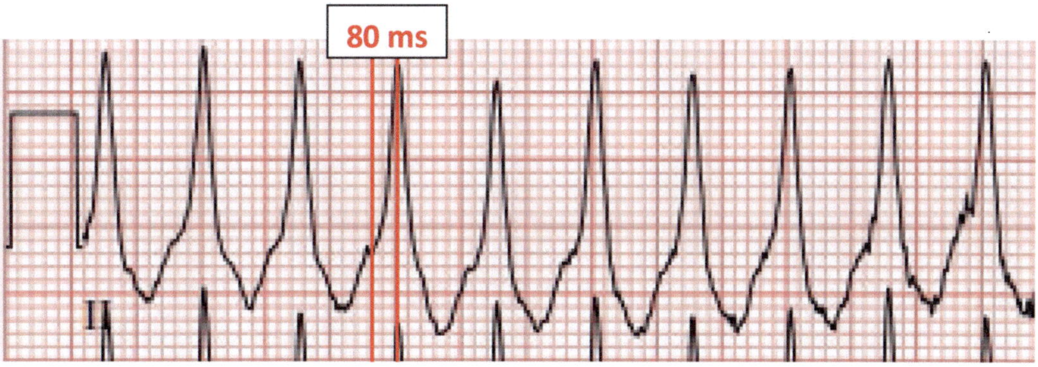

Fig. 7 Lead II from the ECG from Fig. 1 showing the time to first peak of 80 ms, criterion in favor of ventricular tachycardia

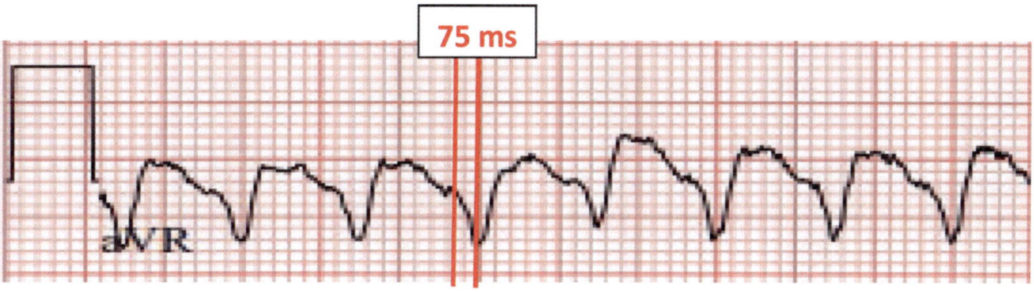

Fig. 8 Lead aVR from the ECG from Fig. 1 showing the time to the first peak of 75 ms, criterion in favor of ventricular tachycardia

References

1. Eckardt L, Breithardt G, Kirchhof P. Approach to wide complex tachycardias in patients without structural heart disease. Heart. 2006;92(5):704–11.
2. Brugada P, Brugada J, Mont L, Smeets J, Andries EW. A new approach to the differential diagnosis of a regular tachycardia with a wide QRS complex. Circulation. 1991;83(5):1649–59.
3. Kindwall KE, Brown J, Josephson ME. Electrocardiographic criteria for ventricular tachycardia in wide complex left bundle branch block morphology tachycardias. Am J Cardiol. 1988;61(15):1279–83.
4. Vereckei A, Duray G, Szenasi G, Altemose GT, Miller JM. Application of a new algorithm in the differential diagnosis of wide QRS complex tachycardia. Eur Heart J. 2007;28(5):589–600.
5. Moccetti F, Yadava M, Latifi Y, Strebel I, Pavlovic N, Knecht S, et al. Simplified integrated clinical and electrocardiographic algorithm for differentiation of wide QRS complex tachycardia: the basel algorithm. JACC Clin Electrophysiol. 2022;8(7):831–9.
6. Kumagai K, Fukuda K, Wakayama Y, Sugai Y, Hirose M, Yamaguchi N, et al. Electrocardiographic characteristics of the variants of idiopathic left ventricular outflow tract ventricular tachyarrhythmias. J Cardiovas Electrophysiol. 2008;19(5):495–501.
7. Anderson RD, Kumar S, Parameswaran R, Wong G, Voskoboinik A, Sugumar H, et al. Differentiating right- and left-sided outflow tract ventricular arrhythmias: classical ECG signatures and prediction algorithms. Circ Arrhythm Electrophysiol. 2019;12(6):e007392.
8. Mariani MV, Piro A, Della Rocca DG, Forleo GB, Pothineni NV, Romero J, et al. Electrocardiographic criteria for differentiating left from right idiopathic outflow tract ventricular arrhythmias. Arrhythm Electrophysiol Rev. 2021;10(1):10–6.
9. Hachiya H, Aonuma K, Yamauchi Y, Harada T, Igawa M, Nogami A, et al. Electrocardiographic characteristics of left ventricular outflow tract tachycardia. Pacing Clin Electrophysiol. 2000;23(11 Pt 2):1930–4.
10. Ouyang F, Mathew S, Wu S, Kamioka M, Metzner A, Xue Y, et al. Ventricular arrhythmias arising from the left ventricular outflow tract below the aortic sinus cusps: mapping and catheter ablation via transseptal approach and electrocardiographic characteristics. Circ Arrhythm Electrophysiol. 2014;7(3):445–55.
11. Yamada T, Doppalapudi H, Maddox WR, McElderry HT, Plumb VJ, Kay GN. Prevalence and electrocardiographic and electrophysiological characteristics of idiopathic ventricular arrhythmias originating from intramural foci in the left ventricular outflow tract. Circ Arrhythm Electrophysiol. 2016;9(9)

ECG 24

Stefan-Lucian Popa

1 Case Presentation

A 57-year-old male patient with a history of ischemic cardiomyopathy with moderate systolic dysfunction (LVEF of 45%), remote inferior myocardial infarction, severe coronary vessel disease (chronic total occlusion of the circumflex coronary artery, severe stenosis of the left anterior descending coronary artery, severe stenosis of the right coronary artery treated with PCI, and stent implantation in the LAD and RCA), and paroxysmal atrial fibrillation is admitted to the Cardiology Department for an episode of palpitations accompanied by dyspnea and anxiety that had occurred several minutes prior to his presentation to the hospital. His ECG recorded in the Cardiology Department is presented in Fig. 1.

Question: What is the nature of the tachycardia presented in Fig. 1?

(a) Ventricular tachycardia originating from the anterior basal LV wall.
(b) Ventricular tachycardia originating from the inferior basal LV wall.
(c) Antidromic tachycardia using a left-sided bypass tract.
(d) Antidromic tachycardia using a right-sided bypass tract.
(e) Supraventricular tachycardia with right bundle branch block.

Hint: A second ECG recorded several minutes later is presented in Fig. 2.

Correct answer: c. Ventricular tachycardia originating from the inferior basal LV wall.

Explanation: The ECG in Fig. 1 shows a regular wide QRS complex tachycardia with a heart rate of 139 bpm and RBBB morphology. The width of the QRS complex is 145 ms. The QRS axis is at +150°. The differential diagnosis of this wide QRS complex tachycardia with RBBB morphology includes: ventricular tachycardia (myocardial-related VT, bundle branch re-entry VT, and fascicular VT), supraventricular tachycardia (atrial fibrillation, atrial flutter, atrial tachycardia, AVNRT, and AVRT) with functional or pre-existing bundle branch block, and antidromic tachycardia (in pre-excitation syndromes).

The ECG from Fig. 2 shows sinus bradycardia with a heart rate of 49 bpm, QRS axis at 0°, absence of LV hypertrophy, negative T waves in leads V5, V6, DI, and aVL, and deep Q waves in leads III and aVF, compatible with inferior necrosis. There are no signs of ventricular pre-excitation

S.-L. Popa (✉)
Department of Internal Medicine, Second Medical Clinic, Cluj-Napoca, Romania
e-mail: popa.stefan@umfcluj.ro

L. Muresan (ed.), *ECG Interpretation of Wide QRS Complex Tachycardia*,
https://doi.org/10.1007/978-3-031-97030-6_25

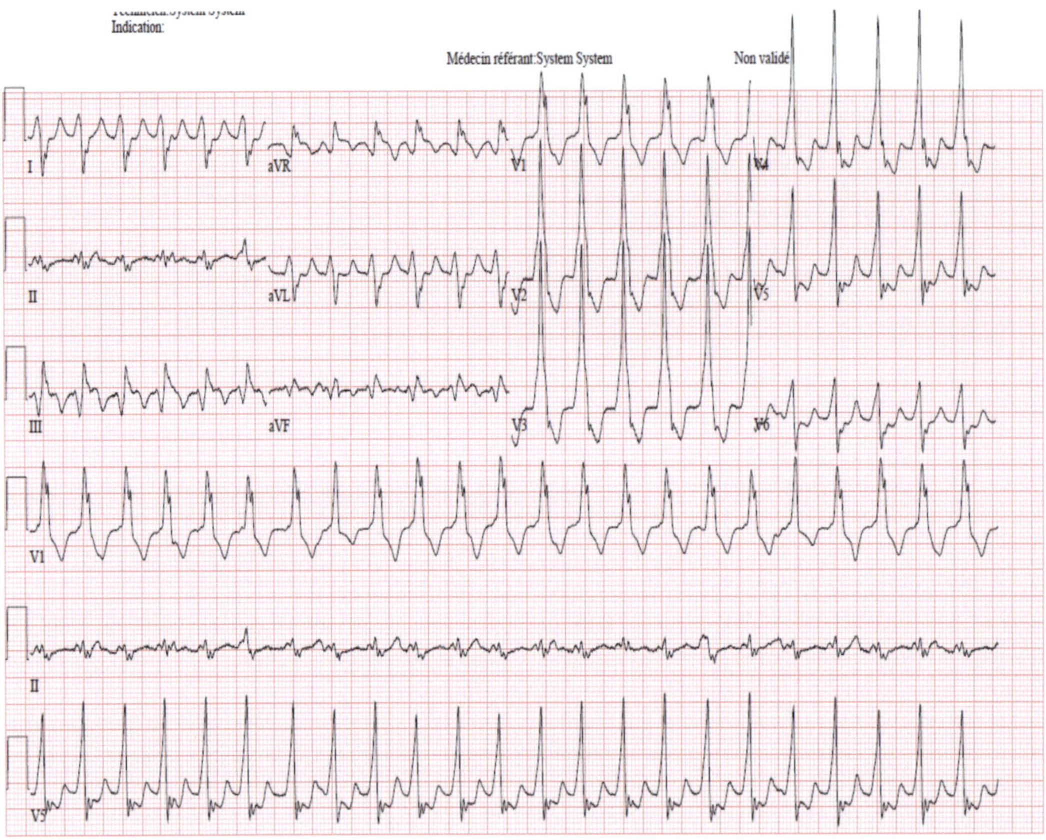

Fig. 1 Twelve-lead ECG recorded at admittance to the Cardiology Department

(no short PR interval and no delta waves), which makes antidromic tachycardia unlikely the correct answer.

The morphology of the right bundle branch block of the QRS complex during tachycardia from Fig. 1 is compatible with that of a typical one [1]: the QRS duration is >120 ms; there is an "RSR'" pattern in lead V1 and an "RS" pattern in leads I, aVL, and V6. So, at this point of the analysis, we cannot say whether this is VT or SVT with RBBB.

Applying the Brugada algorithm [2] to the tachycardia from Fig. 1, it can be seen that: (1) There is no absence of an RS complex in the precordial leads (otherwise said, there are "rS" complexes in leads V4 to V6); we therefore move to the second step of the algorithm: (2) This step analyzes the absence of an R-to-S interval >100 ms in any precordial lead. The RS interval measures 105 ms, criterion in favor of ventricular tachycardia (Fig. 3).

Another argument from the Brugada algorithm in favor of VT is the presence of a taller left peak of the QRS complex in lead V1 (the rabbit ear sign) (Fig. 4).

The Vereckei algorithm [3] for the differential diagnosis of wide QRS complex tachycardias also suggests VT as the correct answer. The first step of the algorithm looks for A–V dissociation, which is not seen on the present ECG. The second step of the algorithm looks for an initial predominant R wave in lead aVR, which, again, is not the case (Fig. 5).

The third step "QRS morphology unlike BBB or fascicular block" might be in favor of SVT with BBB. However, the fourth step of the algorithm, which analyzes the vi/vt index (the amplitude of the first 40 ms of a QRS complex to the amplitude of the last 40 ms of the QRS complex in a lead where the QRS has both an R and an S wave), suggests ventricular tachycardia as the

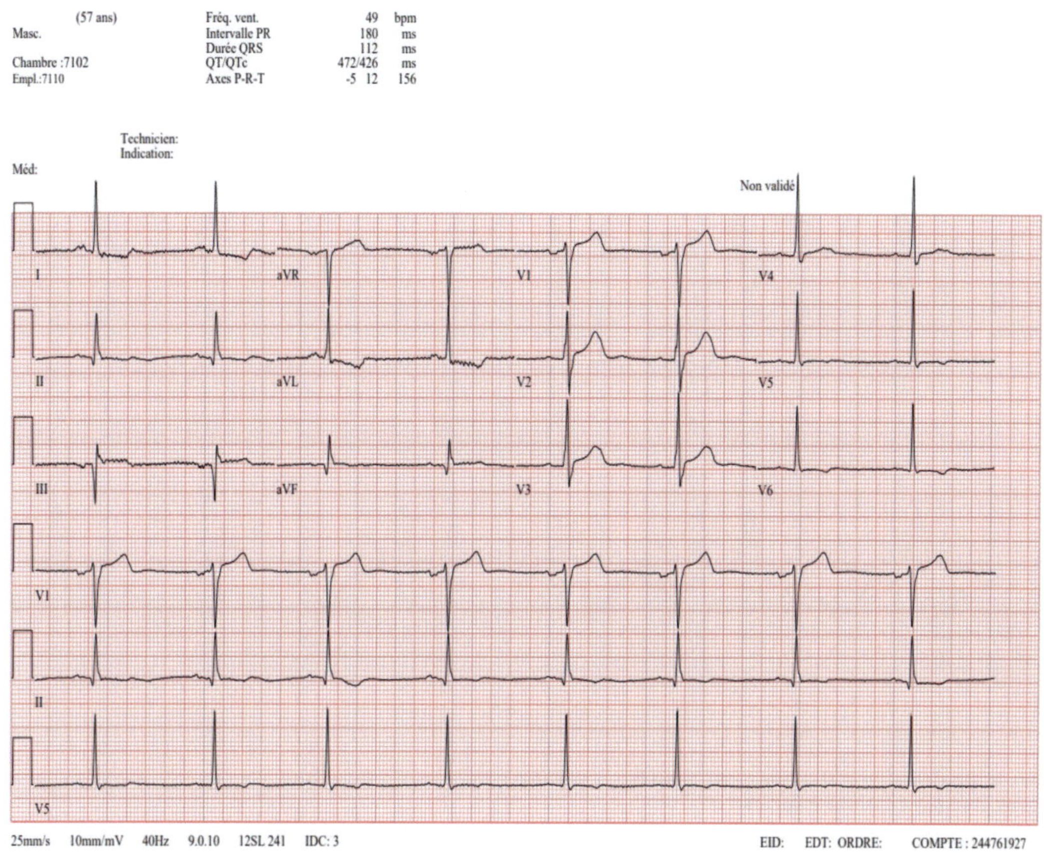

Fig. 2 Twelve-lead ECG recorded after the end of the episode of palpitations

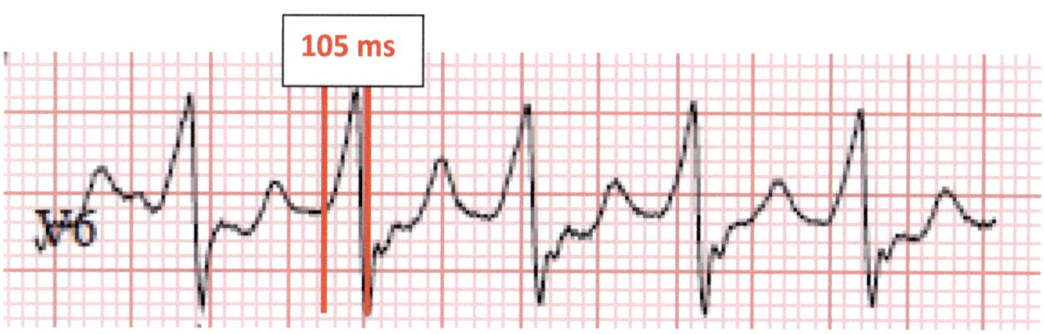

Fig. 3 Lead V6 from the tachycardia presented in Fig. 1 showing an RS duration of 105 ms, argument in favor of ventricular tachycardia

correct answer. In the present case, this is illustrated in Fig. 6.

The Basel algorithm [4] is also in favor of ventricular tachycardia as the right answer. According to this algorithm, a positive diagnosis of VT is established if at least two out of three criteria are present: (1) Structural heart disease (history of myocardial infarction, congestive heart failure (LVEF <35%), and the presence of an ICD and CRT), which the patient has (myocardial infarction). (2) The time to first peak in lead II > 40 ms (Fig. 7), which is not the case. (3)

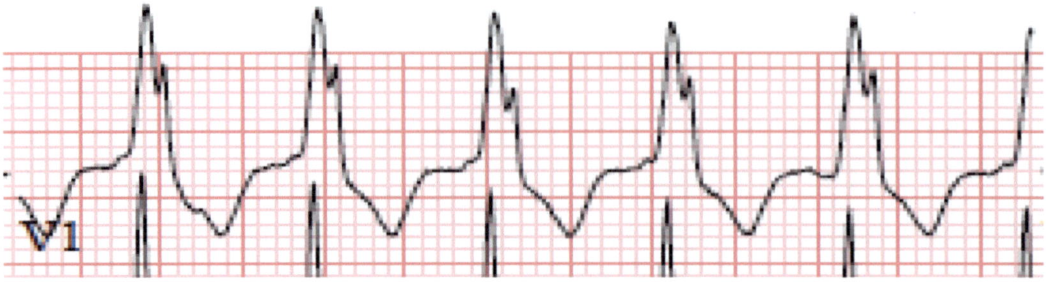

Fig. 4 Lead V1 from the tachycardia from Fig. 1 showing the "rabbit ear sign": the amplitude of the R wave is greater than the amplitude of the R' wave, criterion in favor of ventricular tachycardia

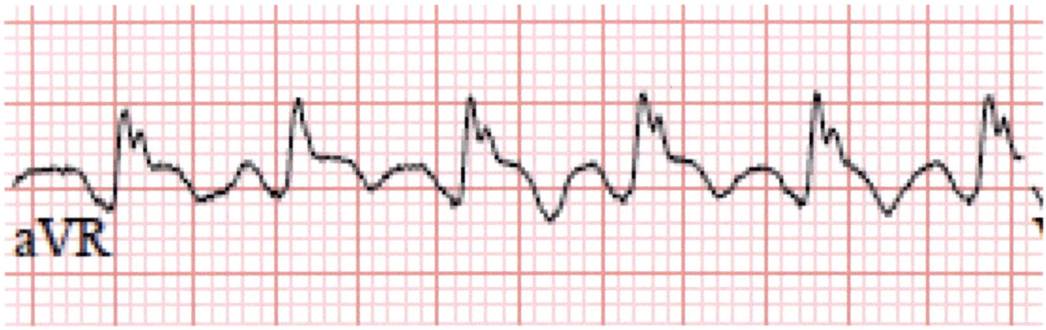

Fig. 5 Lead aVR from the tachycardia from Fig. 1 showing a "qR" pattern, criterion not in favor of ventricular tachycardia (but not excluding it either)

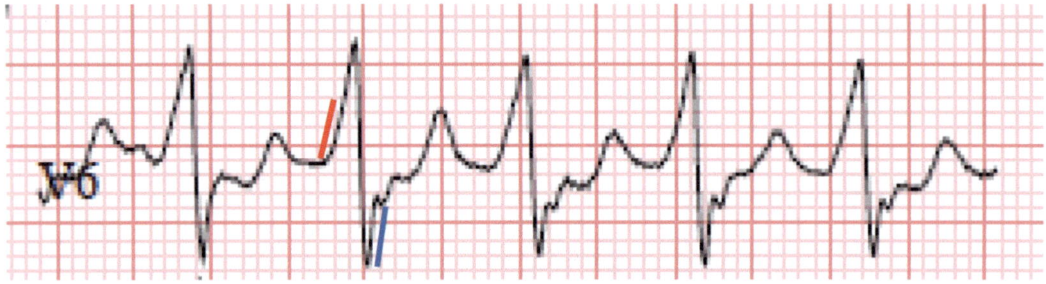

Fig. 6 The vi/vt index from the Vereckei algorithm in lead V1. The ratio of the initial 40 ms and the last 40 ms of the QRS complex is: 4 mV vs 4.5 mV; therefore, 4/4.5 = 0.88, which is <1. This is in favor of ventricular tachycardia

The time to first peak in lead aVR > 40 ms (Fig. 8), which is actually the case [4]. Therefore, according to the Basel algorithm, the diagnosis of VT can be established.

Based on these arguments, the diagnosis of the tachycardia in Fig. 1 is ventricular tachycardia.

The origin of the tachycardia is: in the left ventricle, since the QRS has a RBBB morphology; at the level of the anterior LV wall, since the QRS morphology is predominantly positive in leads II, III, and aVF; basal, since there is a tall R wave from V1 to V6.

The patient underwent an electrophysiological study, which confirmed the diagnosis, and a subsequent radiofrequency catheter ablation procedure.

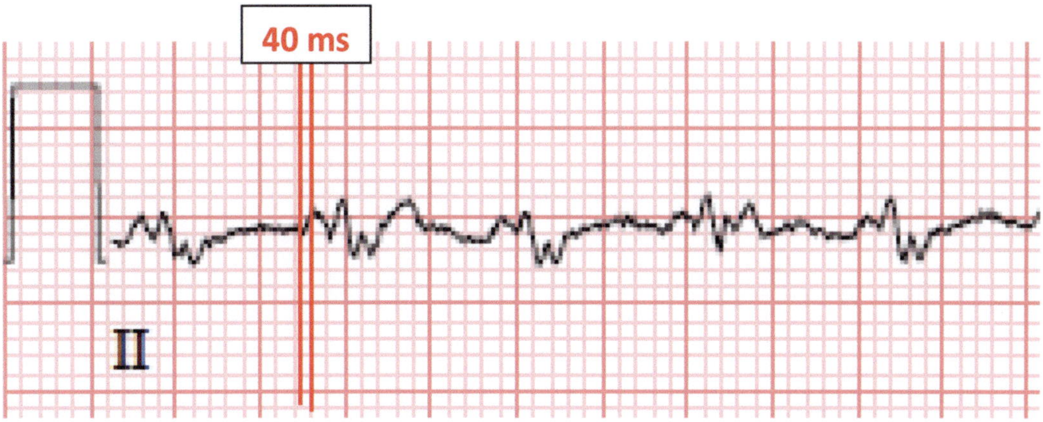

Fig. 7 Lead II from the ECG from Fig. 1 showing the time to first peak of 40 ms, criterion not in favor of ventricular tachycardia

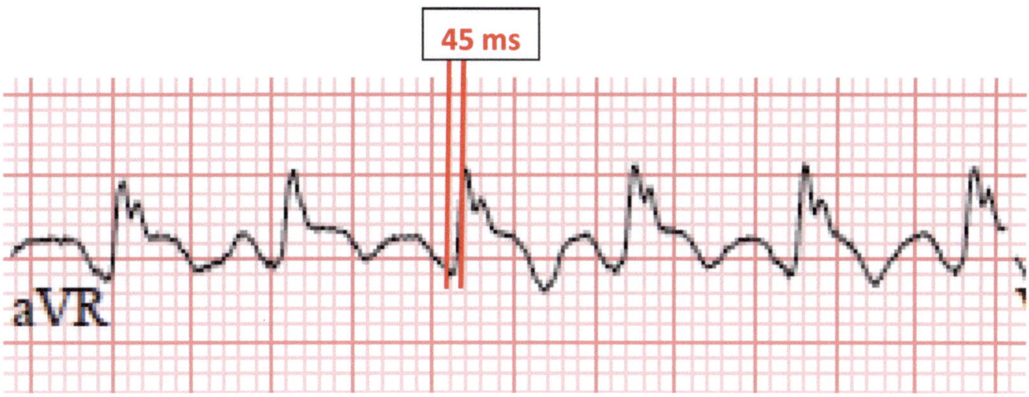

Fig. 8 Lead aVR from the ECG from Fig. 1 showing the time to first peak of 45 ms, criterion in favor of ventricular tachycardia

References

1. Surawicz B, Childers R, Deal BJ, Gettes LS, Bailey JJ, Gorgels A, et al. AHA/ACCF/HRS recommendations for the standardization and interpretation of the electrocardiogram: part III: intraventricular conduction disturbances: a scientific statement from the American Heart Association Electrocardiography and Arrhythmias Committee, Council on Clinical Cardiology; the American College of Cardiology Foundation; and the Heart Rhythm Society. Endorsed by the International Society for Computerized Electrocardiology. J Am Coll Cardiol. 2009;53(11):976–81.
2. Brugada P, Brugada J, Mont L, Smeets J, Andries EW. A new approach to the differential diagnosis of a regular tachycardia with a wide QRS complex. Circulation. 1991;83(5):1649–59.
3. Vereckei A, Duray G, Szenasi G, Altemose GT, Miller JM. Application of a new algorithm in the differential diagnosis of wide QRS complex tachycardia. Eur Heart J. 2007;28(5):589–600.
4. Moccetti F, Yadava M, Latifi Y, Strebel I, Pavlovic N, Knecht S, et al. Simplified integrated clinical and electrocardiographic algorithm for differentiation of wide QRS complex tachycardia: the Basel algorithm. JACC Clinic Electrophysiol. 2022;8(7):831–9.

ECG 25

Razvan Mada

1 Case Presentation

A 71-year-old female patient with a history ischemic cardiomyopathy with moderate systolic dysfunction (LVEF of 43%), remote inferior and inferolateral myocardial infarction, and severe three-vessel disease (chronic total occlusion of the right coronary artery, severe stenosis of the left anterior descending coronary artery, treated with PCI and stent implantation, and moderate stenosis of the circumflex coronary artery) is admitted to the Cardiology Department for an episode of palpitations accompanied by dyspnea and anxiety. Her ECG recorded in the Cardiology Department at her arrival is presented in Fig. 1.

Question: What is the nature of the wide QRS complex tachycardia presented in Fig. 1?

(a) Ventricular tachycardia originating from the anterior septal LV wall.
(b) Ventricular tachycardia originating from the anterior lateral LV wall.
(c) Antidromic tachycardia using a left-sided bypass tract.
(d) Atrial fibrillation with right bundle branch block.
(e) Sinus tachycardia with right bundle branch block.

Hint: A second ECG recorded several minutes later is presented in Fig. 2.

Correct answer: e. Ventricular tachycardia originating from the anterior lateral LV wall.

Explanation: The ECG in Fig. 1 shows a regular wide QRS complex tachycardia with a heart rate of 120 bpm and RBBB morphology. The width of the QRS complex is 142 ms. The QRS axis is at +130°. The differential diagnosis of this regular wide QRS complex tachycardia with RBBB morphology includes: ventricular tachycardia (myocardial-related VT, bundle branch re-entry VT, and fascicular VT), supraventricular tachycardia (atrial fibrillation, atrial flutter, atrial tachycardia, AVNRT, and AVRT) with functional or pre-existing bundle branch block, and antidromic tachycardia (in pre-excitation syndromes).

The ECG from Fig. 2 shows sinus rhythm with a heart rate of 89 bpm, QRS axis at +75°, absence of LV hypertrophy, absence of ischemia, complete RBBB, and five PVCs of which three are isolated and one polymorphic couplet. There are no signs of ventricular pre-excitation (no short PR interval and no delta waves), so the tachycardia from Fig. 1 is unlikely to be antidromic tachycardia.

R. Mada (✉)
Department of Cardiology, "Niculae Stancioiu" Heart Institute, Cluj-Napoca, Romania

L. Muresan (ed.), *ECG Interpretation of Wide QRS Complex Tachycardia*,
https://doi.org/10.1007/978-3-031-97030-6_26

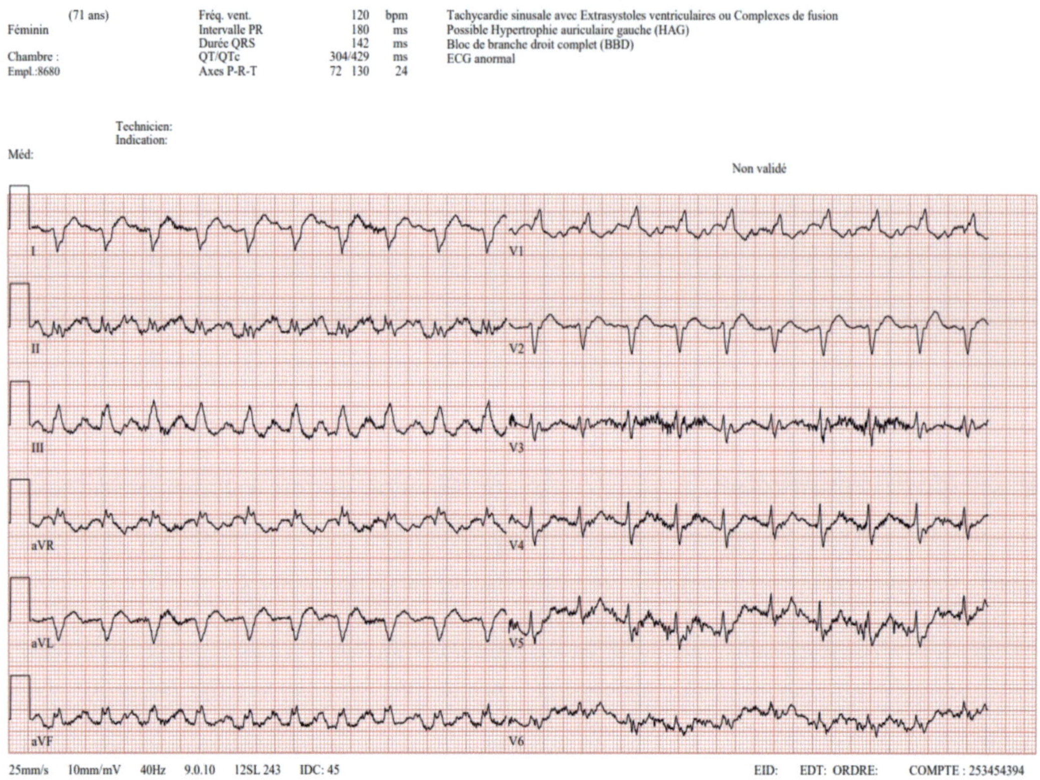

Fig. 1 Twelve-lead ECG recorded at admittance to the Cardiology Department

The morphology of the right bundle branch block of the QRS complex during tachycardia from Fig. 1 suggests that it might be a typical one [1]: the QRS duration is >120 ms; there is an "RSR'" aspect in lead V1, an "rS" aspect in leads I, aVL, and V6. However, there is a double QRS transition in the precordial leads (first from V1 to V2 and then from V2 to V3), which is not characteristic of a typical RBBB.

Applying the Brugada algorithm [2] to the tachycardia from Fig. 1, it can be seen that: (1) There is no absence of an RS complex in the precordial leads (otherwise said, there are rS complexes in leads V2 to V6); we therefore move to the second step of the algorithm: (2) This step analyzes the absence of an R-to-S interval > 100 ms in any precordial lead. This is not the case (Fig. 3).

Step 3 of the algorithm looks for A–V dissociation. There are P waves on the ECG, best visible in lead V1, with a 1:1 A:V relationship (Fig. 4), so there is no A–V dissociation. We therefore need to move to step 4 of the algorithm.

For a RBBB morphology wide QRS complex tachycardia, an argument in favor of VT would be the presence of a taller left peak of the QRS complex in lead V1 (the rabbit ear sign), which is not actually the case, or for biphasic RS or QR complexes, which is not the case. Next, in lead V6, an argument in favor of VT would be the presence of an "rS" complex, which is not the case either. This can also be expressed as a ratio of R/S < 1 in lead V6. So, the algorithm does not suggest VT as the diagnosis for the tachycardia.

The Vereckei algorithm [3] for the differential diagnosis of wide QRS complex tachycardias also suggests SVT as the correct answer. The first step of the algorithm looks for A–V dissociation, which is not seen on the present ECG. The second step of the algorithm looks for an initial predominant R wave in lead aVR, which, again, is not the case (Fig. 5).

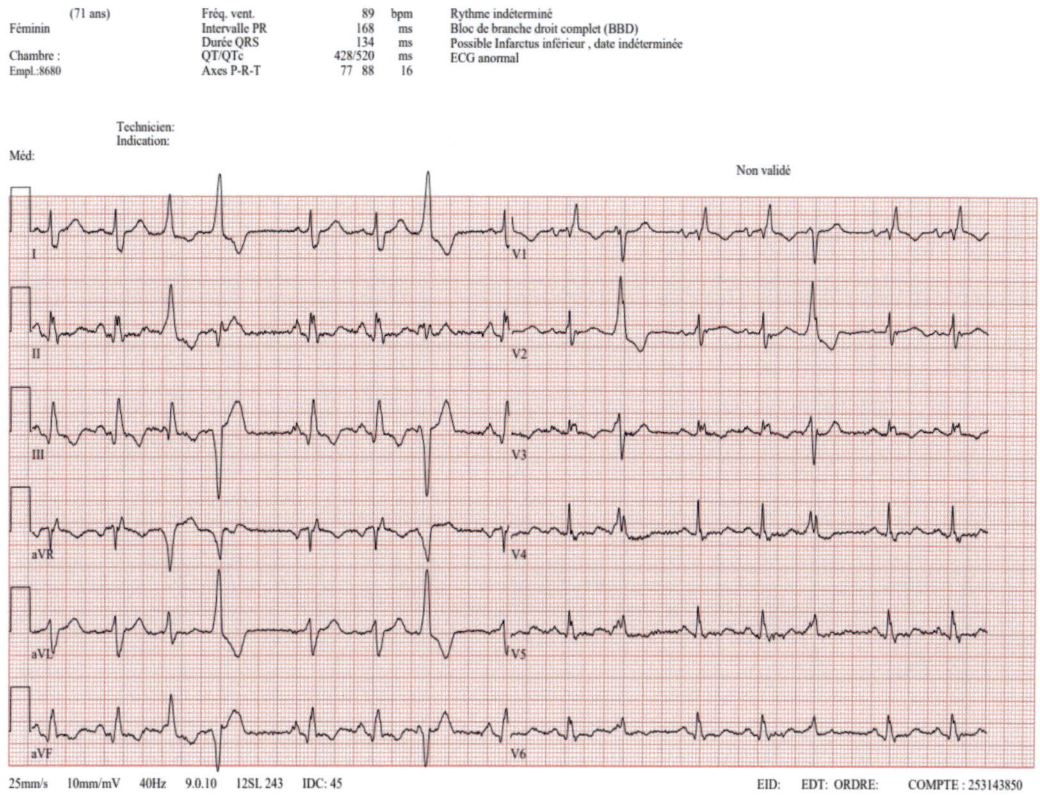

Fig. 2 Twelve-lead ECG recorded after the end of the episode of palpitations

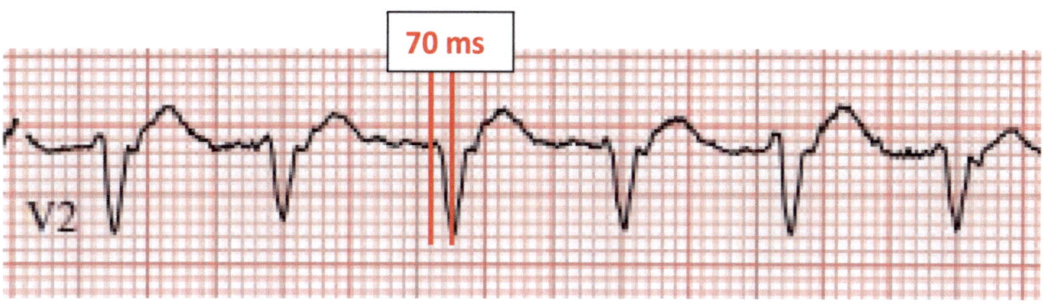

Fig. 3 Lead V2 from the tachycardia presented in Fig. 1 showing an RS interval of 70 ms, argument not in favor of ventricular tachycardia (but not excluding it either)

The third step of the algorithm "QRS morphology unlike BBB or fascicular block" might suggest SVT with BBB, based on the arguments exposed above. However, given the double transition of the QRS complex in the precordial leads, there is doubt concerning the diagnosis.

The fourth step of the algorithm, which analyzes the vi/vt index (the amplitude of the first 40 ms of a QRS complex to the amplitude of the last 40 ms of the QRS complex in a lead where the QRS has both an R and an S wave), suggests supraventricular tachycardia with BBB as the correct answer. In the present case, this is illustrated in Fig. 6.

The Basel algorithm [4] is also in favor of supraventricular tachycardia as the right answer. According to this algorithm, a positive diagnosis of VT is established if at least two out of three

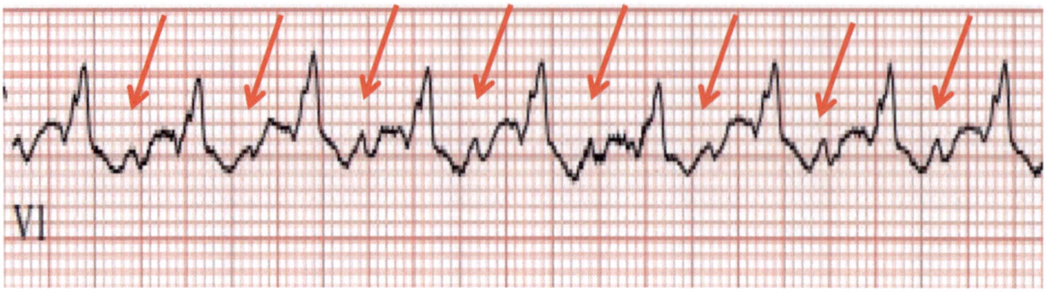

Fig. 4 Lead V1 from the tachycardia from Fig. 1 showing the presence of P waves with a 1 to 1 A:V relationship (see text for discussion)

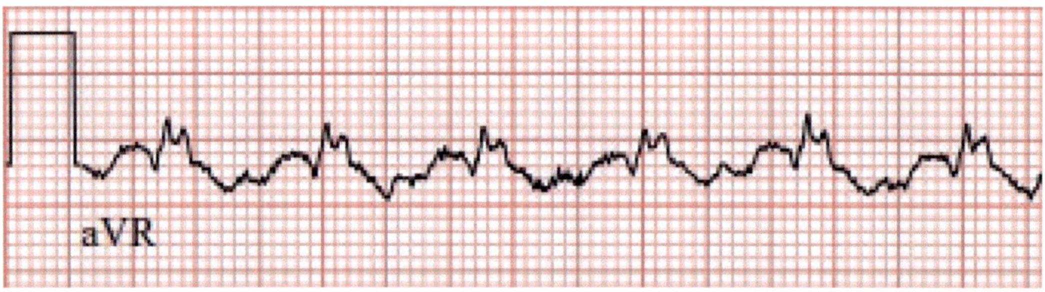

Fig. 5 Lead aVR from the tachycardia presented in Fig. 1 showing a "qR" pattern, argument not in favor of ventricular tachycardia (but not excluding it either)

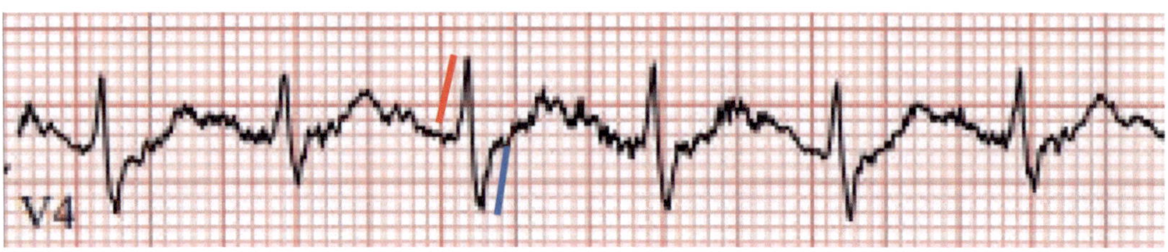

Fig. 6 The vi/vt index from the Vereckei algorithm in lead V1. The ratio of the initial 40 ms and the last 40 ms of the QRS complex is: 5 mV vs 4 mV; therefore, 5/4 = 1.2, which is >1. This is in favor of supraventricular tachycardia

criteria are present: (1) structural heart disease (history of myocardial infarction, congestive heart failure (LVEF <35%), and the presence of an ICD and CRT), which the patient has (myocardial infarction); (2) the time to the first peak in lead II > 40 ms (Fig. 7), which is not the case; and (3) the time to the first peak in lead aVR > 40 ms (Fig. 8), which is also not the case [4]. Therefore, according to the Basel algorithm, the diagnosis of SVT can be established.

Therefore, all the 3 algorithms suggest SVT with right bundle branch block as the correct diagnosis. However, the correct diagnosis can be established by comparing the QRS morphology during tachycardia (Fig. 1) with the QRS morphology during sinus rhythm (Fig. 2). These are

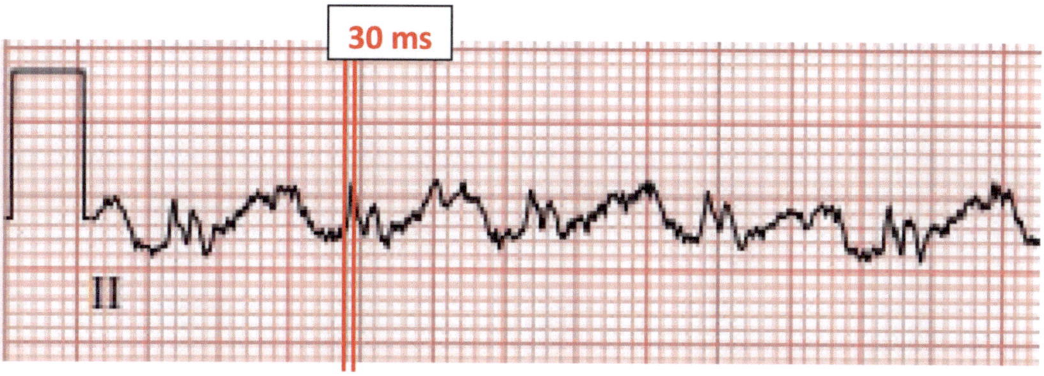

Fig. 7 Lead II from the ECG from Fig. 1 showing the time to the first peak of 30 ms, criterion not in favor of ventricular tachycardia (but not excluding it either)

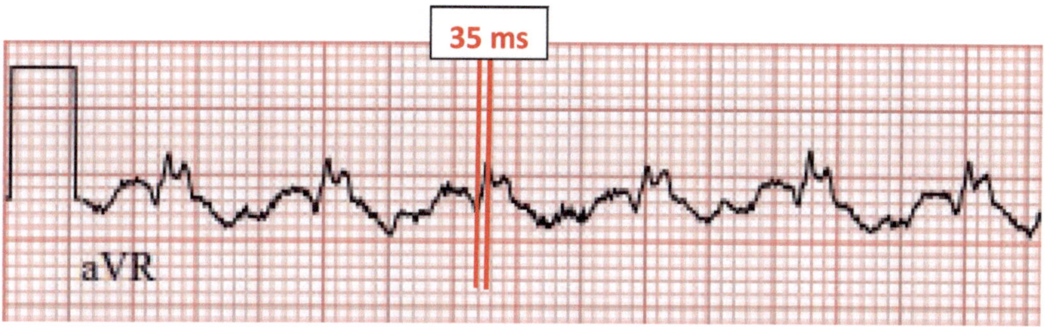

Fig. 8 Lead aVR from the ECG from Fig. 1 showing the time to the first peak of 35 ms, criterion not in favor of ventricular tachycardia (but not excluding it either)

clearly different, best seen in leads I, aVL, and V2. The patient has RBBB during sinus rhythm, with a morphology that is different from the one during tachycardia. This observation, together with the fact that there is a double QRS transition in the precordial leads during tachycardia, makes the diagnosis of VT highly likely.

An interesting observation is that a careful analysis of the atrial rhythm from the ECG recorded during the wide QRS complex tachycardia identifies the presence of P waves. As shown in Fig. 4, there is a 1:1 P-to-QRS relationship. The morphology of the P wave is negative in leads II, III, and aVF, biphasic in lead V1, and positive in lead aVR, different from the P wave morphology during sinus rhythm (Fig. 9). This is most likely compatible with retrograde VA conduction.

This case demonstrates that sometimes the existing algorithms for the differential diagnosis of wide QRS complex tachycardias are not correct and that information provided by the 12-lead ECG recorded during sinus rhythm remains important in establishing the correct diagnosis.

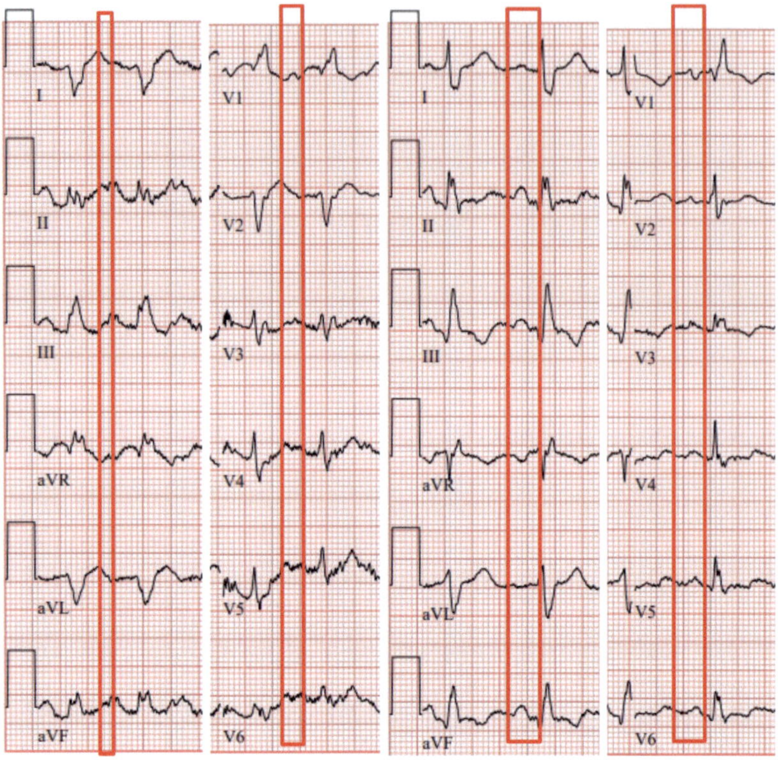

Fig. 9 Twelve-lead ECG showing the morphology of the P wave during the wide QRS complex tachycardia (first two panels) being different to the one recorded in the second ECG (last two panels), the argument in favor of different atrial activation during the wide QRS complex tachycardia and during sinus rhythm, supporting the diagnosis of ventricular tachycardia

References

1. Surawicz B, Childers R, Deal BJ, Gettes LS, Bailey JJ, Gorgels A, et al. AHA/ACCF/HRS recommendations for the standardization and interpretation of the electrocardiogram: part III: intraventricular conduction disturbances: a scientific statement from the American Heart Association Electrocardiography and Arrhythmias Committee, Council on Clinical Cardiology; the American College of Cardiology Foundation; and the Heart Rhythm Society. Endorsed by the International Society for Computerized Electrocardiology. J Am Coll Cardiol. 2009;53(11):976–81.
2. Brugada P, Brugada J, Mont L, Smeets J, Andries EW. A new approach to the differential diagnosis of a regular tachycardia with a wide QRS complex. Circulation. 1991;83(5):1649–59.
3. Vereckei A, Duray G, Szenasi G, Altemose GT, Miller JM. Application of a new algorithm in the differential diagnosis of wide QRS complex tachycardia. Eur Heart J. 2007;28(5):589–600.
4. Moccetti F, Yadava M, Latifi Y, Strebel I, Pavlovic N, Knecht S, et al. Simplified integrated clinical and electrocardiographic algorithm for differentiation of wide QRS complex tachycardia: the Basel algorithm. JACC Clinic Electrophysiol. 2022;8(7):831–9.

ECG 26

Raphael Martins

1 Case Presentation

A 72-year-old male patient with a history of aborted sudden cardiac death (2018), implanted with a Boston Scientific single-chamber ICD for the secondary prevention of SCD, MINOCA (presence of a reduced area of necrosis of the LV anterior wall on cardiac MRI), and LVEF of 50%, is admitted to the Cardiology Department for an episode of palpitations accompanied by anxiety and lightheadedness that had occurred 30 min prior to his presentation to the hospital. The VT detection window of his ICD was programmed between 170 and 230 bpm. His ECG recorded at admittance to the Cardiology Department is presented in Fig. 1.

Question: What is the nature of the tachycardia presented in Fig. 1?

(a) Antidromic tachycardia using a left-sided bypass tract.
(b) AVNRT with functional RBBB.
(c) Ventricular tachycardia originating from the anterior septal LV wall.
(d) Ventricular tachycardia originating from the anterior lateral LV wall.
(e) Ventricular tachycardia originating from the inferior lateral LV wall.

Hint: A second ECG recorded several minutes later is presented in Fig. 2.

Correct answer: d. Ventricular tachycardia originating from the anterior lateral LV wall.

Explanation: The ECG in Fig. 1 shows a regular wide QRS complex tachycardia with a heart rate of 134 bpm and RBBB morphology. The width of the QRS complex is 204 ms. The QRS axis is at +150°. The differential diagnosis of this regular wide QRS complex tachycardia with RBBB morphology includes: ventricular tachycardia (myocardial-related VT and bundle branch re-entry VT), supraventricular tachycardia (atrial fibrillation, atrial flutter, atrial tachycardia, AVNRT, and AVRT) with functional or pre-existing bundle branch block, and antidromic tachycardia (in pre-excitation syndromes).

Antidromic tachycardia is less likely, given the absence of pre-excitation on the ECG in Fig. 2 (no short PR interval, no delta waves present, and normal QRS transition in the precordial leads).

The morphology of the right bundle branch block of the QRS complex during tachycardia from Fig. 1 suggests that it might be that of a typical one [1]: the QRS duration is >120 ms;

R. Martins (✉)
Department of Cardiology, CHU Rennes, Rennes, France
e-mail: raphael.martins@chu-rennes.fr

L. Muresan (ed.), *ECG Interpretation of Wide QRS Complex Tachycardia*,
https://doi.org/10.1007/978-3-031-97030-6_27

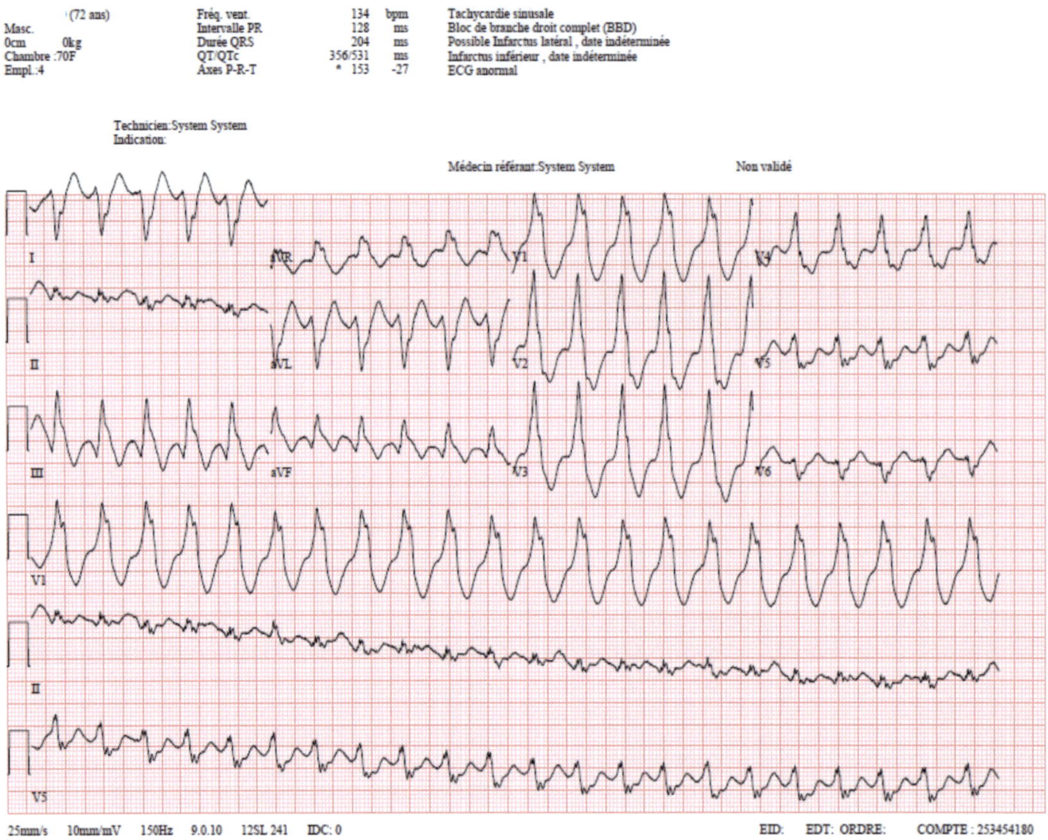

Fig. 1 Twelve-lead ECG recorded at admittance to the Cardiology Department

there is an "RR'" aspect in lead V1 and an "rS" pattern in leads I, aVL, V5, and V6. However, a closer analysis of the ECG points out several details which are not suggestive of a typical RBBB: an R/S ratio < 1 in leads I, aVL, and V6.

Applying the Brugada algorithm [2] to the tachycardia from Fig. 2, it can be seen that: (1) There is no absence of an RS complex in the precordial leads (otherwise said, there are rS complexes in leads V5 and V6); we therefore move to the second step of the algorithm: (2) This step analyzes the absence of an R-to-S interval > 100 ms in any precordial lead. This interval measures 120 ms in lead V5, criterion in favor of ventricular tachycardia (Fig. 3).

Other arguments in favor of ventricular tachycardia from the Brugada algorithm are: (1) the presence of a taller left peak of the QRS complex in lead V1 (the rabbit ear sign) or for biphasic RS or QR complexes, which is actually the case: the amplitude of the R wave is bigger than the amplitude of the R' wave; (2) in lead V6, the presence of an "rS" complex (otherwise said, a ratio of R/S < 1), which is also the case.

The Vereckei algorithm [3] for the differential diagnosis of wide QRS complex tachycardias also suggests VT as the correct answer. The first step of the algorithm looks for A–V dissociation, which is not seen on the present ECG. The second step of the algorithm looks for an initial predominant R wave in lead aVR, which is actually the case (Fig. 4).

The Basel algorithm [4] is also in favor of ventricular tachycardia as the right answer. According to this algorithm, a positive diagnosis of VT is established if at least two out of three criteria are present: (1) Structural heart disease (history of myocardial infarction, congestive heart failure (LVEF <35%), and the presence of an ICD and CRT), which the patient

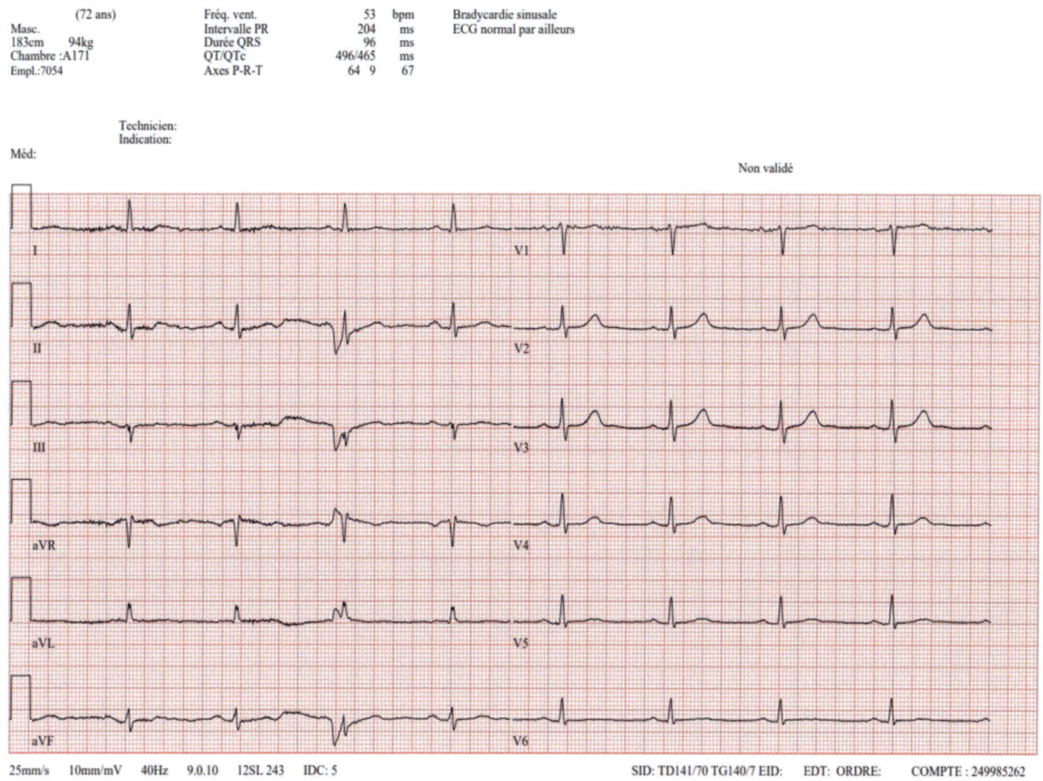

Fig. 2 Twelve-lead ECG recorded after the end of the episode of palpitations

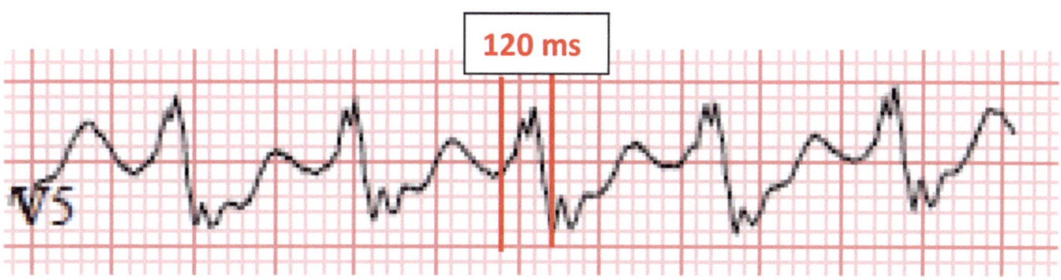

Fig. 3 Lead V2 from the tachycardia presented in Fig. 1 showing an RS interval of 120 ms, argument in favor of ventricular tachycardia

has (ICD implanted in the secondary prevention of SCD). (2) The time to the first peak in lead II > 40 ms (Fig. 5), which is also the case. (3) The time to the first peak in lead aVR > 40 ms (Fig. 6), which is also the case [4]. Therefore, according to the Basel algorithm, the diagnosis of VT can be established.

Another argument in favor of ventricular tachycardia for an RBBB wide QRS complex tachycardia is the QRS width of >140 ms.

Based on these arguments, the diagnosis of ventricular tachycardia was established.

The patient underwent an electrophysiological study which confirmed the ventricular origin of the tachycardia and a subsequent catheter ablation of the VT circuit (the VT was found to have an epicardial origin).

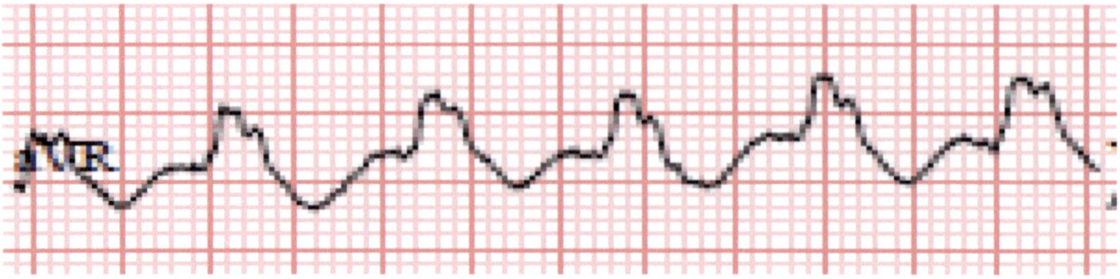

Fig. 4 Lead aVR from the tachycardia presented in Fig. 1 showing a "unique R" pattern, argument in favor of ventricular tachycardia

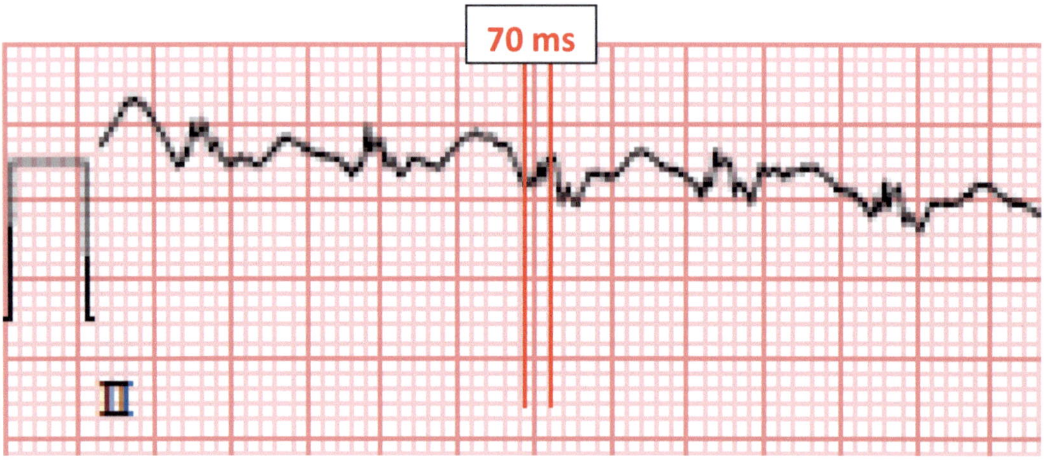

Fig. 5 Lead II from the ECG from Fig. 1 showing the time to the first peak of 70 ms, criterion not in favor of ventricular tachycardia (but not excluding it either)

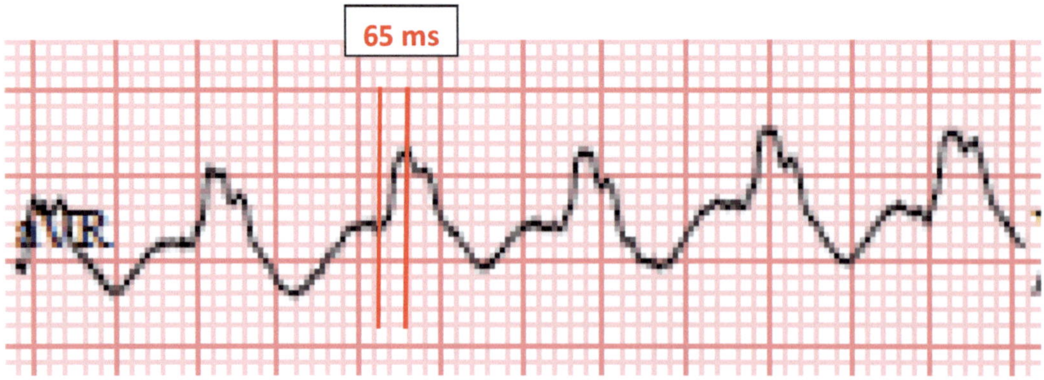

Fig. 6 Lead aVR from the ECG from Fig. 1 showing the time to the first peak of 65 ms, the criterion in favor of ventricular tachycardia

References

1. Surawicz B, Childers R, Deal BJ, Gettes LS, Bailey JJ, Gorgels A, et al. AHA/ACCF/HRS recommendations for the standardization and interpretation of the electrocardiogram: part III: intraventricular conduction disturbances: a scientific statement from the American Heart Association Electrocardiography and Arrhythmias Committee, Council on Clinical Cardiology; the American College of Cardiology Foundation; and the Heart Rhythm Society.

Endorsed by the International Society for Computerized Electrocardiology. J Am Coll Cardiol. 2009;53(11):976–81.
2. Brugada P, Brugada J, Mont L, Smeets J, Andries EW. A new approach to the differential diagnosis of a regular tachycardia with a wide QRS complex. Circulation. 1991;83(5):1649–59.
3. Vereckei A, Duray G, Szenasi G, Altemose GT, Miller JM. Application of a new algorithm in the differential diagnosis of wide QRS complex tachycardia. Eur Heart J. 2007;28(5):589–600.
4. Moccetti F, Yadava M, Latifi Y, Strebel I, Pavlovic N, Knecht S, et al. Simplified integrated clinical and electrocardiographic algorithm for differentiation of wide QRS complex tachycardia: the Basel algorithm. JACC Clinic Electrophysiol. 2022;8(7):831–9.

ECG 27

Ronan Le Bouar

1 Case Presentation

A 74-year-old female patient with a history of arterial hypertension, dyslipidemia, type 2 diabetes mellitus, obstructive sleep apnea, obesity, chronic renal failure, paroxysmal atrial fibrillation, and implanted with a dual-chamber pacemaker for paroxysmal type 2 second degree AV block, is admitted to the Cardiology Department for several episodes of palpitations accompanied by dyspnea and pre-syncope that had occurred several hours prior to her presentation to the hospital. She had presented nausea and repeated episodes of vomiting during the previous 48 h.

At admittance to the Emergency Department, she is hypotensive (BP = 78/65 mmHg), her pulse is rapid around 120 bpm and irregular, her oxygen saturation is 80% breathing room air, and she is in respiratory distress. A blood sample is taken. Her K+ level was found to be 6.5 mmol/L.

The pacemaker was interrogated and found to be programmed in DDD mode at 60 bpm with an upper tracking rate of 130 bpm.

Her ECG recorded at admittance to the Cardiology Department is presented in Fig. 1.

R. Le Bouar (✉)
Department of Cardiology, Emile Muller Hospital, Mulhouse, France
e-mail: LEBOUARR@ghrmsa.fr

Question: What is the nature of the tachycardia presented in the ECG?

(a) Atrial fibrillation with RBBB.
(b) Repetitive nonsustained ventricular tachycardia.
(c) Sinus rhythm with premature atrial contractions and large QRS complexes due to hyperkalemia.
(d) Sinus tachycardia and paced QRS complexes at the upper tracking rate limit of the pacemaker with Wenckebach phenomenon.
(e) Sustained irregular ventricular tachycardia alternating with paced QRS complexes.

Hint: A second ECG recorded 48 h later is presented in Fig. 2.

Correct answer: d. Sinus tachycardia and paced QRS complexes at the upper tracking rate limit of the pacemaker with Wenckebach phenomenon.

Explanation: The ECG in Fig. 1 shows an irregular wide QRS complex tachycardia with a heart rate of around 120 bpm (three RR intervals at 130 bpm, followed by one interval at 86 bpm) (observation: the heart rate of 195 bpm shown by the automatic interpretation of the ECG is incorrect) and RBBB morphology. The width of the QRS complex is 162 ms. The QRS axis is at –75° (the axis at +91° showed by the automatic interpre-

L. Muresan (ed.), *ECG Interpretation of Wide QRS Complex Tachycardia*,
https://doi.org/10.1007/978-3-031-97030-6_28

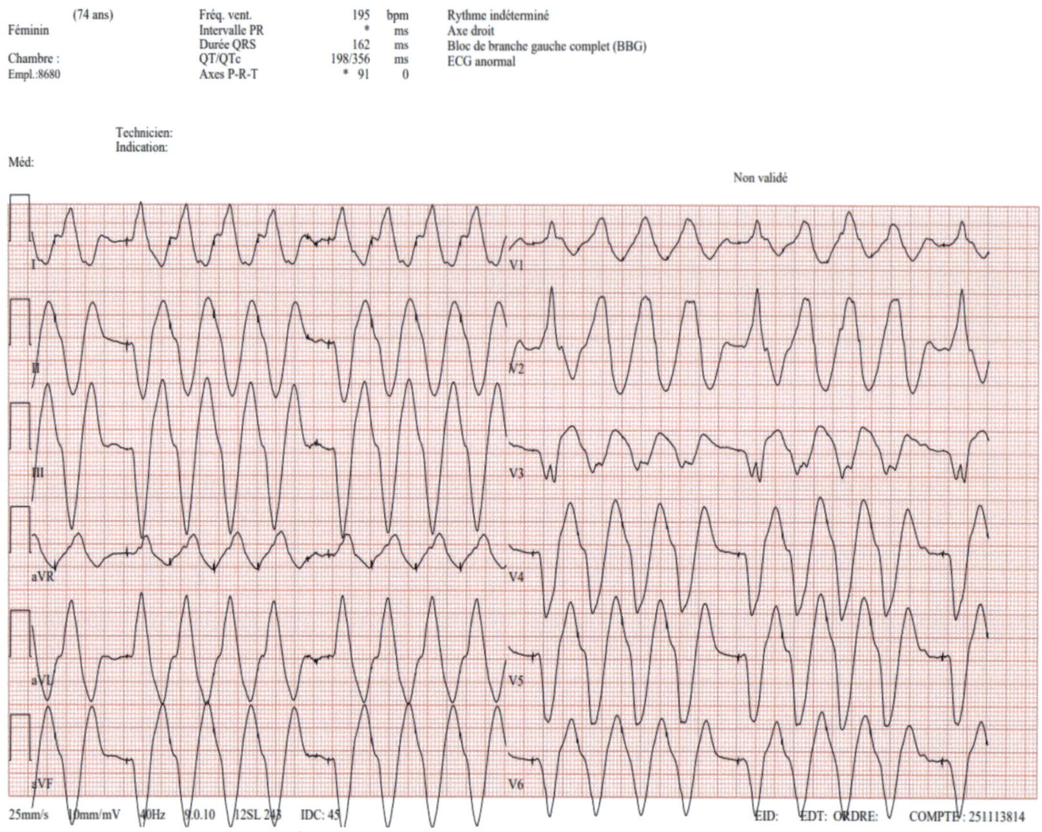

Fig. 1 Twelve-lead ECG recorded at admittance to the cardiology department

tation of the ECG is incorrect). The differential diagnosis of this irregular wide QRS complex tachycardia includes: ventricular tachycardia (myocardial-related VT and bundle branch re-entry VT), supraventricular tachycardia (atrial fibrillation, atrial flutter, atrial tachycardia, AVNRT, and AVRT) with functional or pre-existing bundle branch block, and antidromic tachycardia (in pre-excitation syndromes). However, a careful analysis of the ECG from Fig. 1 shows the presence of a pacing spike before each QRS complex, best visible in leads II, aVR, V5, and V6 (Fig. 2). So, this cannot be ventricular tachycardia, which excludes answers b and e (Fig. 3).

Analysis of the atrial rhythm identifies the presence of P waves, best visible in lead I (Fig. 4). The morphology of the P wave is positive in lead I, compatible with an origin in the right atrium. The presence of P waves excludes answer a—"Atrial fibrillation with RBB".

A careful analysis of the ventricular rhythm identifies grouped beats of four QRS complexes, with a sequence that repeats itself: the first QRS complex on the ECG recorded by the limb leads is followed by a QRS complex with a long RR interval of 700 ms (this first QRS complex is very likely the last QRS complex from a sequence of four), which is followed by four QRS complexes, each having an RR interval of 460 ms. As mentioned before, each QRS complex is preceded by a pacing spike. This, combined with the fact that the atrial rhythm is likely sinus tachycardia and knowing that the patient has a dual-chamber pacemaker, leads to the correct answer: sinus tachycardia and paced QRS complexes at the upper tracking rate limit of the pacemaker with Wenckebach phenomenon (5 to 4). The pacemaker detects the sinus tachycardia, which has a rate of more than 130 bpm, and, in order to maintain the A–V synchrony, tries to pace the ventricle in a 1:1 fashion, the sequence being As–Vp.

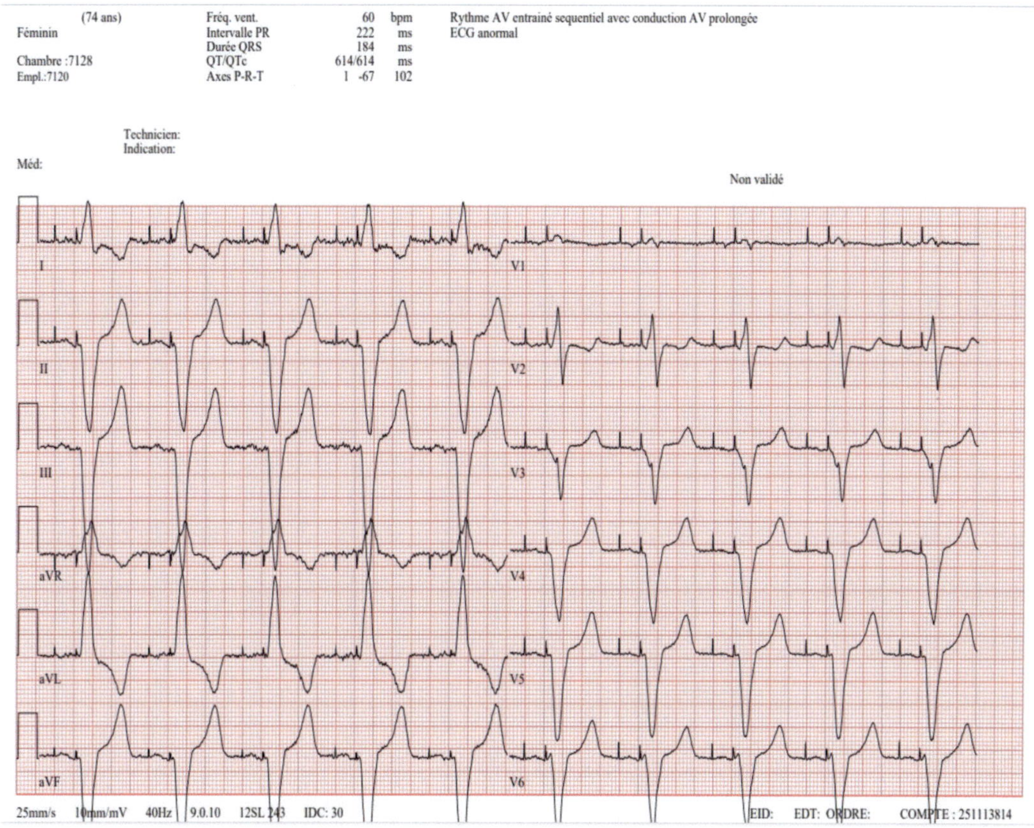

Fig. 2 Twelve-lead ECG recorded after the end of the episode of palpitations

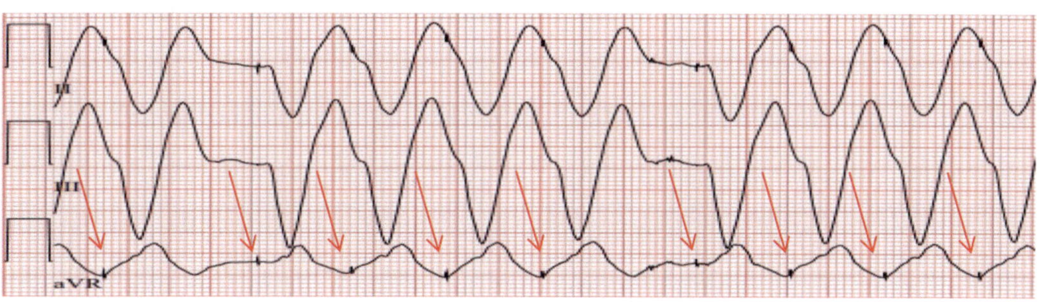

Fig. 3 Leads II, III, and aVR showing the presence of a pacing spike before each QRS complex. This makes the diagnosis of ventricular tachycardia unlikely (see text for explanation)

However, since the rate of the atrial tachycardia exceeds the upper rate limit of the pacemaker (130 bpm), the pacemaker can no longer follow the atrial rate in a 1:1 fashion and drops a ventricular beat every five beats, which explains the regularly irregular rhythm.

The patient's pacemaker interrogation confirmed this hypothesis.

The ECG from Fig. 2 was recorded after iv fluids and correction of hyperkalemia. It shows atrial and ventricular paced rhythms, with a heart rate of 60 bpm. Of note, the morphology of the paced QRS complex is narrower compared to the ECG from Fig. 1. The larger QRS complexes present in the first ECG can be explained by the presence of hyperkalemia at the time of its

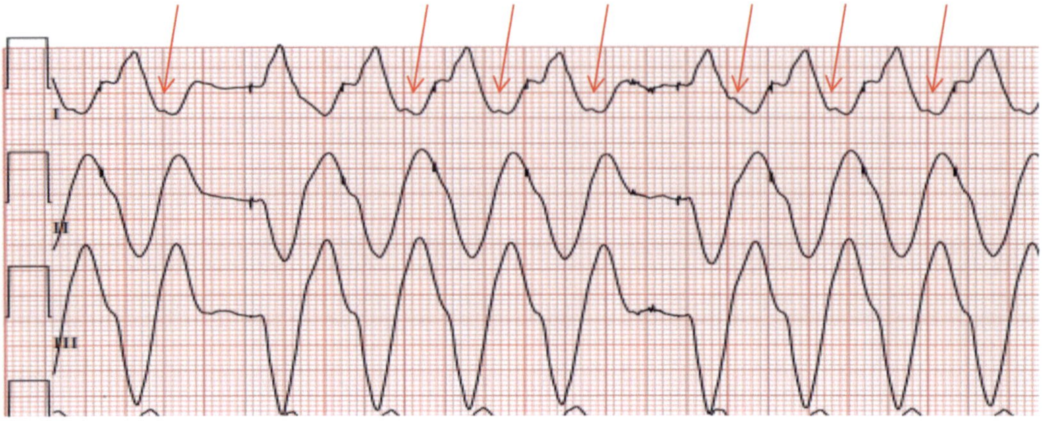

Fig. 4 Leads I, II, and III from the tachycardia presented in Fig. 1. The red arrows point to the visible P waves

Fig. 5 Precordial leads from the tachycardia shown in Fig. 1. The red star identifies a slightly different QRS morphology compared to the rest (see text for explanation)

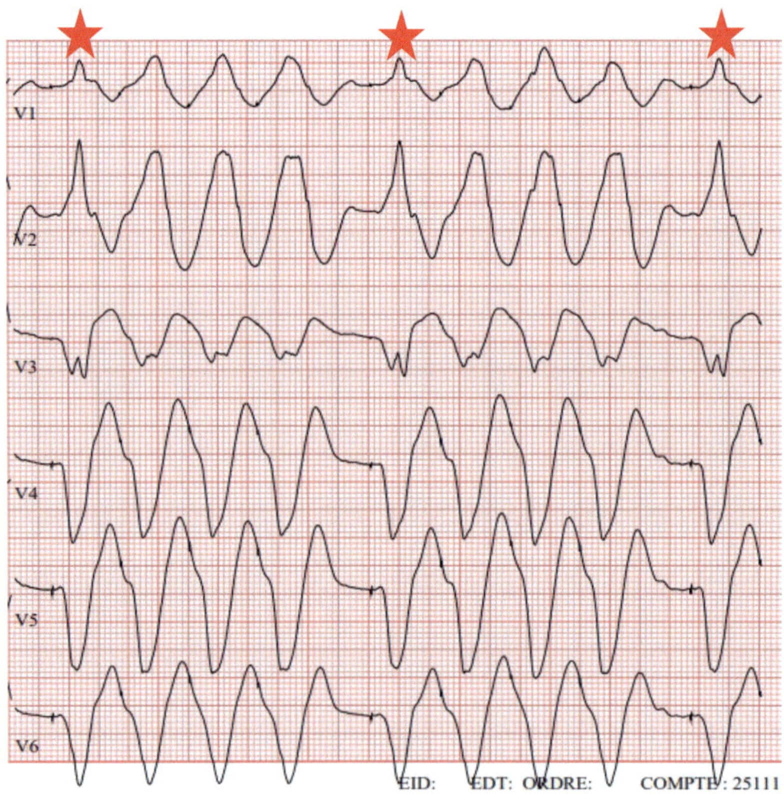

recording, since hyperkalemia can be responsible for the widening of the QRS complexes even for paced rhythms [1–3].

One last observation that merits mentioning is the presence of a slightly different QRS morphology for the QRS complexes that follow a longer RR interval (that of 700 ms), best seen in precordial leads (Fig. 5).

This can be explained by the influence of hyperkalemia and the longer RR interval on the refractory periods of the ventricle. This longer RR interval allows the myocardial tissue to fully recover, and therefore, the first QRS complex after this longer RR interval is narrower compared to the ones preceded by shorter RR intervals. For these shorter RR intervals, the electrical impulses find the ventricle in the relative refractory period, where the myocardial tissue is still excitable but the propagation of the electrical impulse is slower, and therefore the QRS complexes are larger [4].

References

1. Bahl A, Swamy A, Jeevan H, Mahajan R, Talwar KK. ECG changes of hyperkalemia during paced rhythm. Indian Heart J. 2009;61(1):93–4.
2. Barold SS, Herweg B. The effect of hyperkalaemia on cardiac rhythm devices. Europace: European pacing, arrhythmias, and cardiac electrophysiology: journal of the working groups on cardiac pacing, arrhythmias, and cardiac cellular electrophysiology of the European society of. Cardiology. 2014;16(4):467–76.
3. Ortega-Carnicer J, Benezet J, Benezet-Mazuecos J. Hyperkalaemia causing loss of atrial capture and extremely wide QRS complex during DDD pacing. Resuscitation. 2004;62(1):119–20.
4. Parham WA, Mehdirad AA, Biermann KM, Fredman CS. Hyperkalemia revisited. Tex Heart Inst J. 2006;33(1):40–7.

ECG 28

Crina Muresan

1 Case Presentation

An 82-year-old male patient with a history of pericarditis 7 years prior and dyslipidemia is admitted to the Cardiology Department for several episodes of palpitations accompanied by anxiety that had occurred during the past weeks prior to his presentation to the hospital. His ECG recorded during one of the episodes of palpitations at arrival to the Cardiology Department is presented in Fig. 1.

Question: What is the nature of the tachycardia presented in Fig. 1?

(a) Ventricular tachycardia originating from the RVOT.
(b) Ventricular tachycardia originating from the LVOT.
(c) Ventricular tachycardia originating from the left ventricular septum.
(d) Antidromic tachycardia using a right-sided bypass tract.
(e) Orthodromic reciprocating tachycardia with LBBB.

Hint: A second ECG recorded several minutes later is presented in Fig. 2.

C. Muresan (✉)
Department of Cardiology, Emile Muller Hospital, Mulhouse, France
e-mail: crina.muresan@ghrmsa.fr

Correct answer: c. Ventricular tachycardia originating from the left ventricular septum.

Explanation: The ECG in Fig. 1 shows a regular wide QRS complex tachycardia with a heart rate of 177 bpm and LBBB morphology. The width of the QRS complex is 128 ms. The QRS axis is at +80°. The differential diagnosis of this regular wide QRS complex tachycardia with LBBB morphology includes: ventricular tachycardia (myocardial-related VT and upper septal fascicular ventricular tachycardia), supraventricular tachycardia (atrial flutter, atrial tachycardia, AVNRT, and ORT) with functional or pre-existing bundle branch block, and antidromic tachycardia (in pre-excitation syndromes).

The morphology of the left bundle branch block of the QRS complex during tachycardia from Fig. 1 is not that of a typical one [1]: the QRS duration is >120 ms; there is a "QS" pattern in lead V1, and there is ST segment and T wave modification opposite to the major deflection of the QRS complex negative T waves in leads V2 to V6; however, leads I and aVL show an "RS" pattern, which is not common for a typical LBBB; and the QRS transition in the precordial leads takes place in lead V2, which is too early for a typical LBBB (usual transition is in leads V4 and V5). This makes answer e—"Orthodromic reciprocating tachycardia with LBBB"—highly unlikely.

L. Muresan (ed.), *ECG Interpretation of Wide QRS Complex Tachycardia*,
https://doi.org/10.1007/978-3-031-97030-6_29

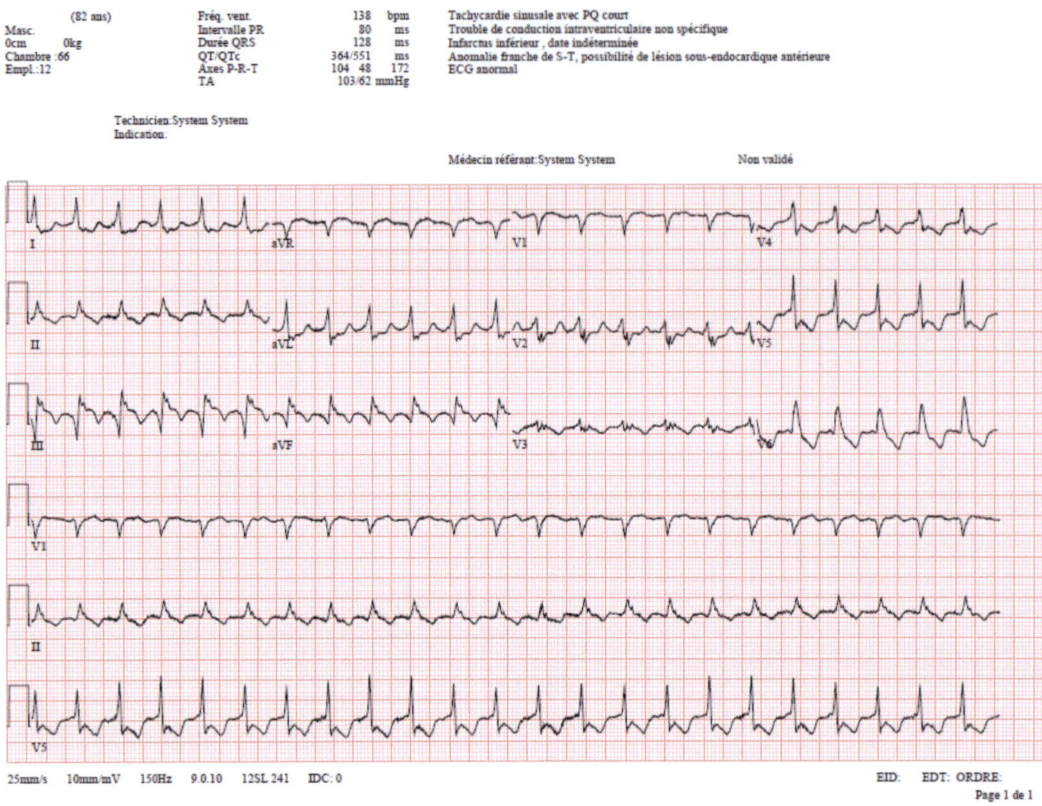

Fig. 1 Twelve-lead ECG recorded at admittance to the Cardiology Department

The ECG from Fig. 2 shows no elements in favor of ventricular pre-excitation: no delta waves, and the PR interval is normal. This makes antidromic tachycardia unlikely.

Applying the Brugada algorithm [2] to the tachycardia from Fig. 1, it can be seen that: (1) There is no absence of an RS complex in the precordial leads (otherwise said, there are rS complexes in leads V2 to V5); we therefore move to the second step of the algorithm: (2) This step analyzes the absence of an R-to-S interval > 100 ms in any precordial lead. This is not the case (Fig. 3).

Step 3 of the algorithm looks for A–V dissociation. P waves are not visible on the ECG. So, we cannot say if there is A–V dissociation. We therefore need to move to step 4 of the algorithm.

For a wide QRS complex tachycardia with LBBB, arguments in favor of VT are: the presence of an "r wave" > 0.04 s in lead V1 or V2, which is actually the case (Fig. 4) [3].

The Vereckei algorithm [4] for the differential diagnosis of wide QRS complex tachycardias also suggests ventricular tachycardia as the correct answer. The first step of the algorithm looks for A–V dissociation, which is not seen on the present ECG. The second step of the algorithm looks for an initial predominant R wave in lead aVR, which, again, is not the case (Fig. 5).

The third step "QRS morphology unlike BBB or fascicular block" suggests the diagnosis of VT on the argument explained above (the presence of a deep S wave in leads I and aVL and early QRS transition in lead V2).

The origin of the tachycardia is at the level of the upper left ventricular septum (relatively narrow QRS complexes, early QRS transition in the precordial leads, predominantly R waves in the inferior leads).

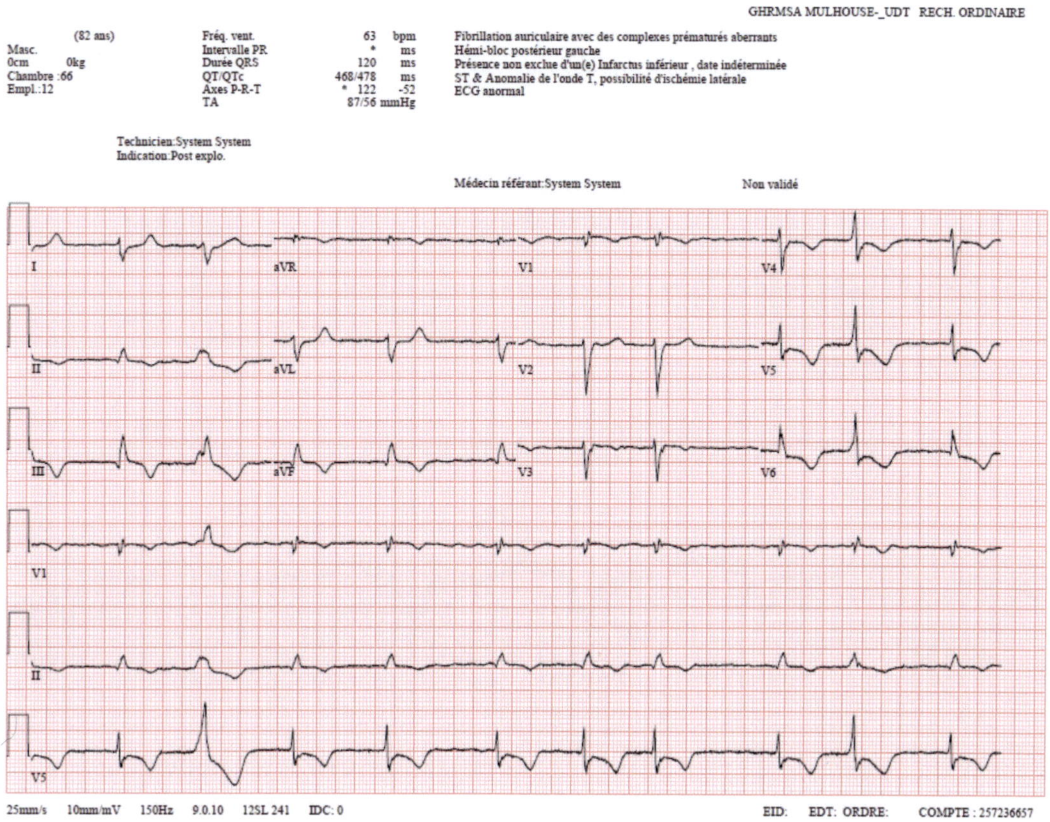

Fig. 2 Twelve-lead ECG recorded after the end of the episode of palpitations

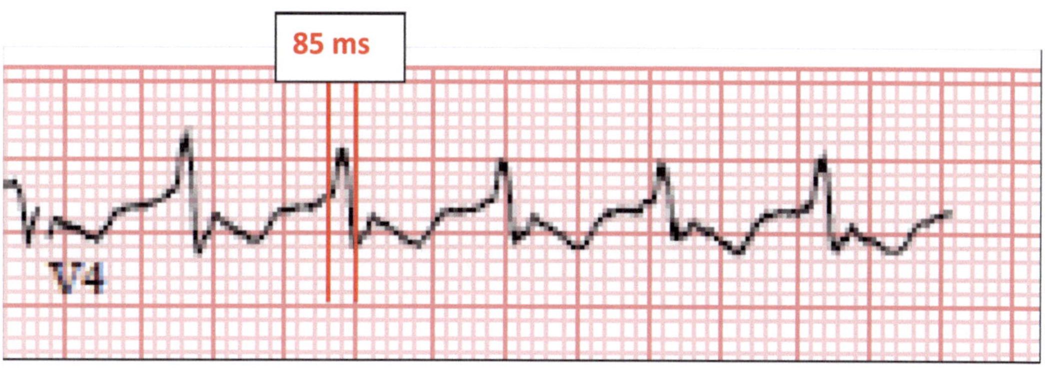

Fig. 3 Lead V4 from the ECG presented in Fig. 1 showing an R-to-S ratio of 85 ms, argument not in favor of ventricular tachycardia (but not excluding it either)

The patient underwent an electrophysiological study, during which the wide QRS complex tachycardia was induced. Three-dimentional mapping with an electro-anatomical system (CARTO, Biosense-Webster) confirmed its origin at the level of the LV septum. The patient underwent catheter ablation with the elimination of ventricular tachycardia.

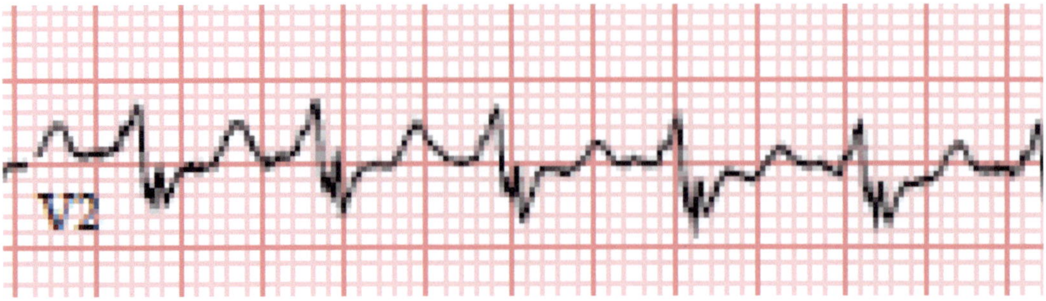

Fig. 4 Lead V2 from the ECG presented in Fig. 1 showing the presence of an "r wave" > 0.04 s, argument in favor of ventricular tachycardia

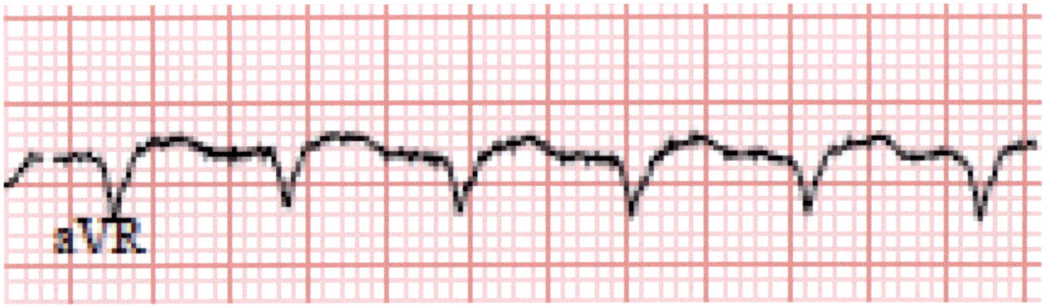

Fig. 5 Lead aVR from the tachycardia presented in Fig. 1, showing the absence of an initial R wave, criterion not in favor of ventricular tachycardia (but not excluding it either)

References

1. Surawicz B, Childers R, Deal BJ, Gettes LS, Bailey JJ, Gorgels A, et al. AHA/ACCF/HRS recommendations for the standardization and interpretation of the electrocardiogram: part III: intraventricular conduction disturbances: a scientific statement from the American Heart Association electrocardiography and arrhythmias committee, council on clinical cardiology; the American College of Cardiology Foundation; and the Heart Rhythm Society. Endorsed by the International Society for Computerized Electrocardiology. J Am Coll Cardiol. 2009;53(11):976–81.
2. Brugada P, Brugada J, Mont L, Smeets J, Andries EW. A new approach to the differential diagnosis of a regular tachycardia with a wide QRS complex. Circulation. 1991;83(5):1649–59.
3. Kindwall KE, Brown J, Josephson ME. Electrocardiographic criteria for ventricular tachycardia in wide complex left bundle branch block morphology tachycardias. Am J Cardiol. 1988;61(15):1279–83.
4. Vereckei A, Duray G, Szenasi G, Altemose GT, Miller JM. Application of a new algorithm in the differential diagnosis of wide QRS complex tachycardia. Eur Heart J. 2007;28(5):589–600.

ECG 29

Jacques Levy

1 Case Presentation

A 55-year-old female patient with a history of repeated episodes of palpitations is admitted to the Cardiology Department for a new episode of palpitations accompanied by chest oppression, dyspnea, anxiety, and lightheadedness that had started 1 h prior to her presentation to the hospital. Her ECG recorded at the admission to the Cardiology Department is presented in Fig. 1.

Question: What is the nature of the tachycardia presented in the ECG?

(a) Ventricular tachycardia originating from the inferior septal LV wall.
(b) Ventricular tachycardia originating from the inferior septal RV wall.
(c) Bundle branch reentry ventricular tachycardia.
(d) Antidromic tachycardia using a right-sided bypass tract.
(e) AVNRT with left bundle branch block.

Hint: A second ECG recorded several minutes later, after the end of palpitations is presented in Fig. 2.

J. Levy (✉)
Department of Cardiology, Emile Muller Hospital, Mulhouse, France
e-mail: LEVYJ@ghrmsa.fr

Correct answer: d. Antidromic tachycardia using a right-sided bypass tract.

Explanation: The ECG in Fig. 1 shows a regular wide QRS complex tachycardia with a heart rate of 252 bpm and LBBB morphology. The width of the QRS complex is 120 ms. The QRS axis is at −60°. The differential diagnosis of this regular wide QRS complex tachycardia with LBBB morphology includes: ventricular tachycardia (myocardial-related VT, bundle branch reentry VT, and fascicular VT), supraventricular tachycardia (atrial fibrillation, atrial flutter, atrial tachycardia, AVNRT, and AVRT) with functional or pre-existing bundle branch block, and antidromic tachycardia (in pre-excitation syndromes).

The morphology of the left bundle branch block of the QRS complex during tachycardia from the figure is not that of a typical one [1]: there are three QRS transitions in the precordial leads: in V2, V4, and V6. This is completely atypical for an SVT with functional BBB. So, answer "e" is highly unlikely to be correct.

The existing algorithm differentiating the nature of wide QRS complex tachycardias perform well in differentiating VT from SVT with aberrancy [2, 3]; however, they perform rather poorly in differentiating pre-excited tachycardia from VT [4, 5].

L. Muresan (ed.), *ECG Interpretation of Wide QRS Complex Tachycardia*,
https://doi.org/10.1007/978-3-031-97030-6_30

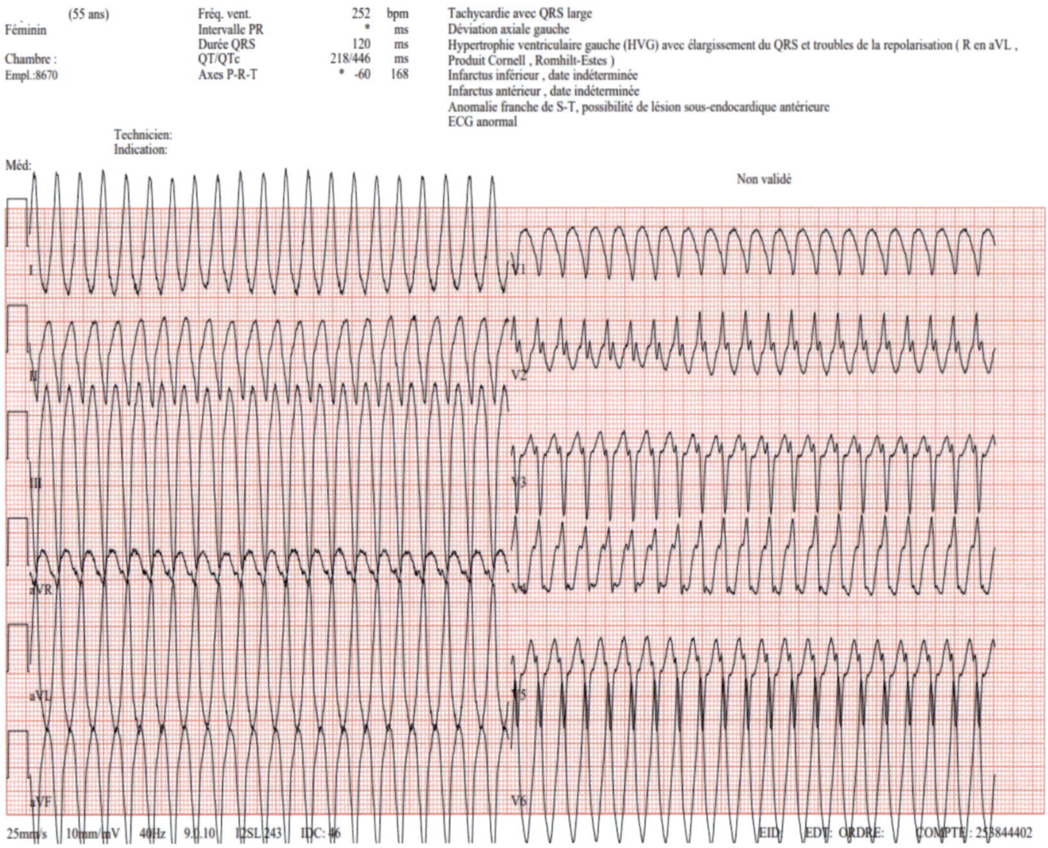

Fig. 1 Twelve-lead ECG recorded at admittance to the Cardiology Department

Applying the Brugada algorithm [6] to the tachycardia from Fig. 1, it can be seen that: (1) There is no absence of an RS complex in the precordial leads (otherwise said, there are rS complexes in leads V3 to V5); we therefore move to the second step of the algorithm: (2) This step analyzes the absence of an R-to-S interval > 100 ms in any precordial lead. This is not the case (Fig. 3).

Step 3 of the algorithm looks for A–V dissociation. If one analyzes the atrial activity, one can see that there are P waves at the end of each QRS complex, best visible in lead V4 (Fig. 4). So, there is no A–V dissociation present. We therefore need to proceed to step 4 of the algorithm.

For a wide QRS complex tachycardia with LBBB, arguments in favor of VT are: the presence of an "r wave" > 0.04 s in lead V1 or V2, which is not the case in the ECG presented in Fig. 1; the presence of a notched S wave in lead V1 or V2, which is also not the case; and the presence of a delayed S nadir >0.06 s in lead V1 or V2, which is also not the case [7]. Therefore, according to the Brugada algorithm, there are no arguments in favor of ventricular tachycardia, and the tachycardia is therefore SVT with BBB.

Another argument in favor of ventricular tachycardia for an LBBB QRS morphology would be a QRS duration of over 160 ms [8], which is also not the case.

The 2023 Vereckei algorithm for the differentiation of regular ventricular and pre-excited tachycardias [9] suggests antidromic tachycardia as the correct answer. The first step of this algorithm looks for A–V dissociation, which is not present on the ECG from Fig. 1 (Fig. 4). The second step of the algorithms analyzes whether in lead avR the onset of the QRS complex is positive and whether the area above the baseline of

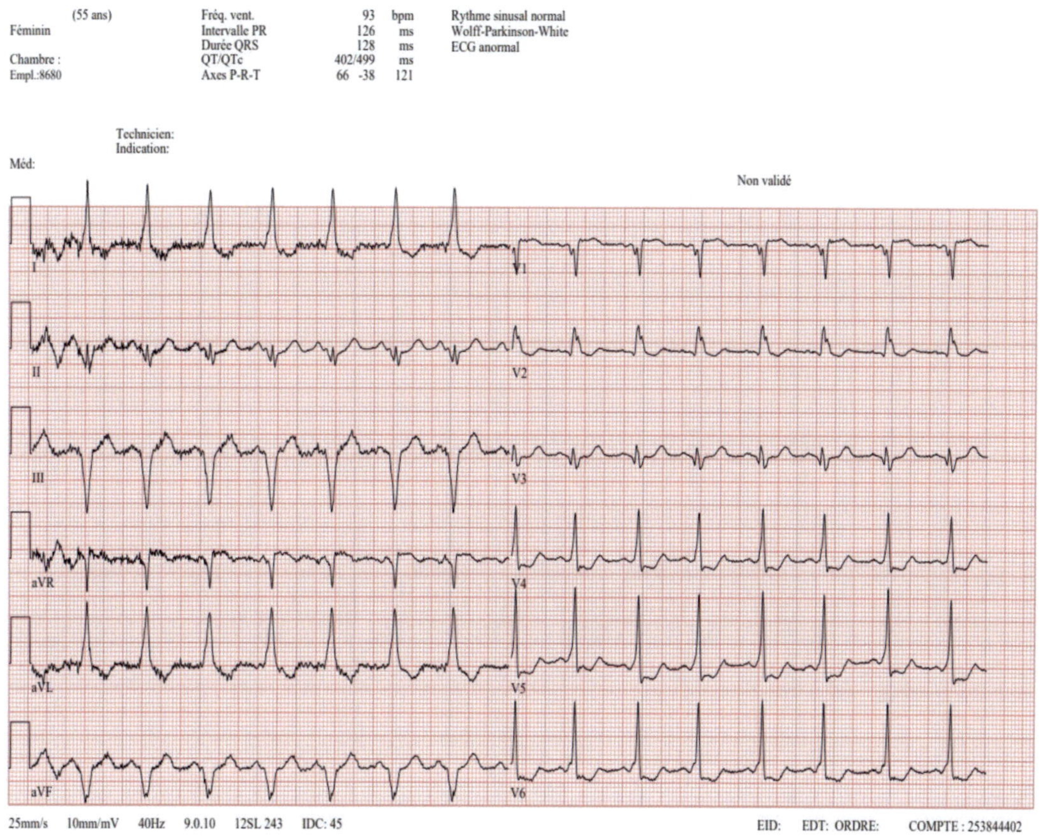

Fig. 2 Twelve-lead ECG recorded after the end of the episode of palpitations

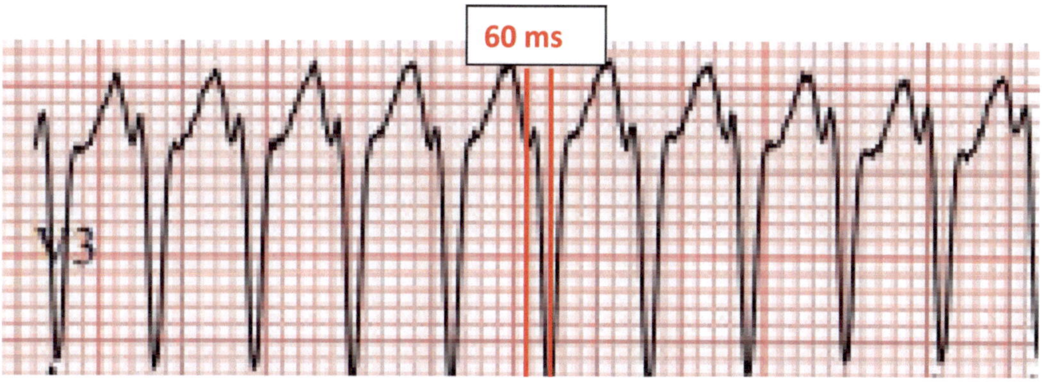

Fig. 3 Lead V3 from the tachycardia presented in Fig. 1 showing an RS interval of 60 ms, argument not in favor of ventricular tachycardia (but not excluding it either)

the QRS complex is greater than the area below the baseline. This is not the case (Fig. 5).

The third step of the algorithm looks for the presence of a "QR" pattern in one or more of the leads V2–V6. This is not the case (Fig. 6).

The fourth and final step of the algorithm looks for predominantly negative QRS complexes in leads V4 to V6. This is not the case, since only V5 records a predominantly negative QRS complex (Fig. 6). Therefore, according to

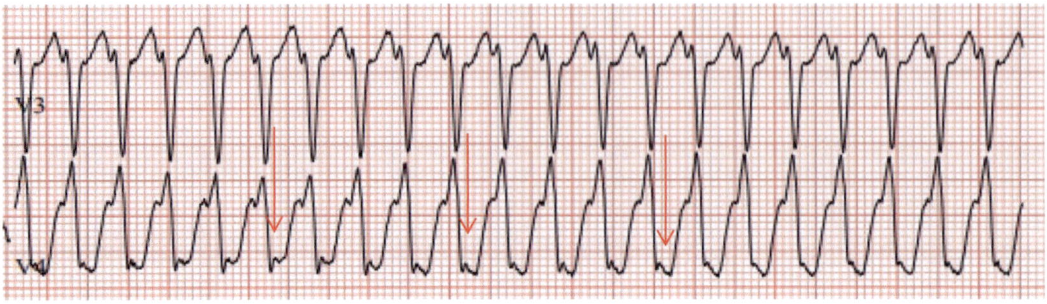

Fig. 4 Leads V3 and V4 from the ECG in Fig. 1 demonstrating the presence of P waves at the end of each QRS complex, with a 1:1 A:V relationship (see text for explanation)

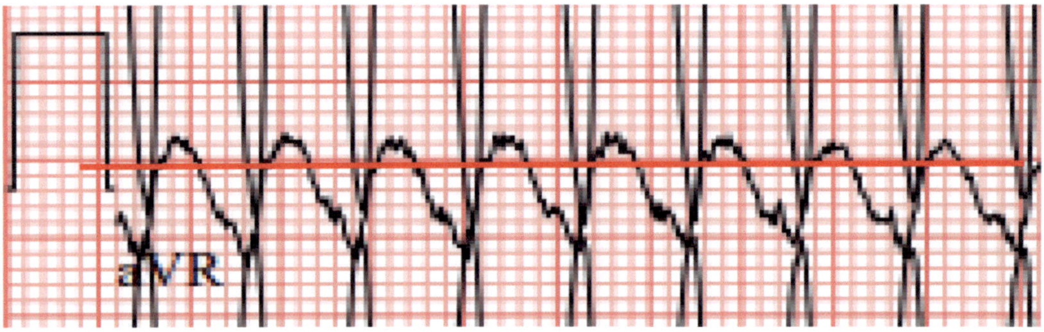

Fig. 5 Lead aVR from the ECG in Fig. 1 not demonstrating an initial positive R wave. The area above the baseline (red horizontal line) is smaller than the area below the baseline, criterion not in favor of VT

the 2023 Vereckei algorithm, the tachycardia is antidromic tachycardia.

A strong argument in favor of antidromic tachycardia comes from the analysis of the ECG recorded during sinus rhythm, presented in Fig. 2. The ECG shows the presence of sinus rhythm with a heart rate of 93 bpm, QRS axis at −40°, with ventricular pre-excitation: short PR interval of 120 ms, negative delta waves in leads II and III, and aVF and V1, positive in DI and aVL and V4 to V6 compatible with a right posteroseptal accessory pathway. The delta waves are best seen in leads V4 to V6 (Fig. 7).

Therefore, the correct answer is d—"antidromic tachycardia using a right-sided bypass tract". The Brugada algorithm was not correct in identifying the tachycardia as SVT with aberrant conduction.

The patient underwent an electrophysiological study which confirmed the diagnosis of ventricular pre-excitation and subsequent successful radiofrequency catheter ablation of the accessory pathway.

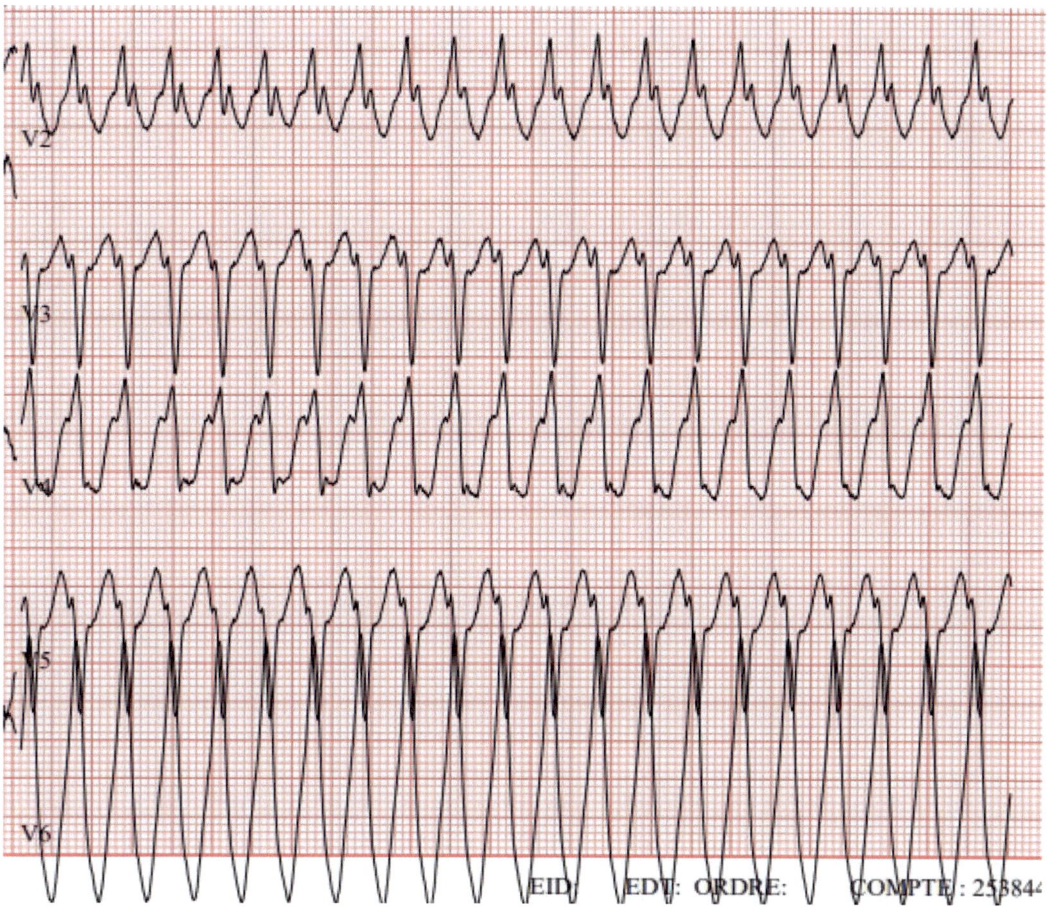

Fig. 6 Leads V2 to V6 from the tachycardia presented in Fig. 1 showing the absence of a "QR" complex, argument not in favor of ventricular tachycardia

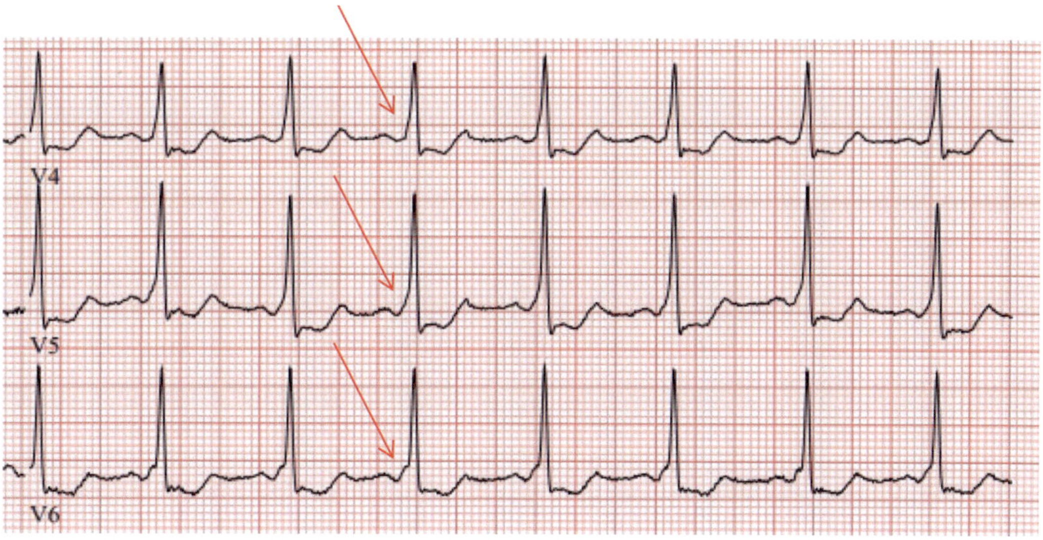

Fig. 7 Leads V4 to V6 from the ECG from Fig. 2 showing delta waves, compatible with ventricular pre-excitation

References

1. Surawicz B, Childers R, Deal BJ, Gettes LS, Bailey JJ, Gorgels A, et al. AHA/ACCF/HRS recommendations for the standardization and interpretation of the electrocardiogram: part III: intraventricular conduction disturbances: a scientific statement from the American Heart Association Electrocardiography and Arrhythmias Committee, Council on Clinical Cardiology; the American College of Cardiology Foundation; and the Heart Rhythm Society. Endorsed by the International Society for Computerized Electrocardiology. J Am Coll Cardiol. 2009;53(11):976–81.
2. Abedin Z. Differential diagnosis of wide QRS tachycardia: a review. J Arrhythmia. 2021;37(5):1162–72.
3. Sun X, Teng Y, Mu S, Wang Y, Chen H. Diagnostic accuracy of different ECG-based algorithms in wide QRS complex tachycardia: a systematic review and meta-analysis. BMJ Open. 2023;13(7):e069273.
4. Vera A, Cecconi A, Nogales-Romo MT, de la Cuerda F, Salamanca J, Jimenez-Borreguero LJ, et al. Wide QRS complex tachycardia: what the algorithms fear. Circulation. 2018;137(13):1407–9.
5. Wellens HJ. Electrophysiology: ventricular tachycardia: diagnosis of broad QRS complex tachycardia. Heart. 2001;86(5):579–85.
6. Brugada P, Brugada J, Mont L, Smeets J, Andries EW. A new approach to the differential diagnosis of a regular tachycardia with a wide QRS complex. Circulation. 1991;83(5):1649–59.
7. Kindwall KE, Brown J, Josephson ME. Electrocardiographic criteria for ventricular tachycardia in wide complex left bundle branch block morphology tachycardias. Am J Cardiol. 1988;61(15):1279–83.
8. Eckardt L, Breithardt G, Kirchhof P. Approach to wide complex tachycardias in patients without structural heart disease. Heart. 2006;92(5):704–11.
9. Vereckei A, Simon A, Szenasi G, Miller JM. The application of a new, modified algorithm for the differentiation of regular ventricular and pre-excited tachycardias. Heart Lung Circ. 2023;32(6):719–25.

ECG 30

Charline Daval

1 Case Presentation

An 18-year-old female patient with a history of tuberous sclerosis and dyslipidemia is admitted to the Cardiology Department for a first episode of palpitations accompanied by chest pain, nausea, vomiting, and anxiety that had occurred 30 min prior to her presentation to the hospital. Her ECG recorded at admittance to the Cardiology Department is presented in Fig. 1.

Question: What is the nature of the tachycardia presented in Fig. 1?

(a) Ventricular tachycardia originating from the anterior lateral RV wall.
(b) Ventricular tachycardia originating from the anterior lateral LV wall.
(c) Bundle branch re-entry ventricular tachycardia.
(d) Antidromic tachycardia using a left-sided bypass tract.
(e) AVNRT with right bundle branch block.

Hint: A second ECG recorded several minutes later is presented in Fig. 2.

Correct answer: b. Ventricular tachycardia originating from the anterior lateral LV wall.

C. Daval (✉)
Department of Cardiology, Emile Muller Hospital, Mulhouse, France
e-mail: charline.daval@ghrmsa.fr

Explanation: The ECG in Fig. 1 shows a regular wide QRS complex tachycardia with a heart rate of 230 bpm and RBBB morphology. The width of the QRS complex is 140 ms. The QRS axis is at +135°. The differential diagnosis of this regular wide QRS complex tachycardia with RBBB morphology includes: ventricular tachycardia (myocardial-related VT, bundle branch re-entry VT, and fascicular VT), supraventricular tachycardia (atrial flutter with 1:1 AV conduction, atrial tachycardia with 1:1 AV conduction, AVNRT, and AVRT) with functional or pre-existing bundle branch block, and antidromic tachycardia (in pre-excitation syndromes).

The ECG from Fig. 2 shows the presence of sinus rhythm with a heart rate of 103 bpm, QRS axis at +60°, absence of LV hypertrophy, and absence of ischemia. Most importantly, there are no elements in favor of ventricular pre-excitation (no short PR interval and no delta waves). Therefore, the probability of the wide QRS complex tachycardia from Fig. 1 to be an antidromic tachycardia is low.

The morphology of the right bundle branch block of the QRS complex during tachycardia from Fig. 1 is not that of a typical one [1]: even though the QRS duration is >120 ms, there is a "QS" pattern in leads I and aVL, and the R-to-S ratio in lead V6 is less than 1. Also, there are several QRS transitions in the precordial leads, the first one taking place in lead V2 (from positive to

L. Muresan (ed.), *ECG Interpretation of Wide QRS Complex Tachycardia*,
https://doi.org/10.1007/978-3-031-97030-6_31

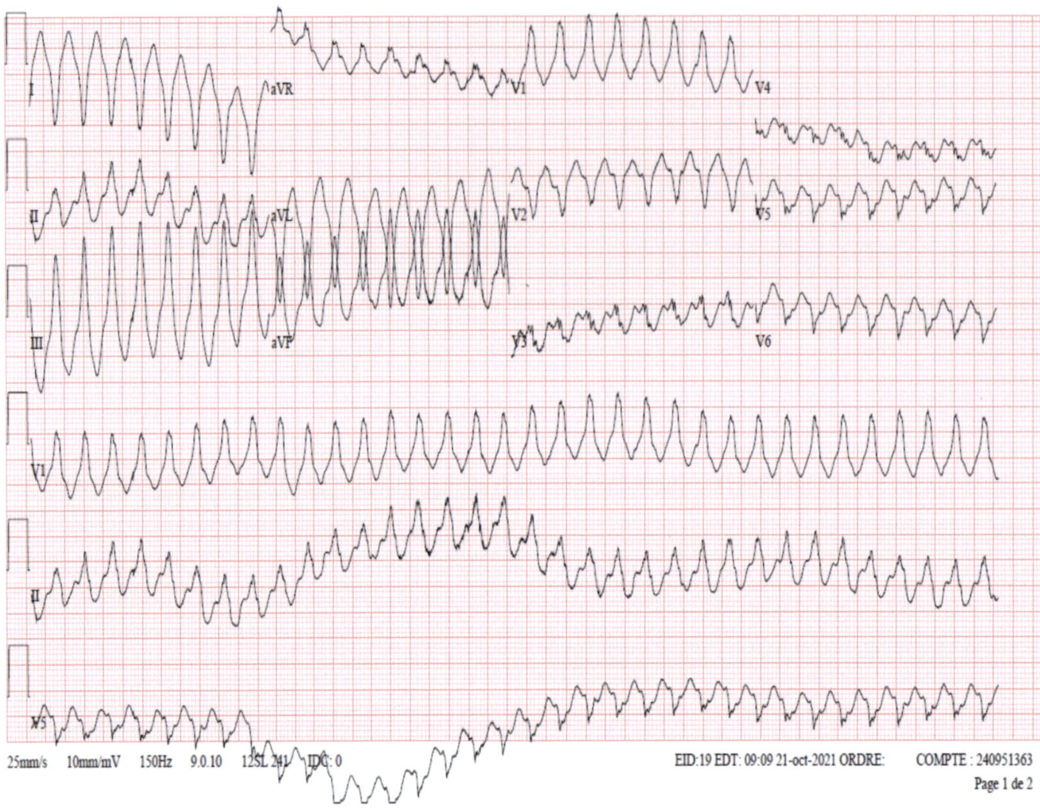

Fig. 1 Twelve-lead ECG recorded at admittance to the Cardiology Department

negative), which, again, is not characteristic for a typical RBBB. The second one takes place in lead V3 (from negative to positive) and then the next one in lead V5 (from positive to negative). This is therefore a strong argument against SVT with functional BBB.

Applying the Brugada algorithm [2] to the tachycardia from Fig. 2, it can be seen that: (1) There is no absence of an RS complex in the precordial leads (otherwise said, there are rS complexes in leads V2 to V6); we therefore move to the second step of the algorithm: (2) This step analyzes the absence of an R-to-S interval > 100 ms in any precordial lead. This is not the case (Fig. 3).

Step 3 of the algorithm looks for A–V dissociation. P waves are not clearly visible on the ECG from Fig. 1, so we cannot say that there is AV dissociation. This takes us to step 4 of the algorithm.

For an RBBB morphology wide QRS complex tachycardia, an argument in favor of VT would be the presence of a taller left peak of the QRS complex in lead V1 (the rabbit ear sign) or for biphasic RS or QR complexes, which is not the case. Next, in lead V6, an argument in favor of VT would be the presence of an "rS" complex, which is actually the case. This is therefore an argument in favor of VT. This can also be expressed as a ratio of R/S < 1 in lead V6 (Fig. 4). Therefore, according to the Brugada algorithm, the tachycardia from Fig. 1 is ventricular tachycardia.

The Vereckei algorithm [3] for the differential diagnosis of wide QRS complex tachycardia also suggests VT as the correct answer. The first step of the algorithm looks for A–V dissociation, which is not seen on the present ECG. The second step of the algorithm looks for an initial pre-

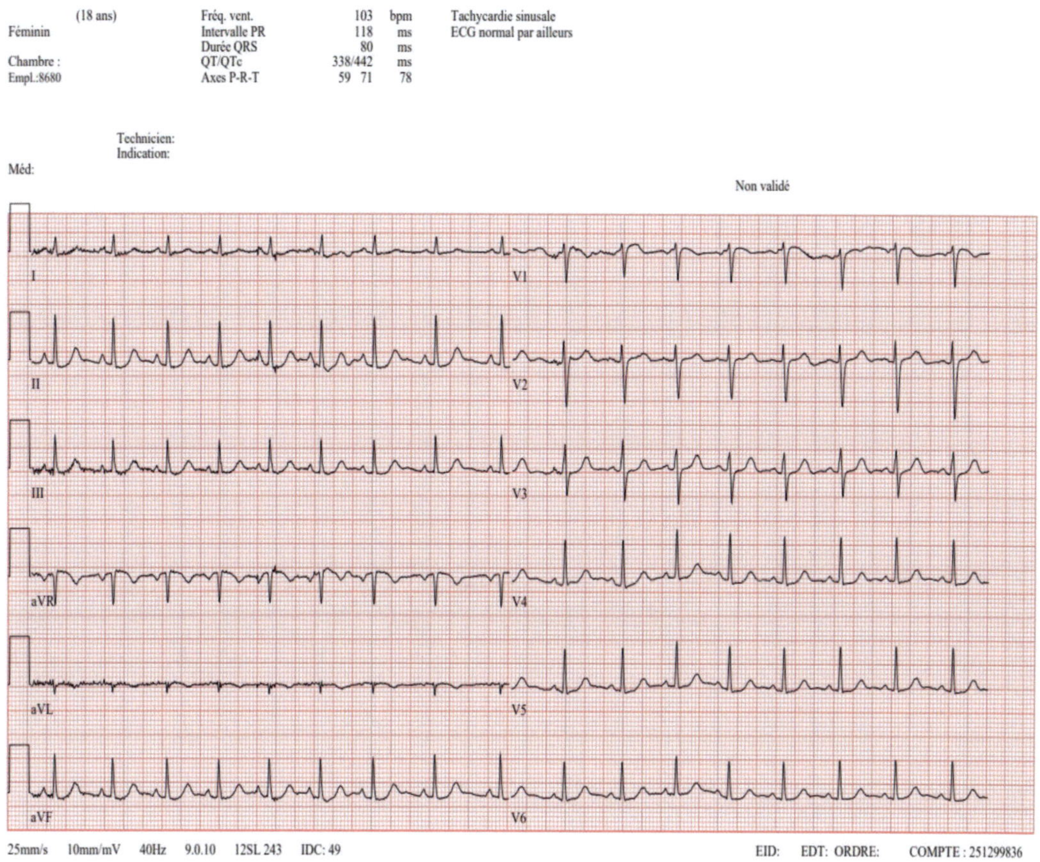

Fig. 2 Twelve-lead ECG recorded after the end of the episode of palpitations

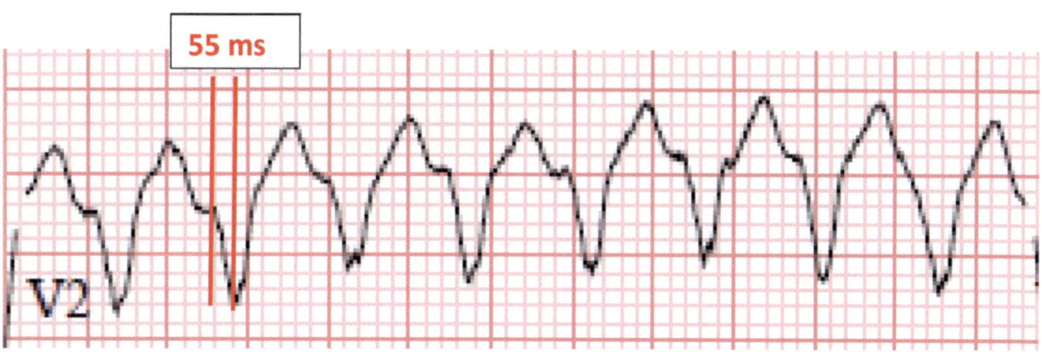

Fig. 3 Lead V2 from the tachycardia presented in Fig. 1, showing an R-to-S interval of 55 ms, criterion not in favor of ventricular tachycardia (but not excluding it either)

dominant R wave in lead aVR, which is actually the case (Fig. 5).

Based on these arguments, the diagnosis of ventricular tachycardia was retained.

The patient underwent an electrophysiological study, which confirmed the ventricular nature of the tachycardia, and a successful catheter ablation procedure.

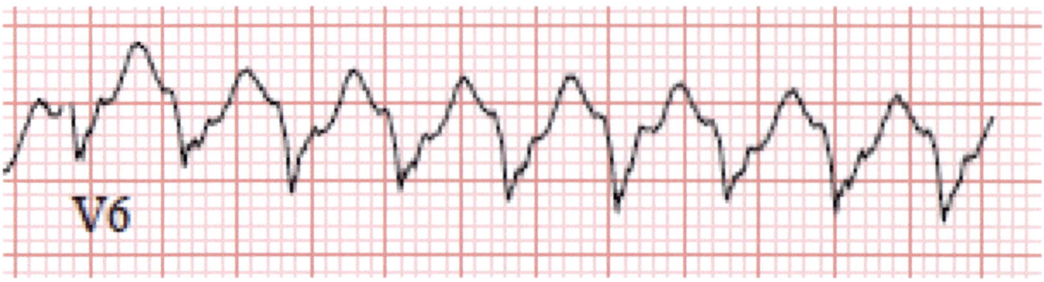

Fig. 4 Lead V6 from the tachycardia presented in Fig. 1, showing an R-to-S ratio of <1, criterion in favor of ventricular tachycardia

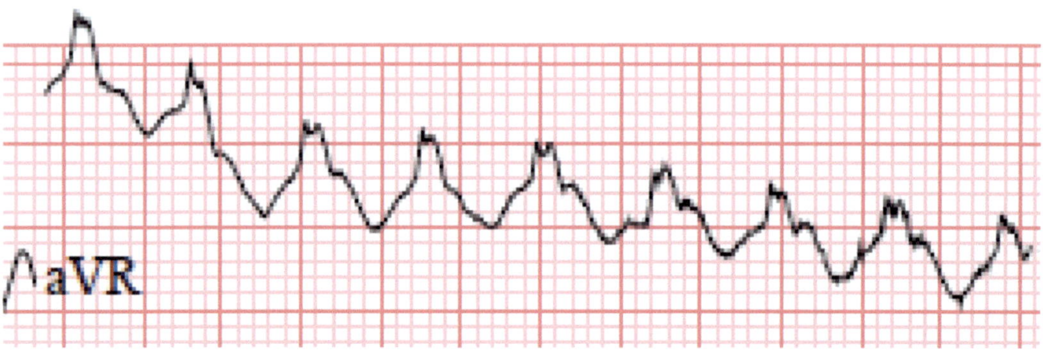

Fig. 5 Lead aVR from the tachycardia presented in Fig. 1, showing the presence of an initial positive tall R wave, criterion in favor of ventricular tachycardia

References

1. Jiang D, Lv J, Han B, Yang X, Zhao L, Yi Y, et al. Electrocardiographic characteristics and catheter ablation of ventricular arrhythmias originating from the moderator band in children. Front Pediatr. 2022;10:740230.
2. Brugada P, Brugada J, Mont L, Smeets J, Andries EW. A new approach to the differential diagnosis of a regular tachycardia with a wide QRS complex. Circulation. 1991;83(5):1649–59.
3. Vereckei A, Duray G, Szenasi G, Altemose GT, Miller JM. Application of a new algorithm in the differential diagnosis of wide QRS complex tachycardia. Eu Heart J. 2007;28(5):589–600.

ECG 31

Serban Schiau

1 Case Presentation

An 86-year-old female patient with a history of systemic sarcoidosis, chronic renal failure, hypothyroidism, and dyslipidemia is admitted to the Cardiology Department for an episode of severe constrictive chest pain with sudden onset, not related to physical effort, irradiating to the left shoulder and left arm, accompanied by diaphoresis and palpitations that occurred 30 min prior to her presentation to the hospital. Her ECG recorded at admittance is presented in Fig. 1.

Question: What is the nature of the tachycardia presented in Fig. 1?

(a) Ventricular tachycardia originating from the lateral RV wall.
(b) Ventricular tachycardia originating from the anterior lateral LV wall.
(c) Atrial fibrillation with right bundle branch block.
(d) Atrial fibrillation with left bundle branch block.
(e) Antidromic tachycardia using a right-sided accessory pathway.

Hint: A second ECG recorded several minutes later is presented in Fig. 2.

S. Schiau (✉)
Department of Cardiology, "Emile Muller" Hospital, Mulhouse, France
e-mail: serban.schiau@ghrmsa.fr

Correct answer: b. Ventricular tachycardia originating from the anterior lateral LV wall.

Explanation: The ECG in Fig. 1 shows an irregular wide QRS complex tachycardia with a heart rate of 133 bpm and an aspect of nonspecific intraventricular conduction delay (neither LBBB nor RBBB). The width of the QRS complex is 170 ms. The QRS axis is at +120°. The differential diagnosis of this irregular wide QRS complex tachycardia with neither LBBB nor RBBB morphology includes: ventricular tachycardia (myocardial-related VT and bundle branch re-entry VT) and supraventricular tachycardia (atrial fibrillation, atrial flutter, and atrial tachycardia) with pre-existing nonspecific intraventricular conduction delay, and antidromic tachycardia (in pre-excitation syndromes).

Supraventricular tachycardia (atrial fibrillation, atrial flutter, atrial tachycardia, AVNRT, and AVRT) with pre-existing bundle branch block is not very likely in this case because the morphology of the QRS complex is not compatible with either the left or right bundle branch block. For a typical left bundle branch block, besides a QRS duration >120 ms, the QRS complex must have a "QS" morphology in lead V1, or an amplitude of the "r wave" of less than 0.04 ms, which is not the case in the ECG from Fig. 1. Also, leads I and aVL must have a unique "R wave" morphology,

L. Muresan (ed.), *ECG Interpretation of Wide QRS Complex Tachycardia*,
https://doi.org/10.1007/978-3-031-97030-6_32

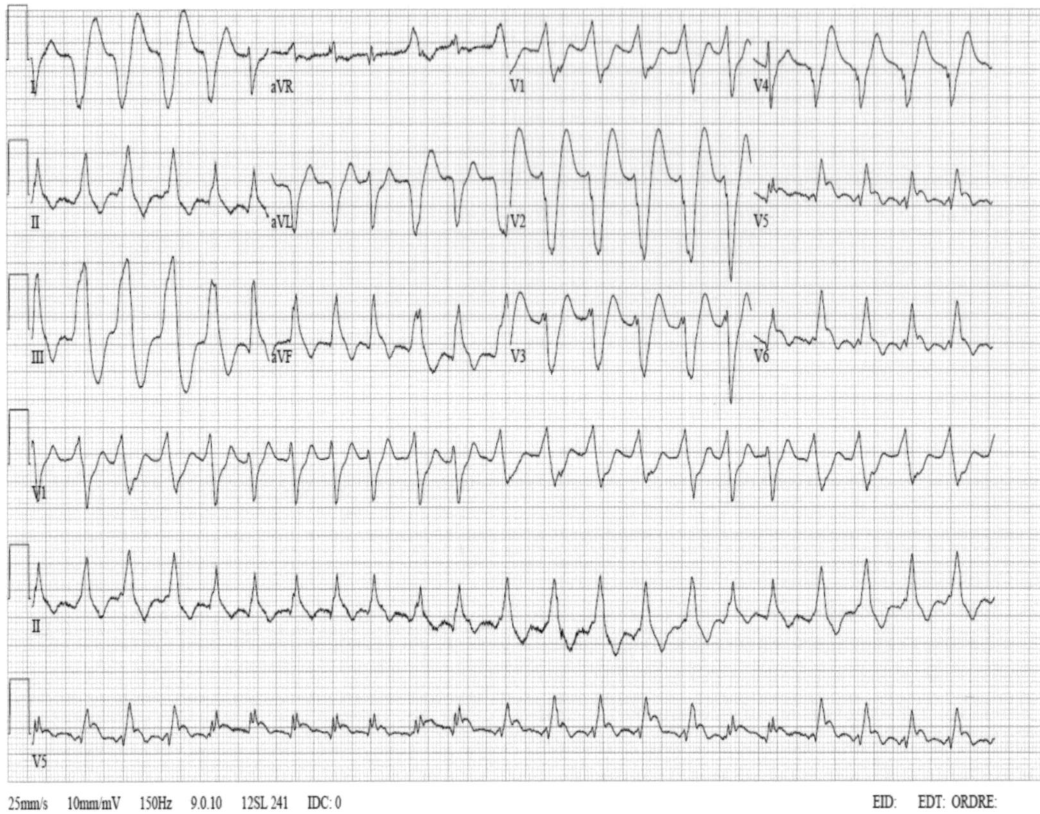

Fig. 1 Twelve-lead ECG recorded at admittance to the Cardiology Department

which is very different from the "QS" morphology on the present ECG [1].

A typical right bundle branch block has an "RSR'" morphology in lead V1 and an "RS" or "rS" morphology in leads V5, V6, I, and aVL, which is not present on this ECG. Therefore, this tachycardia has neither a typical LBBB nor a typical RBBB morphology [1]. SVT with preexisting nonspecific intraventricular conduction delay could be a possibility, if the ECG recorded outside the episode of palpitations (preferably recorded during sinus rhythm) showed the same QRS morphology. However, this is not the case, since the ECG from Fig. 2 shows sinus rhythm with narrow QRS complexes. Therefore, SVT with BBB can be excluded.

Regarding antidromic tachycardia, it is generally regular, and the QRS morphology has a single morphology, which is not the present case (Fig. 3 shows variations in the QRS morphology).

Another argument against antidromic tachycardia would be the absence of ventricular preexcitation on the ECG presented in Fig. 2: no delta waves and no short PR interval. In fact, the ECG from Fig. 2 shows sinus rhythm with a heart rate of 55 bpm, QRS axis at +110°, absence of LV hypertrophy, and subendocardial lesion in the inferolateral territory (II, III, aVF, V5, V6, I, and aVL), in favor of acute myocardial infarction of the inferolateral wall of the LV. Antidromic tachycardia is therefore unlikely in this case.

Applying the Brugada algorithm [2] to the tachycardia from Fig. 1, it can be seen that: (1) There is no absence of an RS complex in the precordial leads (otherwise said, there are RS or rS complexes in leads V1 to V3); we therefore move to the second step of the algorithm: (2) This step

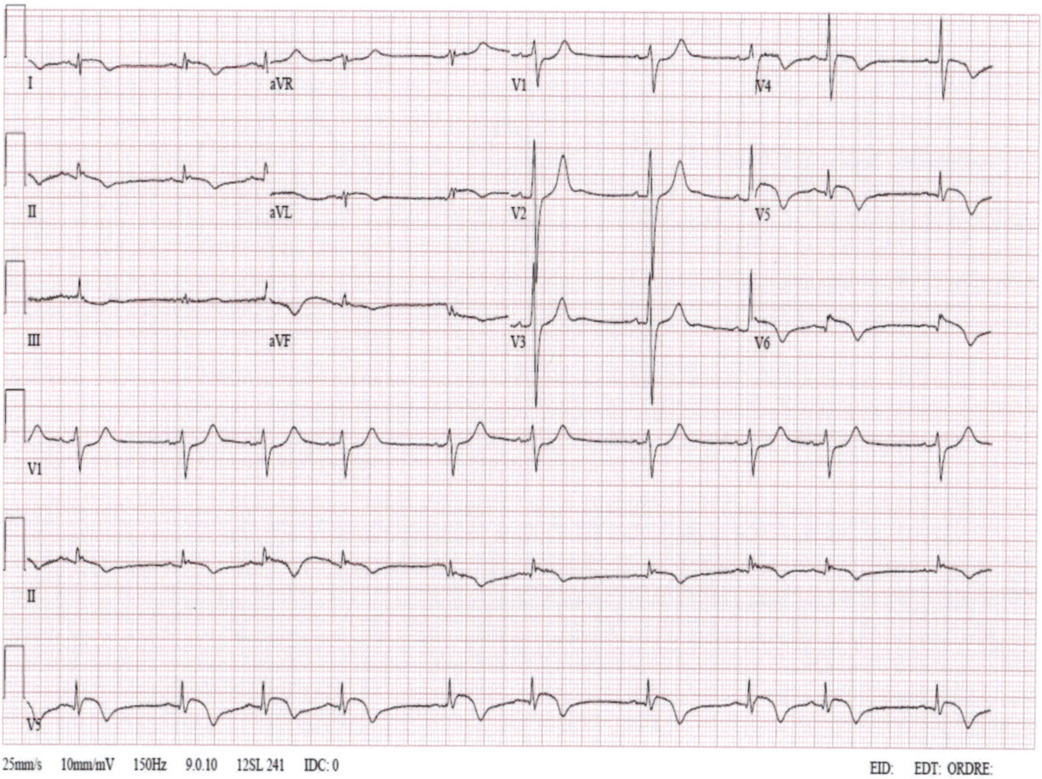

Fig. 2 Twelve-lead ECG recorded after the end of the episode of palpitations

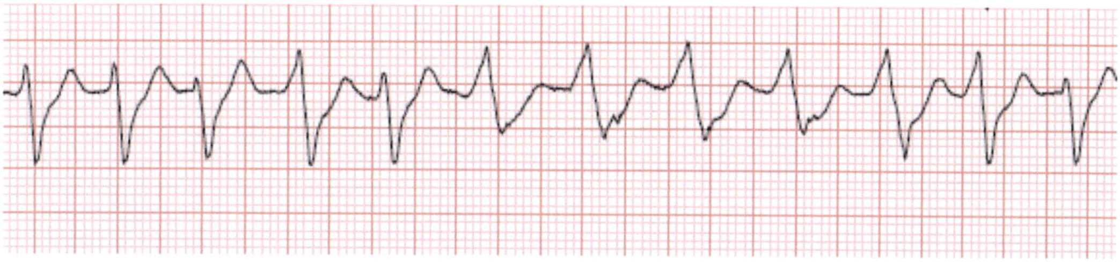

Fig. 3 Lead V1 from the ECG presented in Fig. 1, showing variations in the QRS morphology, argument not in favor of antidromic tachycardia

analyzes the absence of an R-to-S interval > 100 ms in any precordial lead. Analyzing lead V1, we can see that the RS interval is of 165 ms (Fig. 4). This is an argument in favor of VT.

The morphology of the QRS complex in the precordial leads V2 to V6 may be compatible with a typical LBBB (even though, based on the arguments expressed above, this is not a typical LBBB). For an LBBB wide QRS complex tachycardia, other arguments in favor of VT are: the presence of an "r wave" > 0.04 s in lead V1 or V2, which is actually the case (Fig. 5).

The presence of a notched S wave in lead V1 or V2 (Josephson's sign) is also an argument in favor of VT (Fig. 6).

Another argument in favor of ventricular tachycardia is the presence of a delayed S nadir >0.06 s in lead V1 or V2, which is also the case [3] (see Fig. 7).

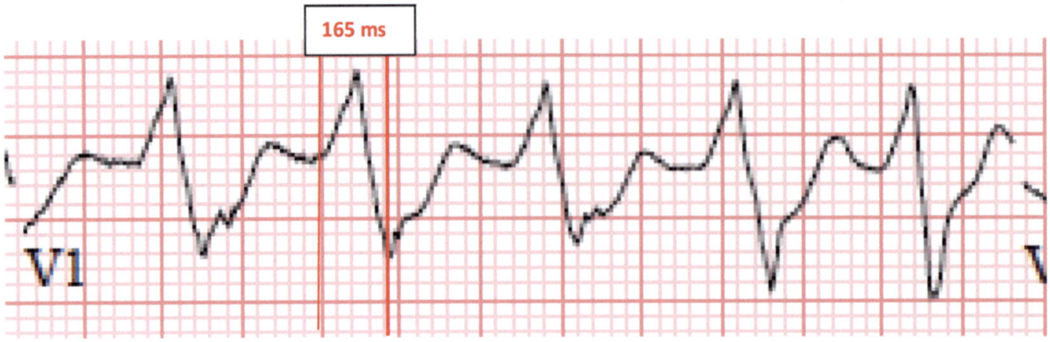

Fig. 4 Lead V1 from the ECG presented in Fig. 1, showing the presence of an RS interval of 165 ms, argument in favor of VT

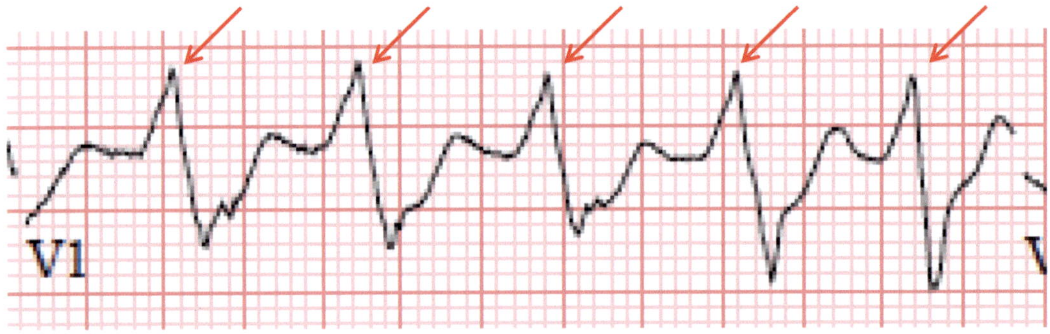

Fig. 5 Lead V1 from the ECG presented in Fig. 1, showing the presence of an R wave >0.04 ms, argument in favor of VT

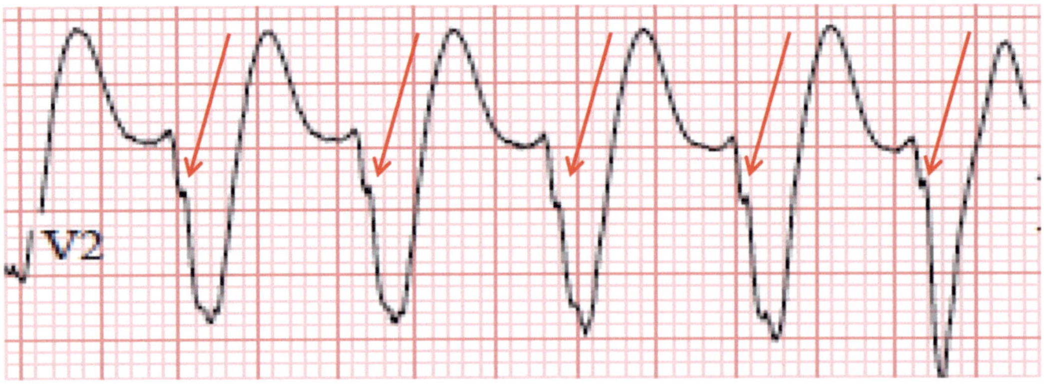

Fig. 6 Lead V2 from the ECG presented in Fig. 1, showing the presence of a notched S wave in lead V2, rgument in favor of VT

Another argument in favor of ventricular tachycardia for an LBBB QRS morphology would be a QRS duration of over 160 ms [4], which is also the case.

Therefore, based on the Brugada algorithm, the wide QRS complex tachycardia presented in Fig. 1 is ventricular tachycardia.

The Vereckei algorithm [5] for the differential diagnosis of wide QRS complex tachycardias

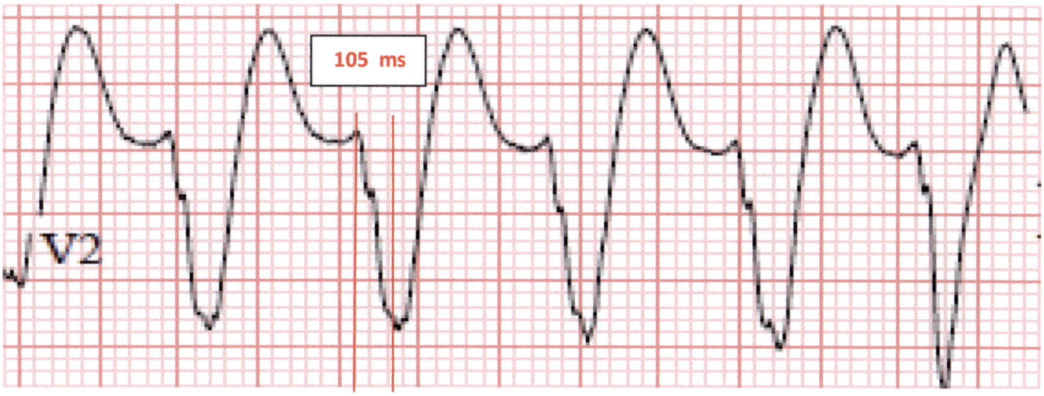

Fig. 7 Lead V2 from the tachycardia presented in Fig. 1, showing the presence of a delayed S nadir >0.06 s in lead V2, argument in favor of ventricular tachycardia

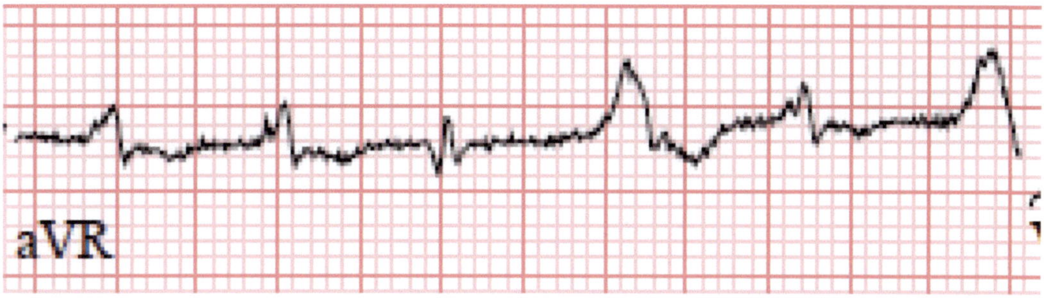

Fig. 8 Lead aVR from the tachycardia presented in Fig. 1, showing the beat-to-beat change in the QRS morphology, making interpretation of the nature of the tachycardia difficult (see text for further comments)

also suggests VT as the correct answer. The first step of the algorithm looks for A–V dissociation, which is not seen on the present ECG. The second step of the algorithm looks for an initial predominant R wave in lead aVR, which is actually hard to say, given the beat-to-beat change in the QRS morphology in this lead (Fig. 8).

The third step "QRS morphology unlike BBB or fascicular block" does not suggest SVT with BBB, based on the arguments explained above. Therefore, based on the Vereckei algorithm, the nature of the tachycardia is also ventricular tachycardia.

What is actually seen in lead aVR (as in the other leads as well) are fusion and capture beats, which represent other arguments in favor of VT. The first, the second, and the fifth QRS complexes in lead aVR are fusion beats (fusion between the QRS complex during VT and the spontaneous QRS depolarization using the His–Purkinje system), the third QRS complex is a capture beat (the QRS morphology is identical to the QRS morphology seen on the ECG from Fig. 2), and the fourth and the sixth beats are VT beats.

Another aspect worth noting is the fact that the VT presented in Fig. 1 is irregular. However, irregularity during ventricular tachycardia has been described before and can be explained by longitudinal dissociation within the re-entry circuit [6].

Both the clinical context and the ECG presented in Fig. 2 support the diagnosis of acute myocardial infarction. The ECG in Fig. 2 shows ST segment elevation in the inferolateral leads.

Concerning the ventricular tachycardia, its origin is in the left ventricle at the level of the lateral wall (negative QRS complexes in leads I and aVL).

The patient underwent coronary angiography, which showed chronic occlusion of the proximal segment of the right coronary artery, acute occlusion of the second marginal coronary artery (responsible for the acute coronary syndrome) and severe (70–90%) stenosis of the proximal LAD. He subsequent underwent stent implantation at the level of the second marginal coronary artery. PTCA of the LAD was done 72 hours later.

References

1. Surawicz B, Childers R, Deal BJ, Gettes LS, Bailey JJ, Gorgels A, et al. AHA/ACCF/HRS recommendations for the standardization and interpretation of the electrocardiogram: part III: intraventricular conduction disturbances: a scientific statement from the American Heart Association Electrocardiography and Arrhythmias Committee, Council on Clinical Cardiology; the American College of Cardiology Foundation; and the Heart Rhythm Society. Endorsed by the International Society for Computerized Electrocardiology. J Am Coll Cardiol. 2009;53(11):976–81.
2. Brugada P, Brugada J, Mont L, Smeets J, Andries EW. A new approach to the differential diagnosis of a regular tachycardia with a wide QRS complex. Circulation. 1991;83(5):1649–59.
3. Kindwall KE, Brown J, Josephson ME. Electrocardiographic criteria for ventricular tachycardia in wide complex left bundle branch block morphology tachycardias. Am J Cardiol. 1988;61(15):1279–83.
4. Eckardt L, Breithardt G, Kirchhof P. Approach to wide complex tachycardias in patients without structural heart disease. Heart. 2006;92(5):704–11.
5. Vereckei A, Duray G, Szenasi G, Altemose GT, Miller JM. Application of a new algorithm in the differential diagnosis of wide QRS complex tachycardia. Eur Heart J. 2007;28(5):589–600.
6. Oreto G, Satullo G, Luzza F, Donato A, Scimone IM, Cavalli A. Irregular ventricular tachycardia: a possible manifestation of longitudinal dissociation within the reentry pathway. Am Heart J. 1992;124(6):1506–11.

ECG 32

Lucien Diene

1 Case Presentation

A 67-year-old female patient with a history of active smoking (50 pack-years), dyslipidemia, and COPD is admitted to the Cardiology Department for an episode of chest pain with irradiation to the upper posterior thorax that had been present for the past 16 h prior to her presentation to the hospital. At home, she was taking Rosuvastatin and a combination of Salmeterol and Fluticasone for her COPD. Her ECG recorded at admittance to the Cardiology Department is presented in Fig. 1.

Question: What is the rhythm presented in Fig. 1?

(a) Sinus tachycardia with ventricular bigemini
(b) Sinus tachycardia with supraventricular bigemini with functional RBBB
(c) Atrial fibrillation with ventricular bigemini
(d) Atrial fibrillation and bidirectional ventricular tachycardia
(e) Bidirectional ventricular tachycardia

Hint: A second ECG recorded several minutes later is presented in Fig. 2.

L. Diene (✉)
Department of Cardiology, Clinique Le Noirmont, Le Noirmont, Switzerland

Correct answer: e. Bidirectional ventricular tachycardia

Explanation: The ECG in Fig. 1 shows an irregular wide QRS complex tachycardia with a heart rate of 128 bpm. There are two types of QRS complexes, both having an RBBB morphology, alternating between each other (to facilitate explanation, the first QRS morphology on the ECG is labeled "morphology A" and the second morphology on the ECG "morphology B") (Fig. 3).

The width of the QRS complex is 140 ms for morphology A and 160 ms for morphology B, as measured in lead III. There is extreme (north-west) axis deviation for the morphology A (QRS axis at −150°) and right (north-west) axis deviation (+120°) for morphology B. Neither of the two QRS morphologies corresponds to the typical right bundle branch block morphology [1]: for morphology A, there is a unique R wave in lead V1, and for morphology B, there is the "rabbit ear sign", with the amplitude of the R wave being greater than the amplitude of the R' wave. For both morphologies, the R/S ratio in lead V6 is <1 [2]. These are arguments in favor of ventricular origin for both morphologies. Therefore, answers a and b are not correct.

Concerning the atrial rhythm, a careful analysis of the ECG from Fig. 1 identifies retrograde P

L. Muresan (ed.), *ECG Interpretation of Wide QRS Complex Tachycardia*,
https://doi.org/10.1007/978-3-031-97030-6_33

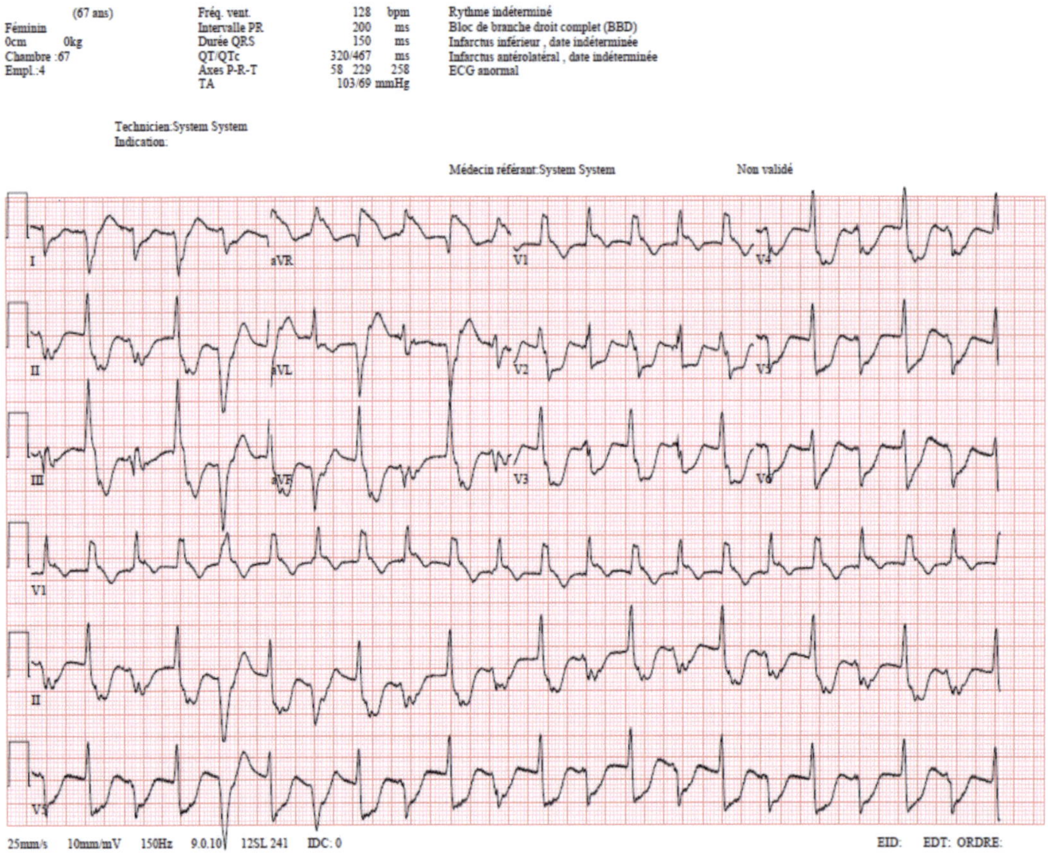

Fig. 1 Twelve-lead ECG recorded at admittance to the Cardiology Department

waves at the end of the B-type QRS complexes, best visible in leads II and V4 (see Fig. 4). Therefore, there is no atrial fibrillation, and answers c and d are not correct either. This leaves answer e—"Bidirectional ventricular tachycardia" as the correct answer.

The ECG in Fig. 2 shows sinus rhythm with a heart rate of 84 bpm, indeterminate QRS axis, and absence of ventricular hypertrophy. There is also an incomplete RBBB (rsr' morphology in lead V1) and a prolonged QTc interval of 531 ms. There is a 1 mm ST segment elevation in lead aVR, accompanied by 0.5 to 1 mm ST segment depression in leads II, III, aVF, and V3–V6, in favor of ongoing myocardial ischemia (high-risk criteria).

The patient underwent coronary angiography which found no significant epicardial coronary artery stenosis. Cardiac MRI was subsequently performed, which did not find arguments in favor

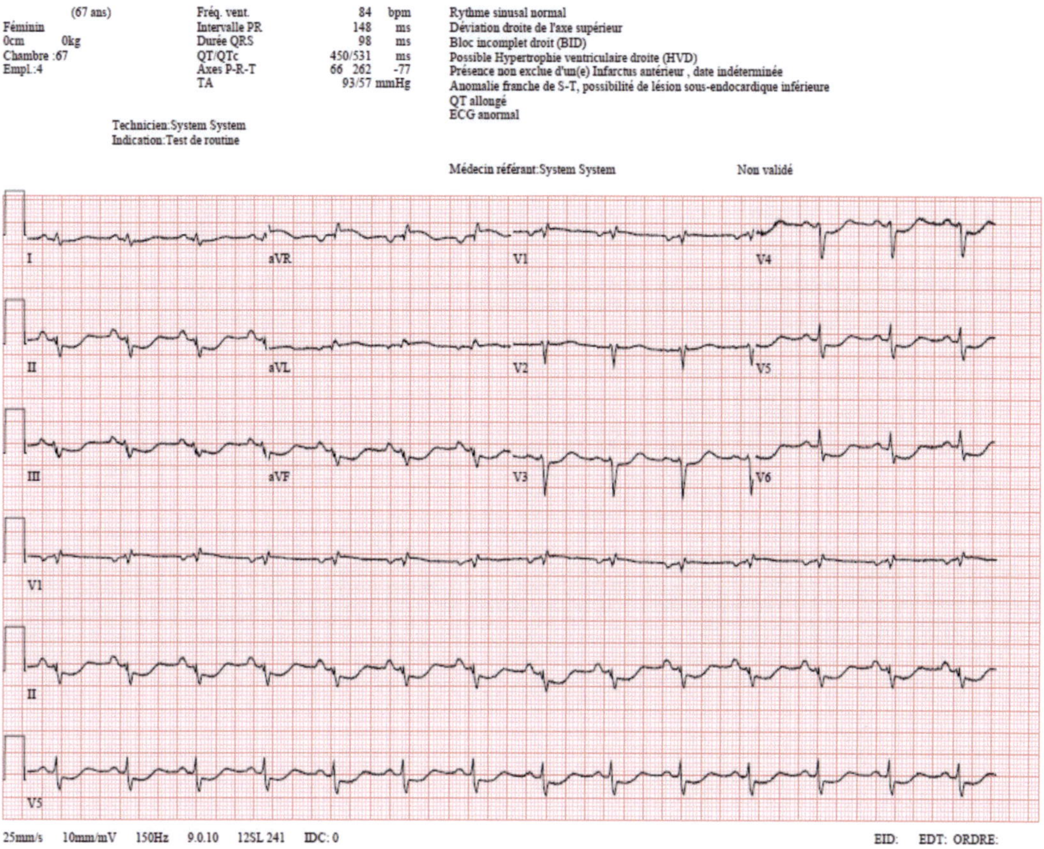

Fig. 2 Twelve-lead ECG recorded after the end of the episode of palpitations

of recent or old myocardial infarction, and supported the diagnosis of nonischemic cardiomyopathy with severe LV systolic dysfunction. It also showed the presence of nonspecific subepicardial fibrosis at the level of the lateral LV wall.

Bidirectional ventricular tachycardia is a special and rare type of ventricular tachycardia that was first described in the context of digoxin intoxication [3, 4], which is usually a hallmark of catecholaminergic polymorphic ventricular tachycardia [5], but that can exist in other clinical scenarios, such as acute myocardial ischemia [6, 7] and myocarditis [8].

The mechanism underlying bidirectional ventricular tachycardia is not fully understood but appears to be related to triggered activity (after depolarization), abnormal automaticity, or reentry. Treatment of this arrhythmia should address the underlying cause. Antiarrhythmic drugs can also be useful.

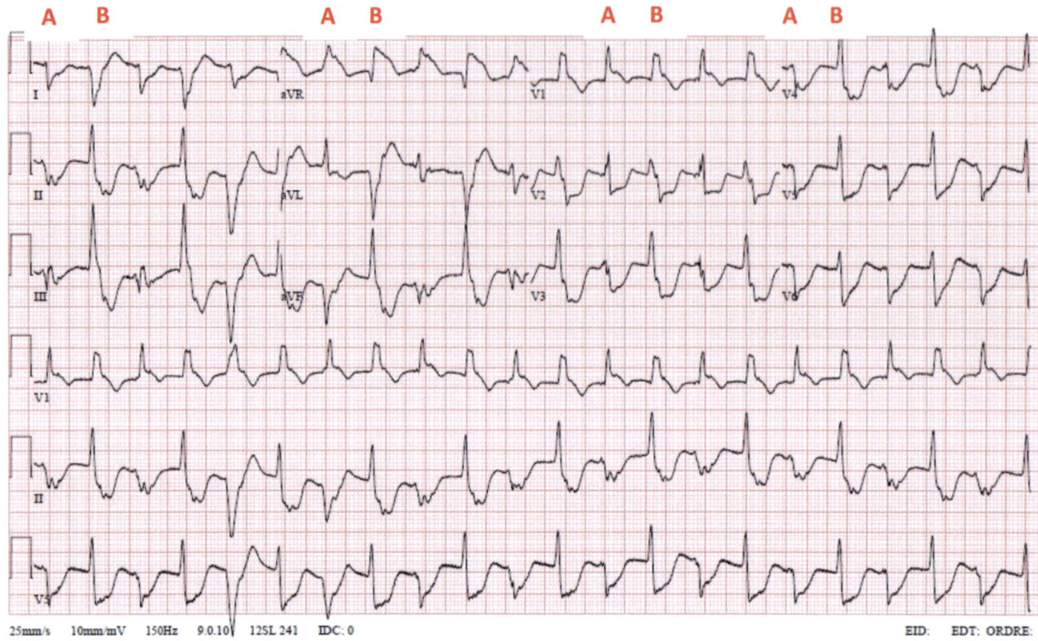

Fig. 3 Annotation of the two alternating QRS morphologies from Fig. 1: A and B

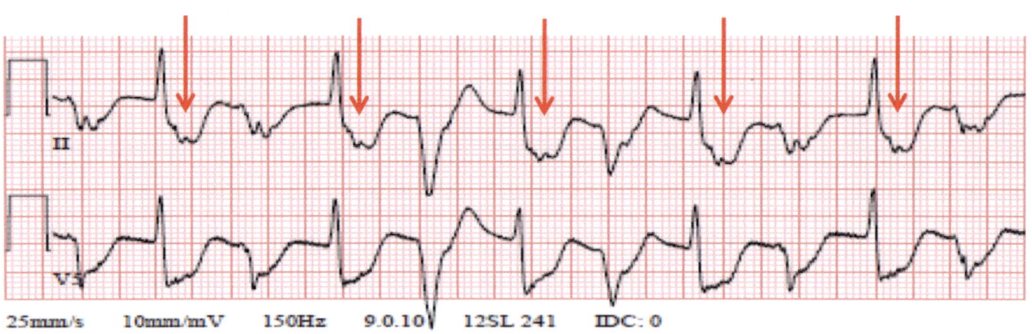

Fig. 4 Leads II and V5 from the tachycardia presented in Fig. 1. The red arrows point to the P waves, each superposed on the preceding T wave

References

1. Surawicz B, Childers R, Deal BJ, Gettes LS, Bailey JJ, Gorgels A, et al. AHA/ACCF/HRS recommendations for the standardization and interpretation of the electrocardiogram: part III: intraventricular conduction disturbances: a scientific statement from the American Heart Association Electrocardiography and Arrhythmias Committee, Council on Clinical Cardiology; the American College of Cardiology Foundation; and the Heart Rhythm Society. Endorsed by the International Society for Computerized Electrocardiology. J Am Coll Cardiol. 2009;53(11):976–81.
2. Brugada P, Brugada J, Mont L, Smeets J, Andries EW. A new approach to the differential diagnosis of a regular tachycardia with a wide QRS complex. Circulation. 1991;83(5):1649–59.
3. Almarzuqi A, Kimber S, Quadros K, Senaratne J. Bidirectional ventricular tachycardia: challenges and solutions. Vasc Health Risk Manag. 2022;18:397–406.
4. Kummer JL, Nair R, Krishnan SC. Images in cardiovascular medicine. Bidirectional ventricular tachycardia caused by digitalis toxicity. Circulation. 2006;113(7):e156–7.
5. Femenia F, Barbosa-Barros R, Sampaio SV, Arce M, Perez-Riera A, Baranchuk A. Bidirectional ventricular tachycardia: a hallmark of catecholaminergic

polymorphic ventricular tachycardia. Indian Pacing Electrophysiol J. 2012;12(2):65–8.
6. Wase A, Masood AM, Garikipati NV, Mufti O, Kabir A. Bidirectional ventricular tachycardia with myocardial infarction: a case report with insight on mechanism and treatment. Indian Heart J. 2014;66(4):466–9.
7. Hsu F, Goh J, Jung A, Patel M, Akel R, Yamamura K. Bidirectional ventricular tachycardia in acute multivessel myocardial infarction. Cureus. 2022;14(6):e25845.
8. Berte B, Eyskens B, Meyfroidt G, Willems R. Bidirectional ventricular tachycardia in fulminant myocarditis. Europace. 2008;10(6):767–8.

ECG 33

Gabriel Gusetu

1 Case Presentation

A 54-year-old female patient presented to the Emergency Department with acute ST segment elevation myocardial infarction of the inferior LV wall. While in the Emergency Department, she presented an episode of cardiac arrest due to ventricular fibrillation. She was treated with defibrillation. She was transfered to the Cardiology Department for urgent coronary angiography. While in the Cardiology Department, before her transfer to the Catheterization Laboratory, she presented another episode of palpitations, and the ECG in Figure 1.

Question: What is the nature of the tachycardia presented in Fig. 1 ?

(a) Atrial fibrillation with ST segment elevation in the inferior leads and RBBB and PVC
(b) Sinus tachycardia with type 1 Mobitz 2 atrioventricular block and ST segment elevation in the inferior leads, RBBB, and PVC
(c) Sinus tachycardia with ST segment elevation in the inferior leads, RBBB, and PVC
(d) Pre-excited atrial fibrillation
(e) Ventricular tachycardia originating from the anterior and septal LV walls

G. Gusetu (✉)
Department of Cardiology, Hôpital Emile Muller, Mulhouse, France

Hint: A second ECG recorded after the administration of 300 mg iv amiodarone is presented in Fig. 2.

Correct answer: a. Atrial fibrillation with ST segment elevation in the inferolateral leads, RBBB, and PVC.

Explanation: The ECG in Fig. 1 shows an irregular wide QRS complex tachycardia with a heart rate of 127 bpm and incomplete RBBB morphology. The width of the QRS complex is 148 ms according to the automatic interpretation of the ECG, but a closer look at QRS complexes can determine that the width of the QRS is between 100 and 120 ms (Fig. 3).

The QRS axis is at +100°. The differential diagnosis of this irregular tachycardia with incomplete RBBB morphology includes: ventricular tachycardia (fascicular VT) and supraventricular tachycardia (atrial fibrillation, atrial tachycardia, and sinus tachycardia with PAC) with functional or pre-existing incomplete right bundle branch block. Antidromic tachycardia (in pre-excitation syndromes) is generally regular, has wide QRS complexes, and is less likely present in this case.

The morphology of the QRS is not identical for all QRS complexes, better seen in precordial leads. There are four different QRS morphologies, all with incomplete RBBB (Fig. 4).

L. Muresan (ed.), *ECG Interpretation of Wide QRS Complex Tachycardia*,
https://doi.org/10.1007/978-3-031-97030-6_34

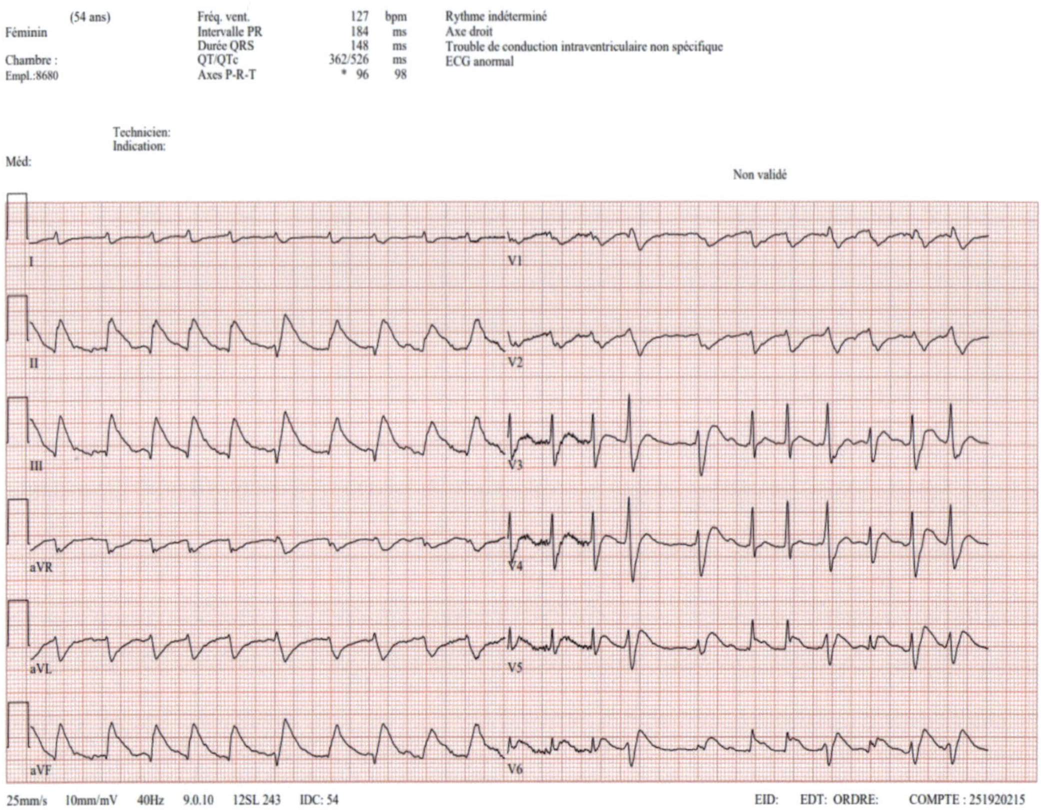

Fig. 1 Twelve-lead ECG recorded in the Cardiology Department

The rhythm is irregular, and there are no P waves preceding the QRS complexes (except for the second and the ninth QRS complexes in the limb leads and for the sixth QRS complex in the precordial leads but of different morphologies). This is therefore atrial fibrillation. Therefore, answers b—"Sinus tachycardia with type 1 Mobitz 2 atrioventricular block and ST segment elevation in the inferior leads, RBBB, and PVC"—and c—"Sinus tachycardia with ST segment elevation in the inferior leads, RBBB, and PVC"—can be excluded.

The variation in the QRS complex morphology can suggest pre-excited atrial fibrillation. However, the QRS complexes are narrow, and there is no sign of ventricular pre-excitation on the ECG from Fig. 2. Therefore, answer d—"Pre-excited atrial fibrillation"—is not correct.

The best explanation for the variation in the QRS morphology is that morphology 1 of the QRS complexes is the baseline QRS complex. In precordial leads, this shows ST segment elevation in leads V5 and V6, compatible with acute inferolateral myocardial infarction. Morphology 2 is ventricular in origin, given the R-to-S ratio < 1 in lead V6 [1]. Morphologies 3 and 4 are fusions between the baseline QRS and the QRS complexes with ventricular origin (morphology 2).

Therefore, the correct answer is a—"Atrial fibrillation with ST segment elevation in the inferolateral leads and RBBB and PVC".

The patient received 300 mg of amiodarone and underwent coronary angiography and PCI of the right coronary artery.

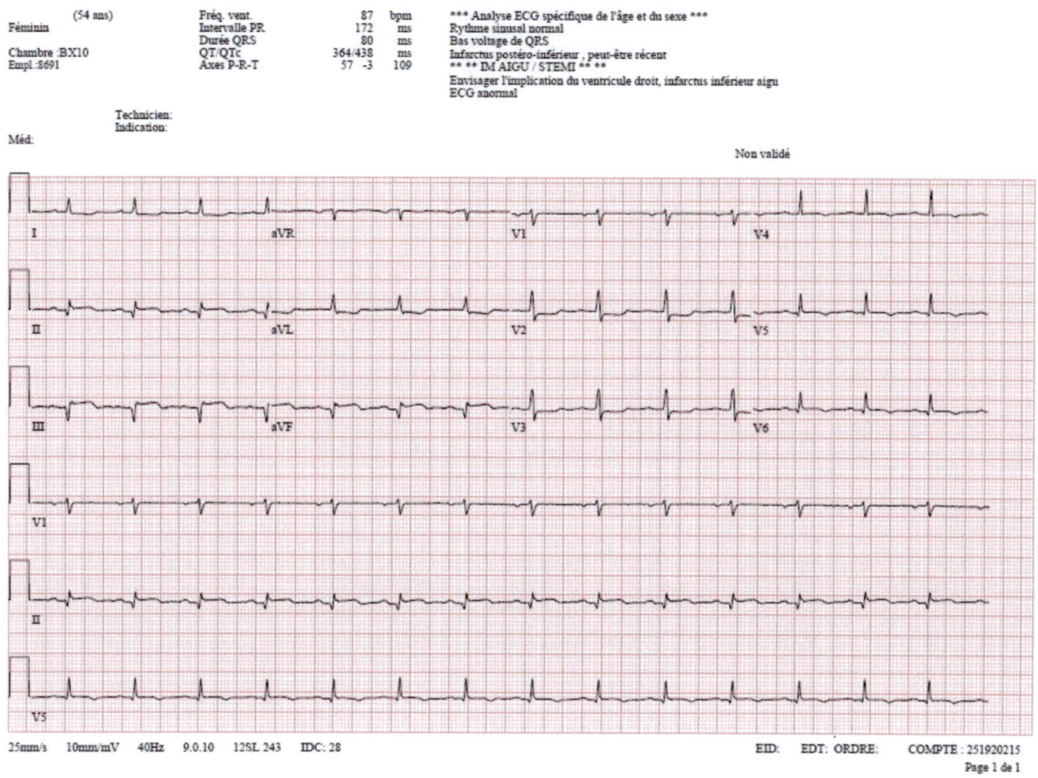

Fig. 2 Twelve-lead ECG recorded after the end of the episode of palpitations

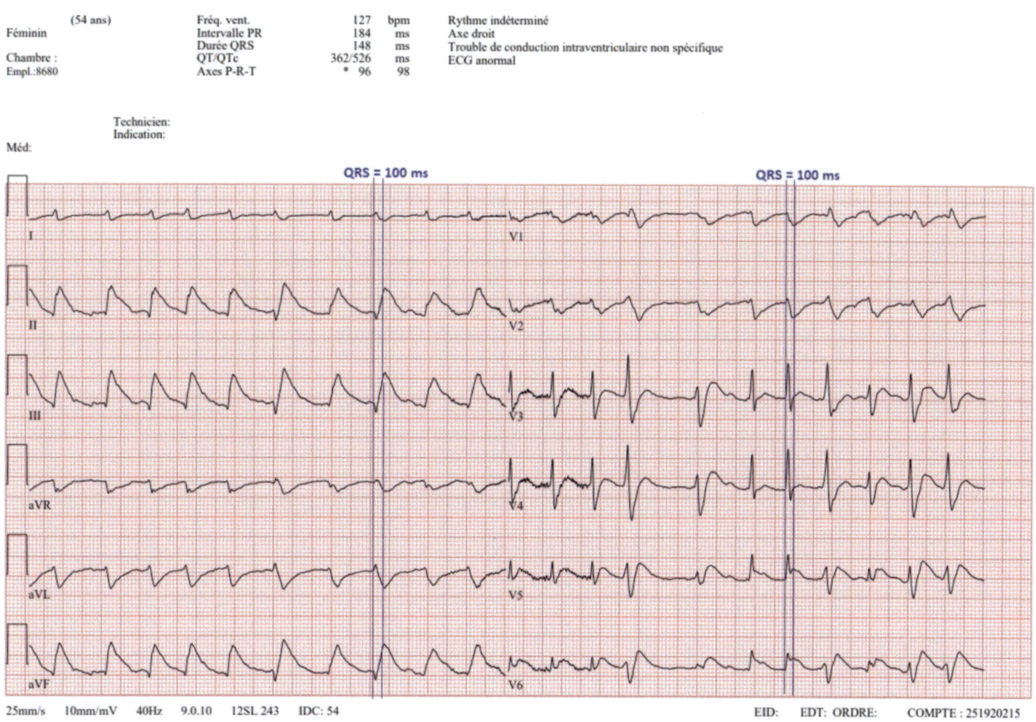

Fig. 3 Same ECG as in Fig. 1; the vertical blue lines delineate the QRS width, which measures 100 ms

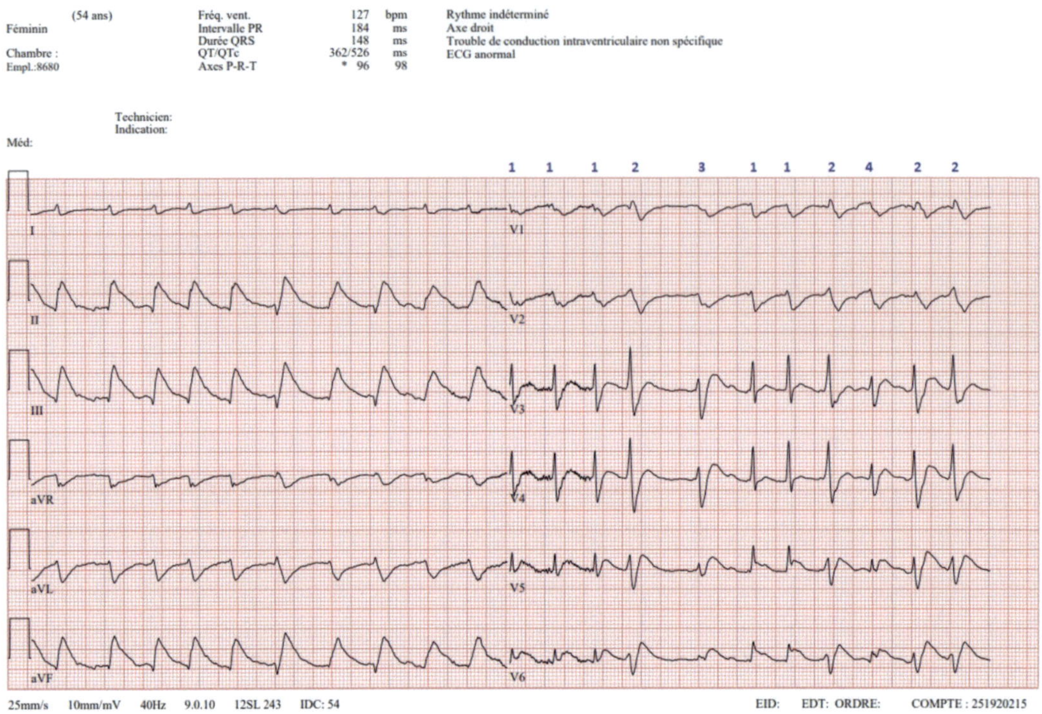

Fig. 4 Same ECG as in Fig. 1. The blue numbers above the QRS complexes in precordial leads indicate four different QRS morphologies (1 = morphology 1, 2 = morphology 2, 3 = morphology 3, and 4 = morphology 4)

Reference

1. Brugada P, Brugada J, Mont L, Smeets J, Andries EW. A new approach to the differential diagnosis of a regular tachycardia with a wide QRS complex. Circulation. 1991;83(5):1649–59.

ECG 34

Gabriel Cismaru

1 Case Presentation

Figure 1 shows the ECG recorded from the same patient presented in case 33, a 54-year-old female patient with acute ST segment elevation myocardial infarction of the inferior LV wall that presented an episode of cardiac arrest due to ventricular fibrillation. While in the Cardiology Department, after PCI of the right coronary artery, she presented the ECG shown in Fig. 1.

Question: What is the nature of the rhythm presented in Fig. 1?

(a) Ventricular tachycardia originating from the right ventricle
(b) Accelerated idioventricular rhythm
(c) Idioventricular escape rhythm
(d) Sinus rhythm with right bundle branch block
(e) Sinus rhythm with ventricular pre-excitation (concertina effect)

Hint: A following ECG recorded 48 h later is presented in Fig. 2.

Correct answer: b. Accelerated idioventricular rhythm.

Explanation: The ECG in Fig. 1 shows a wide QRS complex tachycardia with RBBB morphology, with a heart rate of 103 bpm, QRS axis at +90°, absence of LV hypertrophy, ST segment elevation in inferior leads, compatible with acute inferior myocardial infarction. Of note, the first QRS complex recorded by the limb leads and the first eight QRS complexes recorded by the precordial leads (sequential recording of the limb leads and then the precordial leads) show a different QRS morphology compared to the other recorded QRS complexes: they are not preceded by P waves. The differential diagnosis of this wide QRS complex tachycardia includes: ventricular tachycardia (accelerated idioventricular rhythm), supraventricular tachycardia (atrial tachycardia, AVNRT, and AVRT) with functional right bundle branch block, and antidromic tachycardia (in pre-excitation syndromes).

The ECG in sinus rhythm can sometimes provide valuable clues concerning the most likely and the most unlikely nature of the tachycardia. In the present case, the ECG in Fig. 3 shows sinus rhythm with a heart rate of 53 bpm (sinus bradycardia), QRS axis at +45°, absence of hypertrophy, and q waves in the inferior leads compatible with necrosis of the inferior LV wall. There are no elements in favor of ventricular pre-excitation (no short PR interval or delta waves). The absence of ventricular pre-excitation makes antidromic

G. Cismaru (✉)
Department of Cardiology, Rehabilitation Hospital, Cluj-Napoca, Romania

L. Muresan (ed.), *ECG Interpretation of Wide QRS Complex Tachycardia*,
https://doi.org/10.1007/978-3-031-97030-6_35

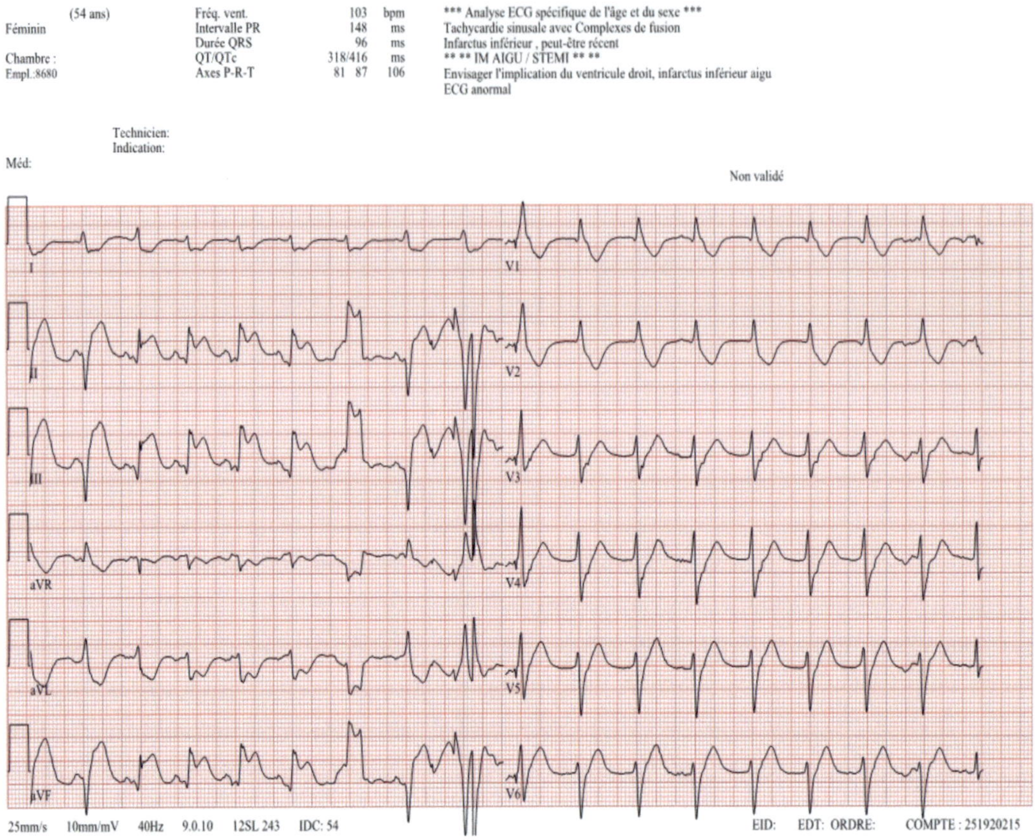

Fig. 1 Twelve-lead ECG recorded after PCI of the right coronary artery

tachycardia less likely There is also no RBBB, in favor of an SVT with pre-existing RBBB.

The morphology of the RBBB tachycardia from Fig. 1 is not that of a typical one [1]: even though the QRS complexes are large, the R-to-S ratio in lead V6 is <1, which is not common for a typical RBBB.

Applying the Brugada algorithm [2], it can be seen that: 1. There is no absence of an RS complex in the precordial leads (otherwise said, there are RS complexes in leads V3 to V6). 2. There is no R-to-S interval > 100 ms in any precordial lead (Fig. 3). 3. There is no AV dissociation visible. Therefore, we need to move to the fourth step of the algorithm and analyze the morphology of the QRS complexes during tachycardia.

For an RBBB morphology wide QRS complex tachycardia, an argument in favor of VT would be the presence of a taller left peak of the QRS complex in lead V1 (the rabbit ear sign) or for biphasic RS or QR complexes. Lead V1 shows a "qR" aspect, argument in favor of ventricular tachycardia. Next, in lead V6, an argument in favor of VT would be the presence of an "rS" complex, which is the case. This can also be expressed as a ratio of R/S < 1 in lead V6 (Fig. 4).

Therefore, according to this algorithm, the diagnosis is ventricular tachycardia. Given the heart rate of 103 bpm and the clinical context (acute myocardial infarction), the correct answer is accelerated idioventricular rhythm. A (passive) escape idioventricular rhythm would have a heart rate of less than 60 bpm, which makes answer c—"Idioventricular escape rhythm"—incorrect.

Idioventricular rhythm, also called "the reperfusion rhythm", is frequent in patients with myocardial ischemia, after coronary revascularization (spontaneous reperfusion, thrombolysis, or PCI) [3–10].

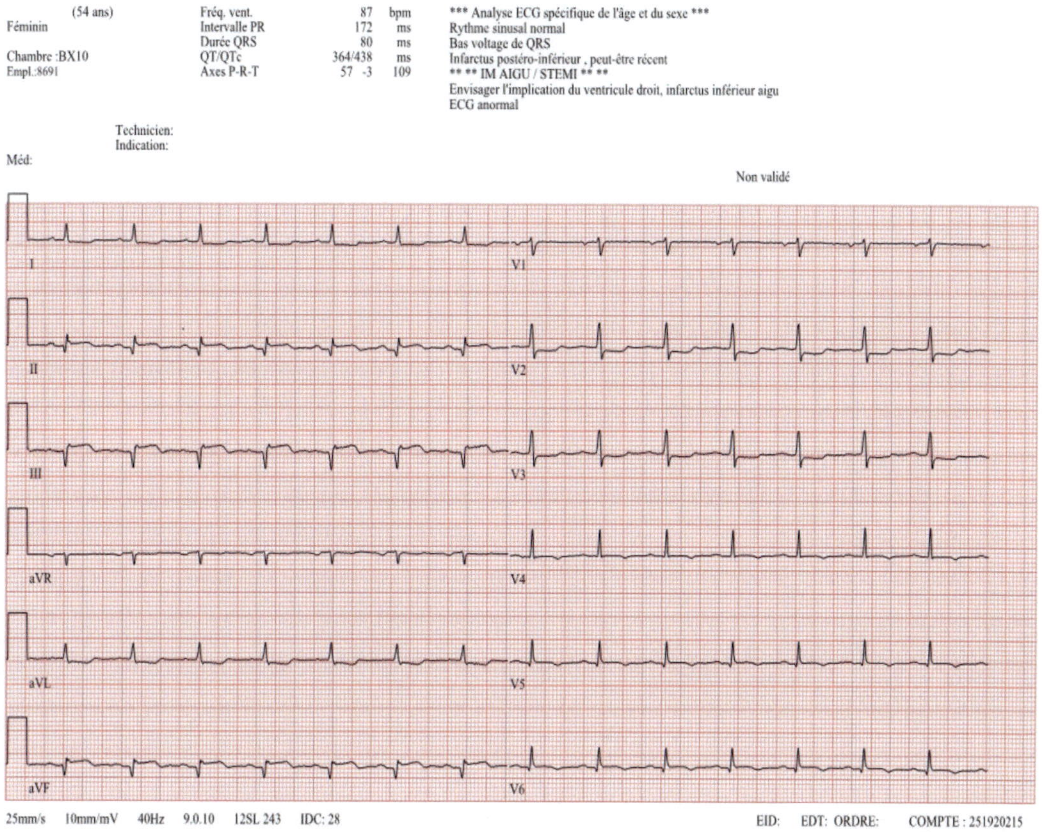

Fig. 2 Twelve-lead ECG recorded after the end of the episode of palpitations

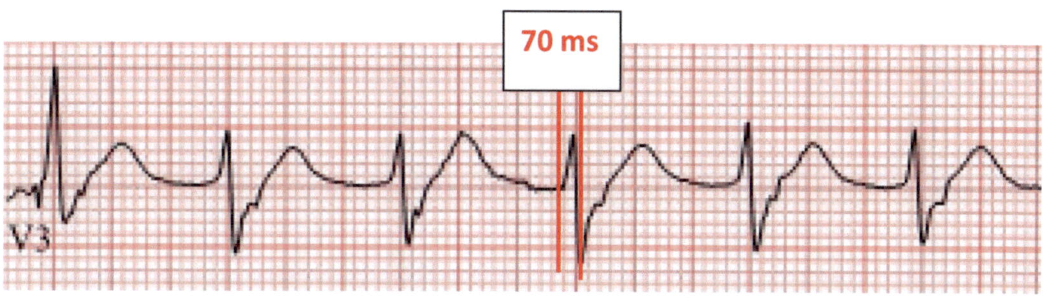

Fig. 3 Lead V3 from the ECG presented in Fig. 1 showing an R-to-S interval of 70 ms, argument not in favor of ventricular tachycardia (but not excluding it either)

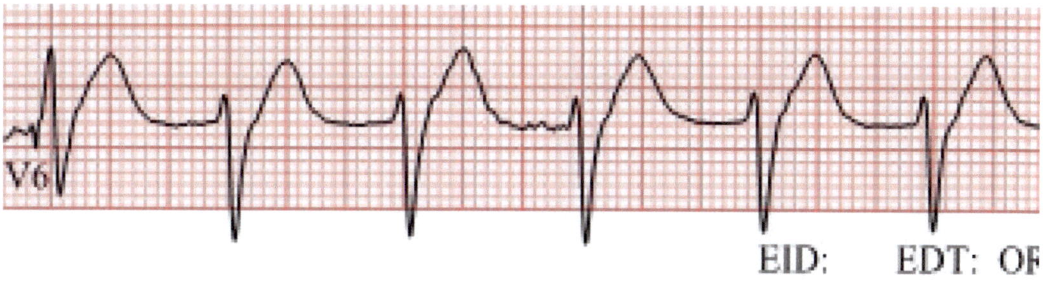

Fig. 4 Lead V6 from the ECG presented in Fig. 1 showing an R-to-S interval ratio < 1, argument in favor of ventricular tachycardia

References

1. Surawicz B, Childers R, Deal BJ, Gettes LS, Bailey JJ, Gorgels A, et al. AHA/ACCF/HRS recommendations for the standardization and interpretation of the electrocardiogram: part III: intraventricular conduction disturbances: a scientific statement from the American Heart Association Electrocardiography and Arrhythmias Committee, Council on Clinical Cardiology; the American College of Cardiology Foundation; and the Heart Rhythm Society. Endorsed by the International Society for Computerized Electrocardiology. J Am Coll Cardiol. 2009;53(11):976–81.
2. Brugada P, Brugada J, Mont L, Smeets J, Andries EW. A new approach to the differential diagnosis of a regular tachycardia with a wide QRS complex. Circulation. 1991;83(5):1649–59.
3. Hutchinson RG. Accelerated idioventricular rhythm after recovery from myocardial infarction. Angiology. 1977;28(9):579–82.
4. Shirayama T, Nakagawa M. Accelerated idioventricular rhythm. Ryoikibetsu Shokogun Shirizu. 1996;12:458–60.
5. Negrusz-Kawecka M, Gajek J. Idioventricular rhythm in patients with acute myocardial infarction: an indicator of perfusion or ischemic symptom. Pol Merkur Lekarski. 2000;8(44):80–3.
6. Terkelsen CJ, Sorensen JT, Kaltoft AK, Nielsen SS, Thuesen L, Botker HE, et al. Prevalence and significance of accelerated idioventricular rhythm in patients with ST-elevation myocardial infarction treated with primary percutaneous coronary intervention. Am J Cardiol. 2009;104(12):1641–6.
7. Riera AR, Barros RB, de Sousa FD, Baranchuk A. Accelerated idioventricular rhythm: history and chronology of the main discoveries. Indian Pacing Electrophysiol J. 2010;10(1):40–8.
8. Gildea TH, Levis JT. ECG diagnosis: accelerated idioventricular rhythm. Perm J. 2018;22:17–173.
9. Jakkoju A, Jakkoju R, Subramaniam PN, Glancy DL. Accelerated idioventricular rhythm. Proceedings. 2018;31(4):506–7.
10. Morita Y, Endo A, Tanabe K. Accelerated Idioventricular rhythm following Transcatheter self-expandable aortic valve implantation. Circ Rep. 2021;3(7):421–2.

ECG 35

Radu Rosu

1 Case Presentation

A 45-year-old male patient with no significant past medical history is admitted to the Intensive Care Unit for an episode of aborted sudden cardiac death that had occurred during a physical effort (football match), 45 min before his admittance to the hospital. After being resuscitated by the Mobile Emergency Team, he was intubated; he received iv adrenaline and noradrenaline and was taken to the Catheterization Laboratory. An urgent coronary angiography was performed which demonstrated acute occlusion of the left anterior descending coronary artery. He was treated with PTCA and stent implantation. In the ICU, his first echocardiography showed an LVEF of 20%. An ECG was recorded and is presented in Fig. 1.

Question: What is the nature of the tachycardia presented in Fig. 1?

(a) Sinus tachycardia in a patient with Brugada syndrome
(b) Ventricular tachycardia originating from the left ventricle in the context of acute STEMI
(c) Atrial tachycardia with right bundle branch block
(d) Antidromic tachycardia using a left-sided bypass tract
(e) Atypical AVNRT with right bundle branch block

Hint: A second ECG recorded several minutes later is presented in Fig. 2.

Correct answer: b. Ventricular tachycardia originating from the left ventricle in the context of acute STEMI

Explanation: The ECG in Fig. 1 shows the sudden onset of a wide QRS complex tachycardia, which is present only in the precordial leads. The tachycardia is regular and has a heart rate of 180 bpm and RBBB morphology. The width of the QRS complex is 120 ms (Fig. 3).

The context in which the tachycardia occurred, suggestive of acute myocardial infarction (leads V1 to V3 show the first QRS complex which has a "QS" morphology with a slight ST segment elevation, compatible with STEMI), is strongly in favor of ventricular tachycardia. In fact, any wide QRS complex tachycardia in the setting of myocardial infarction should be considered ventricular in nature, until proven otherwise [1, 2]. However, supraventricular tachycardia with a functional right bundle branch block and antidromic tachycardia, even though less likely, are still possible options at this point of the analysis.

R. Rosu (✉)
Department of Cardiology, Rehabilitation Hospital, Cluj-Napoca, Romania

L. Muresan (ed.), *ECG Interpretation of Wide QRS Complex Tachycardia*,
https://doi.org/10.1007/978-3-031-97030-6_36

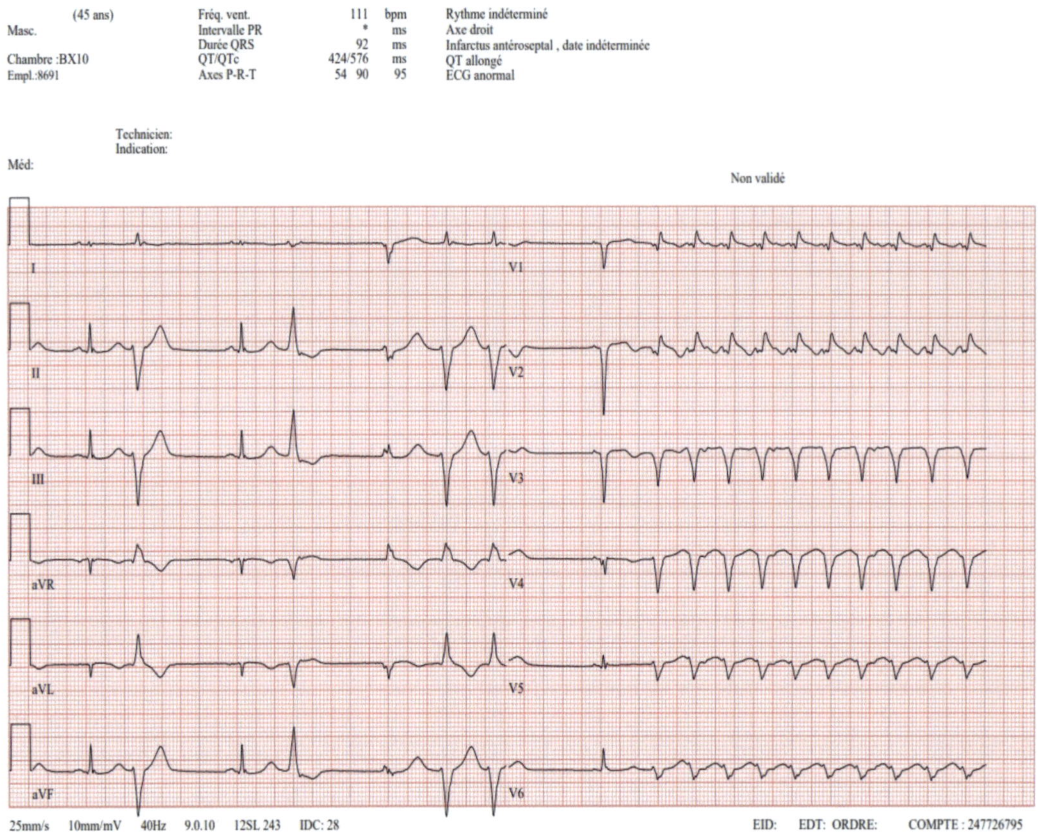

Fig. 1 Twelve-lead ECG recorded in the Intensive Care Unit

There is no argument in favor of ventricular pre-excitation, neither on the first nor on the second ECG: no short PR interval and no delta waves. Answer d—"antidromic tachycardia using a left-sided bypass tract"—is therefore highly unlikely.

The morphology of the right bundle branch block of the QRS complex during tachycardia from Fig. 1 is not that of a typical one [3]. Even though the QRS duration is 120 ms, and even though the QRS complex has an rsR' pattern in lead V1, there is a "QS" morphology in lead V3 and V4, which is not characteristic of a typical RBBB. Therefore, SVT (AVNRT or atrial tachycardia) with RBBB is unlikely.

The morphology of the QRS complex in leads V1 and V2 during tachycardia might suggest that this is actually Brugada syndrome. At a first glance, it seems that P waves are present, best visible in leads V1 and V2, with one P wave preceding each QRS complex (Fig. 4). However, a careful analysis demonstrates that these possible P waves are actually low-amplitude r waves, part of the QRS complex, which has an rsR' morphology, as evidenced in Fig. 3. So, answer a—"sinus tachycardia in a patient with Brugada syndrome"—is therefore not correct.

Applying the Brugada algorithm [4] to the tachycardia from Fig. 1, it can be seen that: 1. There is no absence of an RS complex in the precordial leads (otherwise said, there are rS complexes present, in leads V5 and V6); we can therefore move to the second step of the algorithm: 2. This step analyzes the absence of an R-to-S interval > 100 ms in any precordial lead. There is no R-to-S interval greater than 100 ms (Fig. 5); we can therefore move to the next step of the algorithm.

Step 3 looks for A–V dissociation. As previously mentioned, what seem to be P waves in

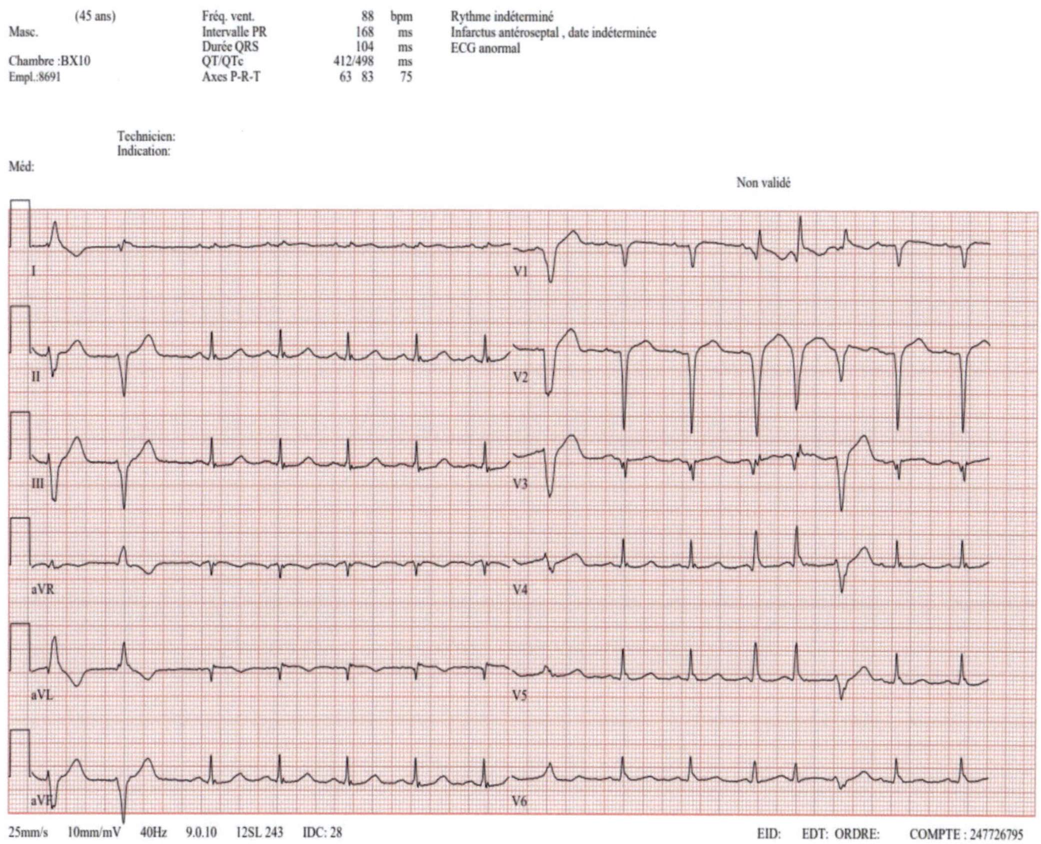

Fig. 2 Twelve-lead ECG recorded several minutes after the first ECG

leads V1 and V2 are actually r waves. These are not to be mistaken with P waves. However, a careful analysis of leads V3 and V4 identifies the presence of P waves, with A–V dissociation being present (Fig. 6). This is a strong argument in favor of ventricular tachycardia.

Another argument from the Brugada algorithm in favor of ventricular tachycardia is the r-to-S ratio of less than 1 in lead V6.

The Vereckei algorithm [5] for the differential diagnosis of wide QRS complex tachycardias also suggests VT as the correct answer. The first step of the algorithm looks for A–V dissociation, which, as previously mentioned, is present on the ECG from Fig. 1 (see Fig. 5). We could stop here and conclude that the tachycardia present in Fig. 1 is actually ventricular tachycardia. However, continuing to the next steps of the algorithms finds further arguments in favor of ventricular tachycardia. The second step of the algorithm looks for an initial predominant R wave in lead aVR. The tachycardia from Fig. 1 is recorded only in the precordial leads, so this step is not helpful in establishing the correct diagnosis. The third step of the algorithm "QRS morphology unlike BBB or fascicular block" also suggests VT as the correct diagnosis, for the reasons explained above (the QRS complex has a "QS" morphology in leads V3 and V4, which is not typical for an RBBB [3]). The fourth step of the algorithm analyzes the vi/vt index. This index compares the amplitude of the first 40 ms of a QRS complex to the amplitude of the last 40 ms of the QRS complex in a lead where the QRS has both an R and an S wave. In the present case, this is illustrated in Fig. 7.

Based on all these arguments, the diagnosis of ventricular tachcyardia can be established.

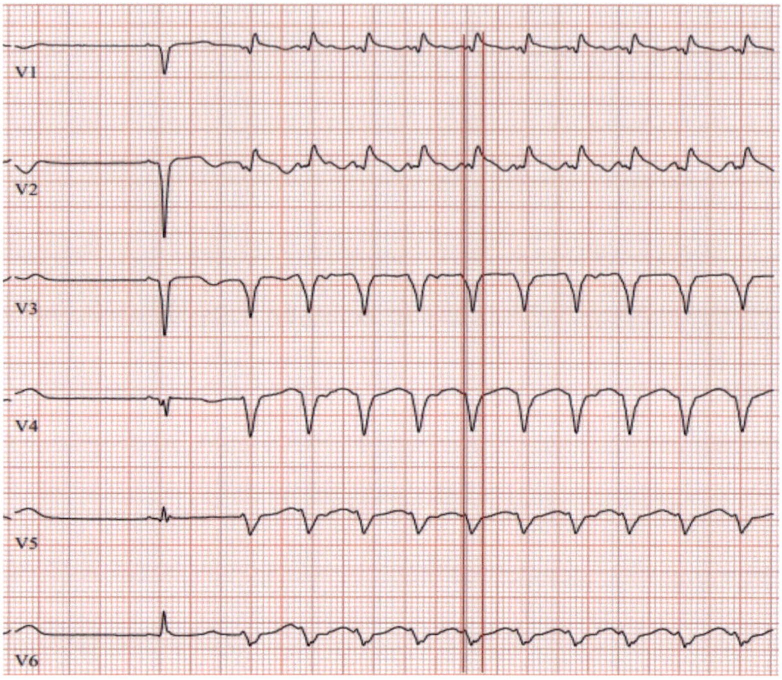

Fig. 3 Leads V1 to V6 showing the sudden onset of a wide QRS complex tachycardia. The vertical red lines delineate the QRS complex, which has a duration of 120 ms

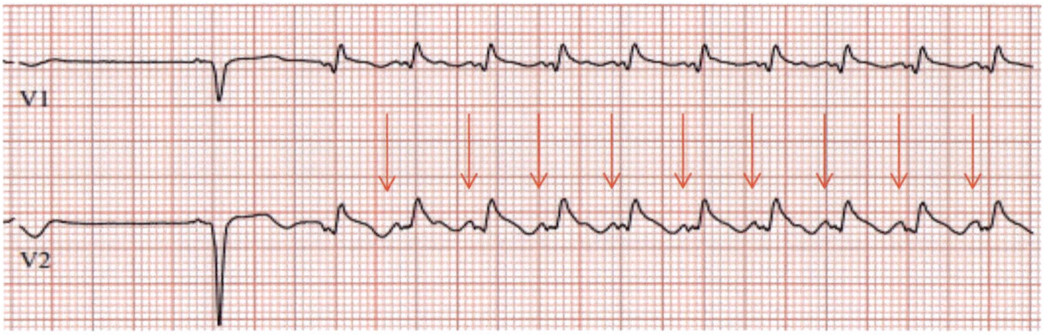

Fig. 4 Leads V1 and V2 from Fig. 1. The red vertical arrows point to what might be interpreted as P waves (see text for further explanation)

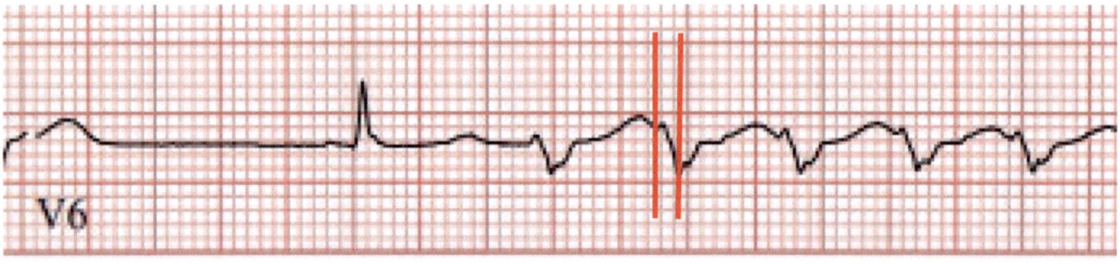

Fig. 5 Lead V6 from the tachycardia presented in Fig. 1 showing an R-to-S interval of 60 ms, argument not in favor of ventricular tachycardia (but not excluding it either)

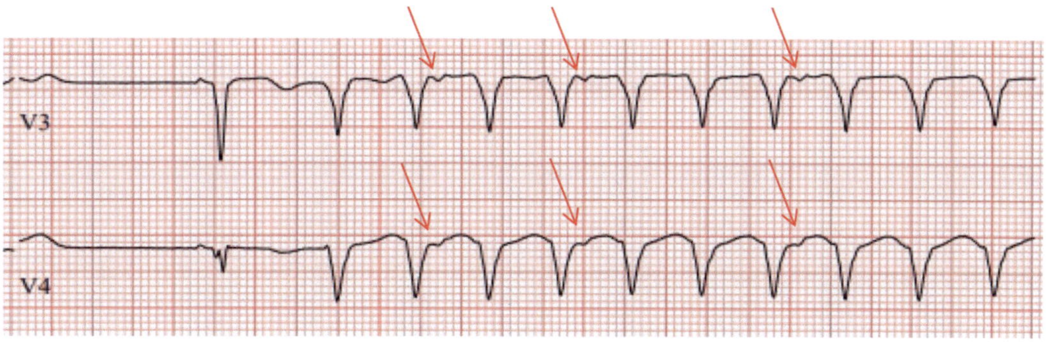

Fig. 6 Leads V3 and V4 from the ECG in Fig. 1 showing the onset of the wide QRS complex tachycardia. The red arrows point to the P waves. There is atrioventricular dissociation, an argument in favor of ventricular tachycardia

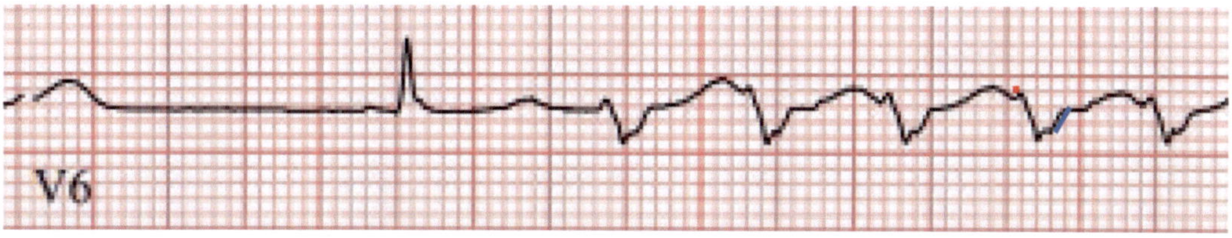

Fig. 7 The vi/vt index from the Vereckei algorithm in lead V1. The ratio of the initial 40 ms and the last 40 ms of the QRS complex is analyzed using the fourth QRS complex during tachycardia: 1 mV vs 2 mV; therefore, 1/2 = 0.5, which is <1. This is in favor of ventricular tachycardia

Therefore, the correct answer is b—"Ventricular tachycardia originating from the left ventricle in the context of acute STEMI".

An urgent coronary angiography was performed which demonstrated acute occlusion of the left anterior descending coronary artery. This was treated with PTCA and stent implantation.

References

1. Steinman RT, Herrera C, Schuger CD, Lehmann MH. Wide QRS tachycardia in the conscious adult. Ventricular tachycardia is the most frequent cause. JAMA. 1989;261(7):1013–6.
2. Garner JB, Miller JM. Wide complex tachycardia – ventricular tachycardia or not ventricular tachycardia, that remains the question. Arrhythmia Electrophysiol Rev. 2013;2(1):23–9.
3. Surawicz B, Childers R, Deal BJ, Gettes LS, Bailey JJ, Gorgels A, et al. AHA/ACCF/HRS recommendations for the standardization and interpretation of the electrocardiogram: part III: intraventricular conduction disturbances: a scientific statement from the American Heart Association Electrocardiography and Arrhythmias Committee, Council on Clinical Cardiology; the American College of Cardiology Foundation; and the Heart Rhythm Society. Endorsed by the International Society for Computerized Electrocardiology. J Am Coll Cardiol. 2009;53(11):976–81.
4. Brugada P, Brugada J, Mont L, Smeets J, Andries EW. A new approach to the differential diagnosis of a regular tachycardia with a wide QRS complex. Circulation. 1991;83(5):1649–59.
5. Vereckei A, Duray G, Szenasi G, Altemose GT, Miller JM. Application of a new algorithm in the differential diagnosis of wide QRS complex tachycardia. Eur Heart J. 2007;28(5):589–600.

ECG 36

Mihai Puiu

1 Case Presentation

Figure 1 shows the ECG recorded in the same patient presented in case 35: a 45-year old male patient with a history of active smoking (30 pack-years) but without any other significant past medical history is admitted to the hospital for an episode of aborted sudden cardiac death that occurred during a football match. The first ECG recorded by the Mobile Emergency Team showed the presence of ST segment elevation in the anterior leads. The diagnosis of STEMI was established, and the patient underwent urgent coronary angiography, which demonstrated the presence of acute thrombotic occlusion of the proximal left anterior descending coronary artery. PTCA + stent implantation was performed, and the patient was transferred to the Coronary Care Unit. An ECG was recorded by the nurse at arrival (Fig. 1), who is worried and quickly presents it to the junior doctor.

Question: What is the nature of the tachycardia presented in Fig. 1?

(a) Atrial flutter with right bundle branch block
(b) Accelerated idioventricular rhythm (AIVR)
(c) Atrial fibrillation with intermittent right bundle branch block
(d) Sinus node dysfunction with intermittent right bundle branch block
(e) Atrial fibrillation with misplaced ECG limb leads

Hint: A second ECG recorded several minutes later is presented in Fig. 2.

Correct answer: b. Accelerated idioventricular rhythm (AIVR).

Explanation: The ECG in Fig. 1 shows an irregular wide QRS complex tachycardia with a heart rate of 102 bpm and RBBB morphology. The width of the QRS complex is 122 ms. There is extreme (north-west) QRS axis deviation. The differential diagnosis of this irregular wide QRS complex tachycardia with RBBB morphology includes: automatic ventricular tachycardia and supraventricular tachycardia (atrial fibrillation, atrial flutter, atrial tachycardia, and AVNRT) with a functional or pre-existing bundle branch block. Antidromic tachycardia (in pre-excitation syndromes) is generally regular and is less likely present in this case, given the absence of pre-excitation on the ECG in sinus rhythm from Fig. 2: no short PR interval and no delta waves.

The morphology of the right bundle branch block of the QRS complex during tachycardia

M. Puiu (✉)
Department of Cardiology, Rehabilitation Hospital, Cluj-Napoca, Romania

L. Muresan (ed.), *ECG Interpretation of Wide QRS Complex Tachycardia*,
https://doi.org/10.1007/978-3-031-97030-6_37

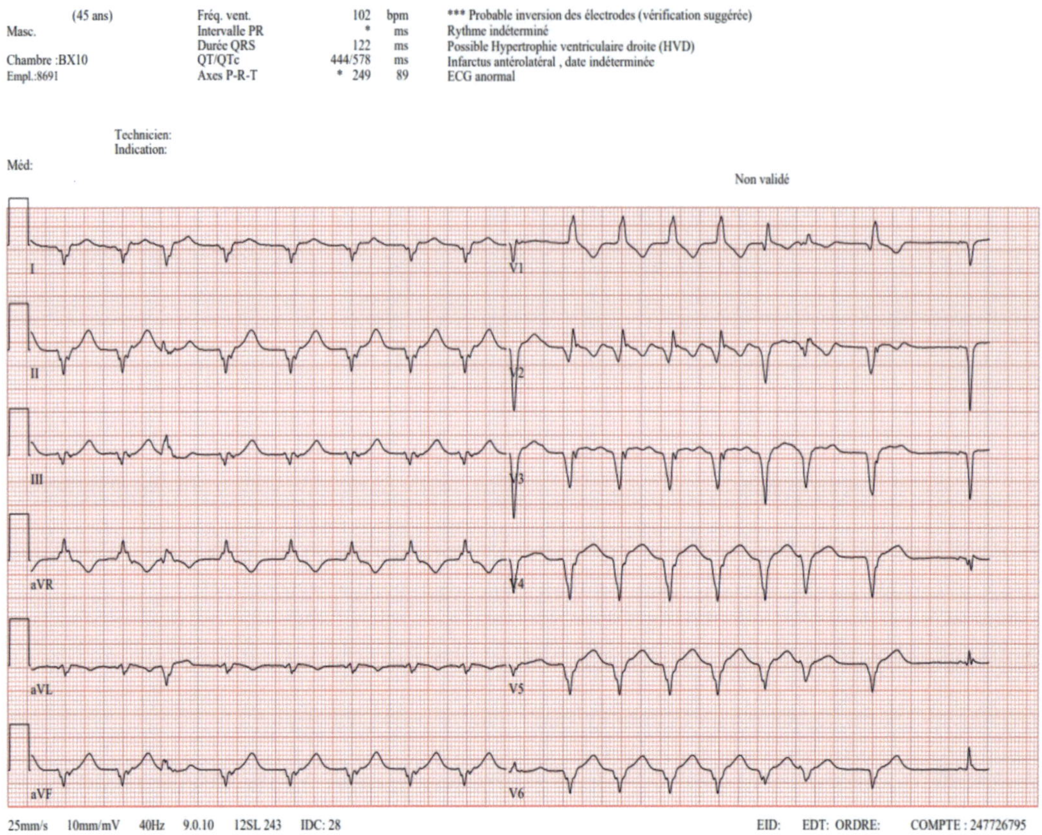

Fig. 1 Twelve-lead ECG recorded at admittance to the Cardiology Department

from Fig. 1 is not that of a typical one [1]: even though the QRS duration is >120 ms, there is a monomorphic R wave in lead I; the QRS complex has a "QS" morphology in leads I and aVF; and the R-to-S ratio in lead V6 is less than 1 (there is actually a "QS" aspect in lead V6). Even more, the morphology of the fifth and sixth QRS complexes in precordial leads is different from the first four beats, which, again, is not typical for an SVT with BBB.

Applying the Brugada algorithm [2] to the tachycardia from Fig. 1, it can be seen that: 1. There is an absence of an RS complex in the precordial leads (otherwise said, there is no "rS" complexes in any precordial lead: the QRS complex in lead V1 shows a unique R wave, in lead V2 a "QR" aspect, and from V3 to V6, there is a "QS" aspect); therefore, according to this algorithm, the diagnosis is ventricular tachycardia.

The Vereckei algorithm [3] for the differential diagnosis of wide QRS complex tachycardias also suggests VT as the correct answer. The first step of the algorithm looks for A–V dissociation, which is not seen on the present ECG. The second step of the algorithm looks for an initial predominant R wave in lead aVR, which is actually the case (Fig. 3). So, according to this algorithm, the correct diagnosis is also ventricular tachycardia.

The clinical context of the patient, with acute ST segment elevation myocardial infarction, treated with PTCA + stent implantation, is also suggestive of a ventricular rhythm, notably accelerated idioventricular rhythm (also called reperfusion rhythm). The fifth and sixth QRS complexes recorded by the precordial leads during the wide QRS complex tachycardia from Fig. 1 are likely fusion complexes between the

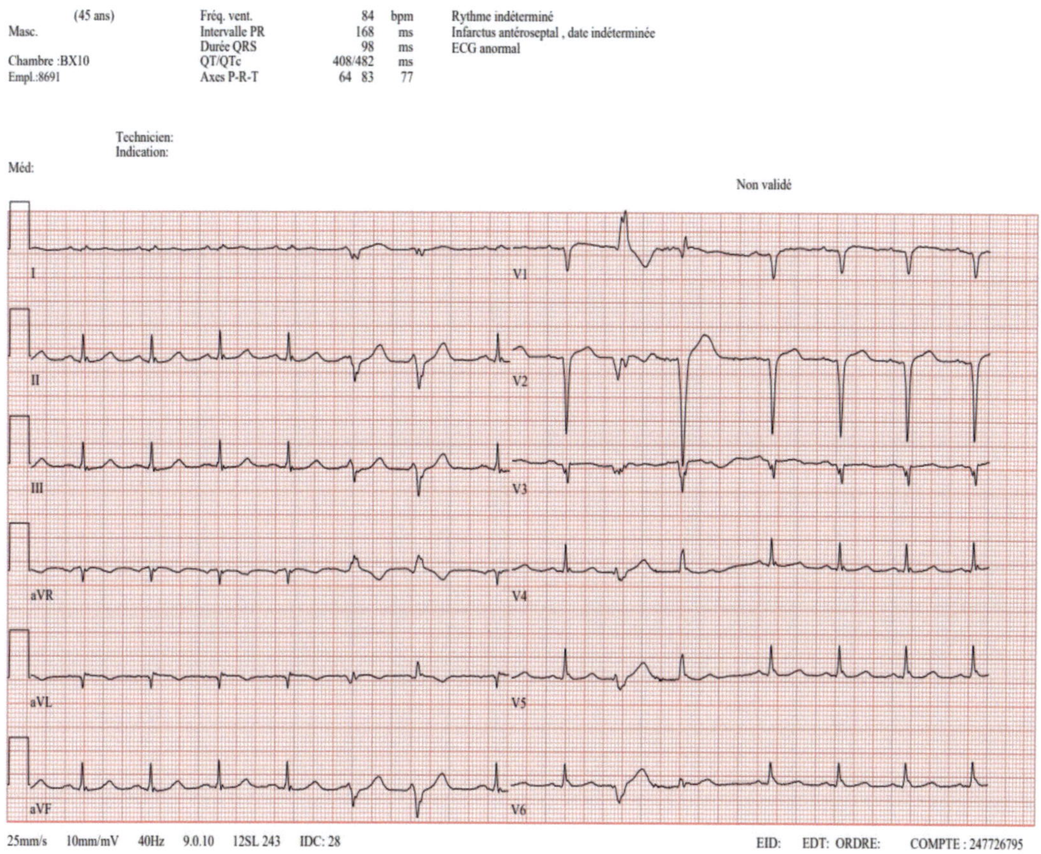

Fig. 2 Twelve-lead ECG recorded several minutes after the first ECG

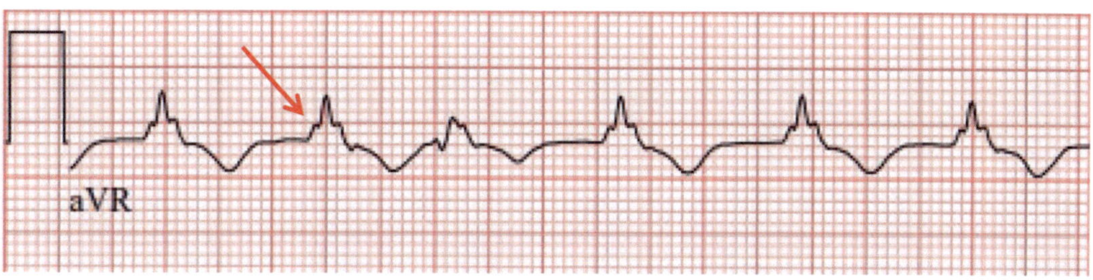

Fig. 3 Lead aVR from the ECG from Fig. 1 during tachycardia, showing a predominant initial R wave, argument in favor of ventricular tachycardia

sinus QRS complex and the AIVR (the morphology is neither that of any of the two but a mix of the two) (Fig. 4). The extreme left-axis deviation is also an argument in favor of ventricular origin of the tachycardia.

The ECG from Fig. 2 shows sinus rhythm with a heart rate of 84 bpm, with a "QS" morphology in leads V1 to V3, compatible with anterior myocardial necrosis.

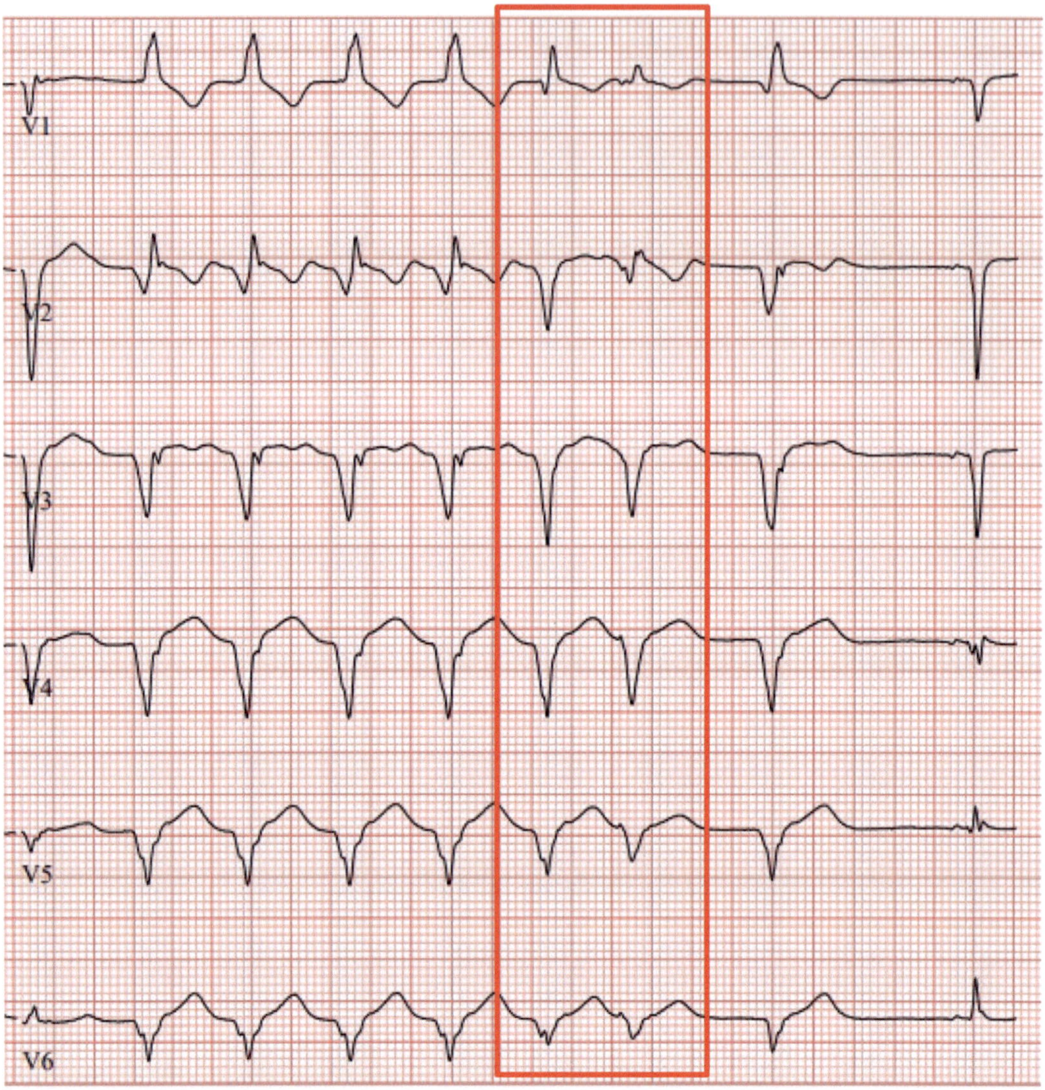

Fig. 4 Limb leads from the ECG from Fig. 1. The sixth and the seventh QRS complexes (red rectangle) have different morphologies and represent fusion beats between the AIVR and the sinus QRS complexes, argument in favor of a ventricular origin of the wide QRS complex tachycardia (see text for explanation)

References

1. Surawicz B, Childers R, Deal BJ, Gettes LS, Bailey JJ, Gorgels A, et al. AHA/ACCF/HRS recommendations for the standardization and interpretation of the electrocardiogram: part III: intraventricular conduction disturbances: a scientific statement from the American Heart Association Electrocardiography and Arrhythmias Committee, Council on Clinical Cardiology; the American College of Cardiology Foundation; and the Heart Rhythm Society. Endorsed by the International Society for Computerized Electrocardiology. J Am Coll Cardiol. 2009;53(11):976–81.
2. Brugada P, Brugada J, Mont L, Smeets J, Andries EW. A new approach to the differential diagnosis of a regular tachycardia with a wide QRS complex. Circulation. 1991;83(5):1649–59.
3. Vereckei A, Duray G, Szenasi G, Altemose GT, Miller JM. Application of a new algorithm in the differential diagnosis of wide QRS complex tachycardia. Eur Heart J. 2007;28(5):589–600.

ECG 37

Stefan-Lucian Popa

1 Case Presentation

A 66-year-old female patient with no significant past medical history presents to the Emergency Department for an episode of chest pain of moderate intensity accompanied by palpitations and malaise that had started 30 min prior to her presentation to the hospital. Her ECG recorded at admittance is presented in Fig. 1.

Twenty milligrams of triphosadenine was administered intravenously, with no effect on the tachycardia. Electrical cardioversion was performed, and a second ECG was then recorded (Fig. 2).

Question: What is the nature of the tachycardia presented in Fig. 1?

(a) Ventricular tachycardia originating from the inferior septal LV wall
(b) Ventricular tachycardia originating from the inferior septal RV wall
(c) Ventricular tachycardia originating from the anterior septal LV wall
(d) Antidromic tachycardia using a right-sided bypass tract
(e) AVNRT with right bundle branch block

S.-L. Popa (✉)
Department of Internal Medicine, Second Medical Clinic, Cluj-Napoca, Romania
e-mail: popa.stefan@umfcluj.ro

Hint: The ECG recorded several minutes later is presented in Fig. 2.

Correct answer: a. Ventricular tachycardia originating from the inferior septal LV wall.

Explanation: The ECG in Fig. 1 shows a regular wide QRS complex tachycardia with a heart rate of 211 bpm and RBBB morphology. The width of the QRS complex is 192 ms. The QRS axis is at −60°. The differential diagnosis of this regular wide QRS complex tachycardia with RBBB morphology includes: ventricular tachycardia (myocardial-related VT, bundle branch reentry VT, and fascicular VT), supraventricular tachycardia (atrial fibrillation, atrial flutter, atrial tachycardia, AVNRT, and AVRT) with functional or pre-existing bundle branch block, and antidromic tachycardia (in pre-excitation syndromes).

The ECG from Fig. 2 shows sinus rhythm with a heart rate of 96 bpm, with typical complete LBBB, with no signs of ventricular pre-excitation (no short PR interval and no delta waves). Therefore, antidromic tachycardia is not likely to be the correct answer for the tachycardia from Fig. 1.

The morphology of the right bundle branch block of the QRS complex during tachycardia from Fig. 1 is clearly not that of a typical one [1]:

L. Muresan (ed.), *ECG Interpretation of Wide QRS Complex Tachycardia*,
https://doi.org/10.1007/978-3-031-97030-6_38

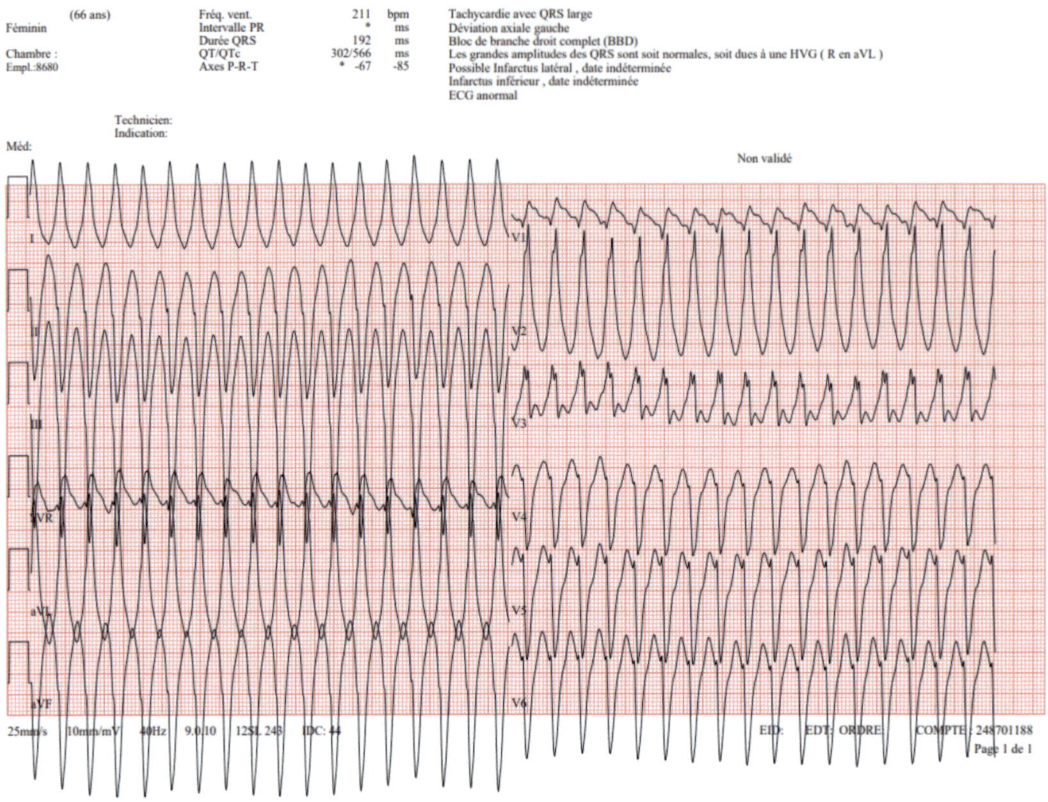

Fig. 1 Twelve-lead ECG recorded at admittance to the Emergency Department

even though the QRS duration is >120 ms, there is a monomorphic R wave in leads I and aVL, with an R-to-S ratio of less than 1 in lead V6 (Fig. 3). So, answer e—"AVNRT with right bundle branch block"—is not correct.

Applying the Brugada algorithm [2] to the tachycardia from Fig. 1, it can be seen that: 1. There is no absence of an RS complex in the precordial leads (otherwise said, there are rS complexes in leads V3 to V6); we therefore move to the second step of the algorithm: 2. This step analyzes the absence of an R-to-S interval > 100 ms in any precordial lead. If we measure this interval in lead V3, we can see that it exceeds 100 ms (Fig. 4). So, according to this algorithm, ventricular tachycardia is the correct answer.

The Vereckei algorithm [3] for the differential diagnosis of wide QRS complex tachycardias also suggests VT as the correct answer. The first step of the algorithm looks for A–V dissociation, which is not seen on the present ECG. The second step of the algorithm looks for an initial predominant R wave in lead aVR, which, again, is not the case. The third step "QRS morphology unlike BBB or fascicular block" does not suggest SVT with BBB, given the elements discussed above: the presence of a monomorphic R wave in leads I and aVL, with an R-to-S ratio of less than 1 in lead V6 [1]. Therefore, according to this algorithm, the correct answer is also ventricular tachycardia.

Another argument in favor of ventricular tachycardia is the presence of a QRS complex duration of more than 140 ms for an RBBB wide QRS complex tachycardia [4].

Based on these arguments, the diagnosis of ventricular tachycardia can be retained.

The origin of the tachycardia is in the left ventricle (the VT shows an RBBB morphology), at the level of the inferior LV wall ("QS"

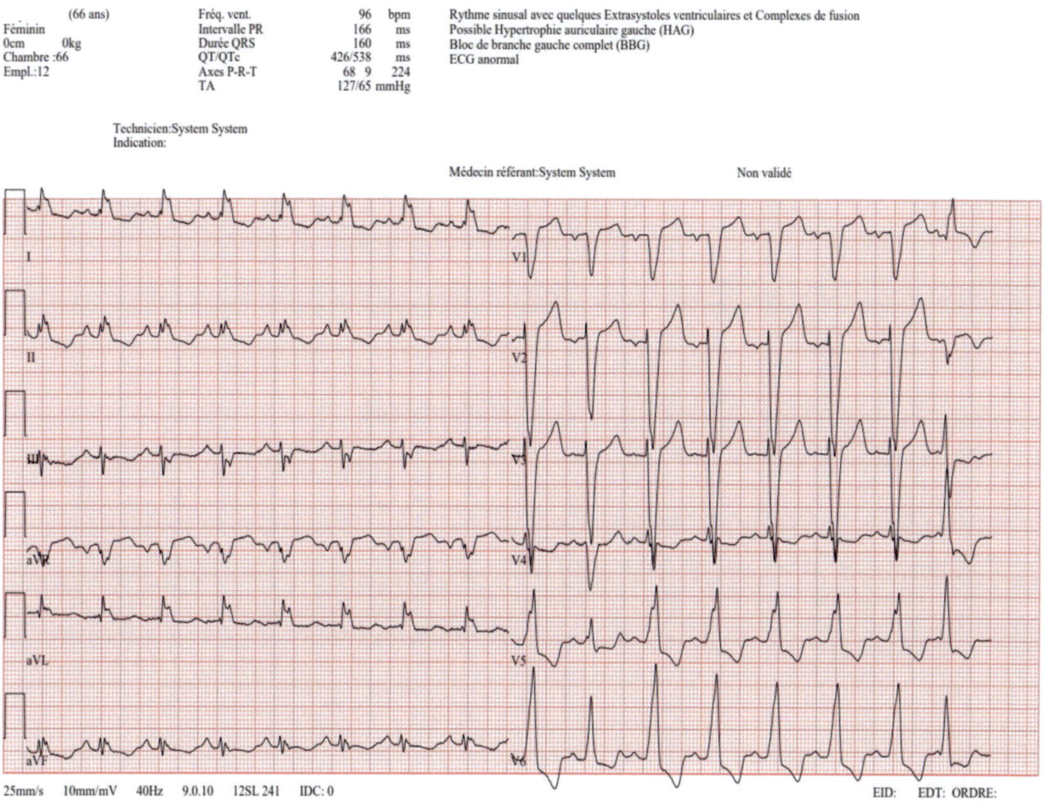

Fig. 2 Twelve-lead ECG recorded after the end of the episode of palpitations

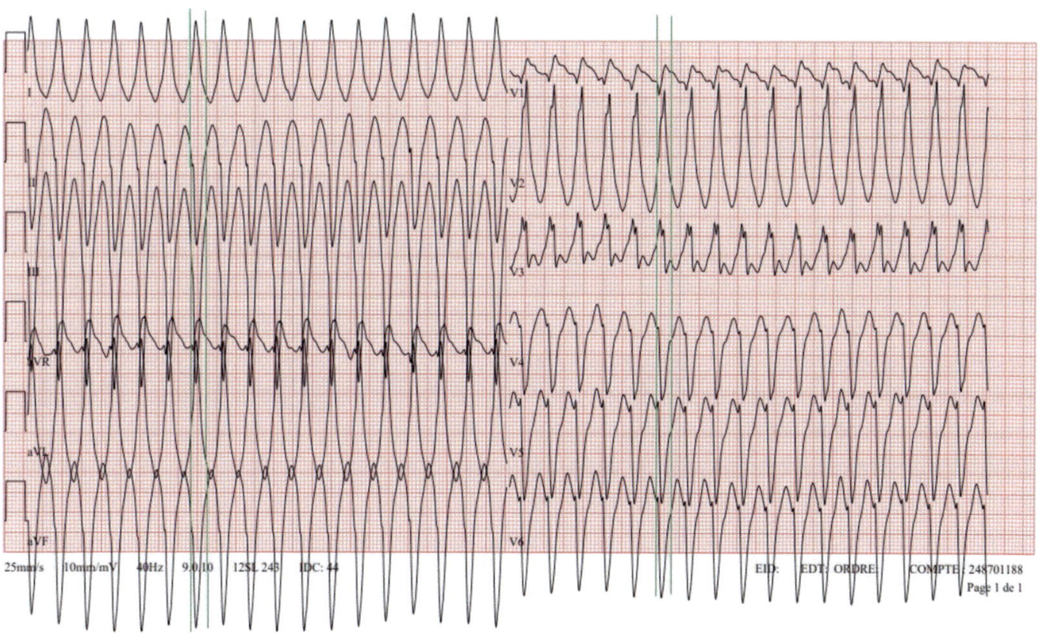

Fig. 3 Delimitation of the QRS complex during the wide QRS complex tachycardia from Fig. 1

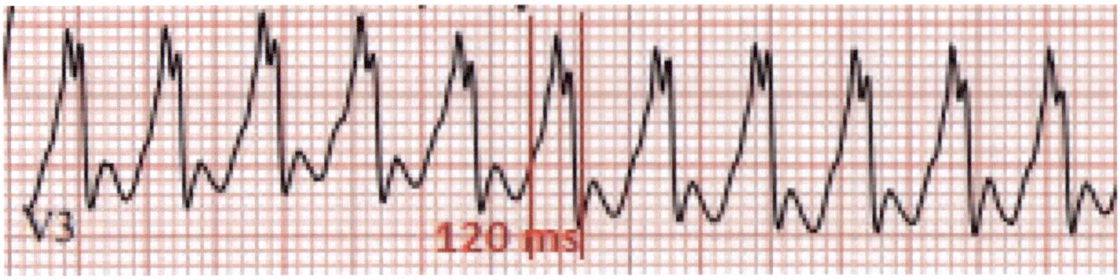

Fig. 4 Lead V3 from the ECG from Fig. 1 demonstrating the presence of an R-to-S interval of 120 ms, argument in favor of ventricular tachycardia

morphology in leads II, III, and aVF) and septal LV wall (unique "R" wave in leads I and aVL). Therefore, the correct answer is a—"Ventricular tachycardia originating from the inferior septal LV wall".

2 Aditional Comments

Blood sample analysis showed the presence of elevated T troponine levels of 98,488 ng/L. Echocardiography showed a dilated left ventricle (end-diastolic diameter of 71 mm) with severe global hypokinesia and with severe LV systolic dysfunction (LVEF of 19%). Coronary angiography was performed, which did not show obstruction of any major epicardial coronary artery. Cardiac MRI was then performed, which confirmed the severe LV dilation and the severe LV systolic dysfunction (LVEF of 20%). It also showed the presence of moderate RV dysfunction (RVEF of 39%) and the presence of a small area of subendocardial fibrosis, compatible with a very limited area of focal myocardial infarction at the level of the inferior and apical LV walls (1 segment out of 17), which did not explain the severe LV systolic dysfunction.

In order to elucidate the VT mechanism (focal, localized re-entry, macro-re-entry, or bundle branch re-entry [5–9]), an electrophysiological study was considered necessary and offered to the patient, but the patient did not agree. Therefore, the exact mechanism of the VT was not established.

References

1. Surawicz B, Childers R, Deal BJ, Gettes LS, Bailey JJ, Gorgels A, et al. AHA/ACCF/HRS recommendations for the standardization and interpretation of the electrocardiogram: part III: intraventricular conduction disturbances: a scientific statement from the American Heart Association Electrocardiography and Arrhythmias Committee, Council on Clinical Cardiology; the American College of Cardiology Foundation; and the Heart Rhythm Society. Endorsed by the International Society for Computerized Electrocardiology. J Am Coll Cardiol. 2009;53(11):976–81.
2. Brugada P, Brugada J, Mont L, Smeets J, Andries EW. A new approach to the differential diagnosis of a regular tachycardia with a wide QRS complex. Circulation. 1991;83(5):1649–59.
3. Vereckei A, Duray G, Szenasi G, Altemose GT, Miller JM. Application of a new algorithm in the differential diagnosis of wide QRS complex tachycardia. Eur Heart J. 2007;28(5):589–600.
4. Garner JB, Miller JM. Wide complex tachycardia – ventricular tachycardia or not ventricular tachycardia, that remains the question. Arrhythmia Electrophysiol Rev. 2013;2(1):23–9.
5. Blanck Z, Jazayeri M, Dhala A, Deshpande S, Sra J, Akhtar M. Bundle branch reentry: a mechanism of ventricular tachycardia in the absence of myocardial or valvular dysfunction. J Am Coll Cardiol. 1993;22(6):1718–22.
6. Lloyd EA, Zipes DP, Heger JJ, Prystowsky EN. Sustained ventricular tachycardia due to bundle branch reentry. Am Heart J. 1982;104(5 Pt 1):1095–7.
7. Mizusawa Y, Sakurada H, Nishizaki M, Ueda-Tatsumoto A, Fukamizu S, Hiraoka M. Characteristics of bundle branch reentrant ventricular tachycardia with a right bundle branch block configuration: feasibility of atrial pacing. Europace. 2009;11(9):1208–13.
8. Tchou P, Mehdirad AA. Bundle branch reentry ventricular tachycardia. Pacing Clin Electrophysiol. 1995;18(7):1427–37.
9. Touboul P, Kirkorian G, Atallah G, Moleur P. Bundle branch reentry: a possible mechanism of ventricular tachycardia. Circulation. 1983;67(3):674–80.

ECG 38

Razvan Mada

1 Case Presentation

A 73-year-old male patient with a past medical history of typical atrial flutter treated with catheter ablation of the CTI at the age of 67, recurrent symptomatic paroxysmal atrial fibrillation and atypical atrial flutter treated with catheter ablation 1 week prior to his presentation to the hospital, and amiodarone-induced hyperthyroidism was admitted to the Cardiology Department complaining of palpitations accompanied by asthenia and dyspnea on exertion, symptoms that had started 3 h prior to his presentation to the Emergency Department. The patient was on chronic antiarrhythmic treatment with Flecainide 200 mg/day, which was continued after the catheter ablation procedure. His GFR at admittance was 35 mL/min, compared to 55 mL/min 1 week prior. Transthoracic echocardiography showed an LVEF of 50%.

His ECG recorded at admittance to the Cardiology Department is presented in Fig. 1.

Question: What is the nature of the rhythm presented in Fig. 1?

(a) Ventricular tachycardia originating from the inferior lateral LV wall
(b) Ventricular tachycardia originating from the inferior septal LV wall
(c) Bundle branch re-entry ventricular tachycardia
(d) Antidromic tachycardia using a right-sided bypass tract
(e) Atrial tachycardia with 2:1 atrioventricular conduction and left bundle branch block

Hint: A second ECG recorded 24 h later is presented in Fig. 2.

Correct answer: e. Atrial tachycardia with 2:1 atrioventricular conduction and left bundle branch block.

Explanation: The ECG in Fig. 1 shows a regular wide QRS complex tachycardia with a heart rate of 152 bpm and LBBB morphology. The width of the QRS complex is 220 ms (contrary to what is automatically measured as 140 ms) (Fig. 3). The QRS axis is at −60°.

The differential diagnosis of this regular wide QRS complex tachycardia with LBBB morphology includes: ventricular tachycardia (myocardial-related VT and bundle branch re-entry VT), supraventricular tachycardia (atrial flutter, atrial tachycardia, AVNRT, and AVRT) with functional or pre-existing bundle branch block, and antidromic tachycardia (in pre-excitation syndromes).

R. Mada (✉)
Department of Cardiology, "Niculae Stancioiu" Heart Institute, Cluj-Napoca, Romania

L. Muresan (ed.), *ECG Interpretation of Wide QRS Complex Tachycardia*,
https://doi.org/10.1007/978-3-031-97030-6_39

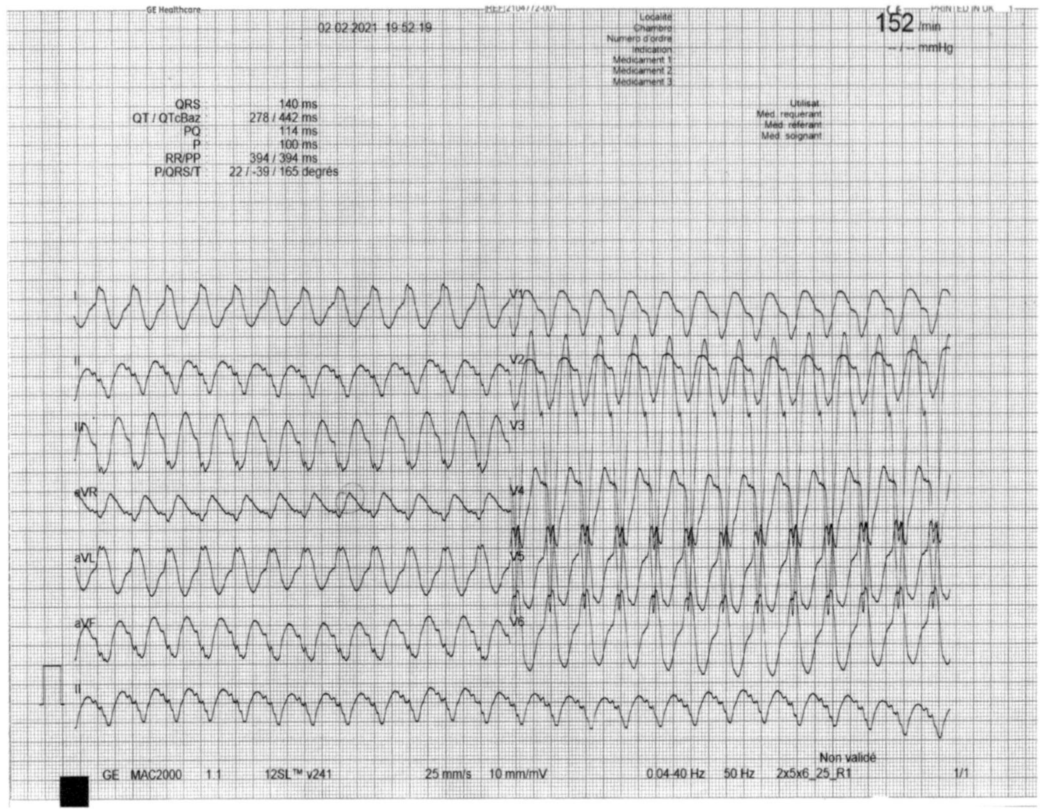

Fig. 1 Twelve-lead ECG recorded at admittance to the Cardiology Department

The morphology of the left bundle branch block of the QRS complex during tachycardia from Fig. 1 is that of a typical one [1]: the QRS duration is >120 ms; the QRS has a "QS'" pattern in lead V1 and a unique notched R wave in leads I and aVL; there is a "notched unique R wave" in leads V5 and V6. Therefore, at this point of the analysis, we cannot say whether this is VT, SVT with BBB, or antidromic tachycardia.

The ECG from Fig. 2 shows atrial tachycardia with an atrial rate close to 300 bpm, with variable atrioventricular conduction and a ventricular rate of 92 bpm. The QRS complexes are narrow. There are no signs of ventricular pre-excitation. This makes antidromic tachycardia unlikely as the correct diagnosis for the tachycardia from Fig. 1.

Applying the Brugada algorithm [2] to the tachycardia from Fig. 1, it can be seen that: 1. There is no absence of an RS complex in the precordial leads (otherwise said, there are rS complexes in leads V2 to V4); we therefore move to the second step of the algorithm: 2. This step analyzes the absence of an R-to-S interval > 100 ms in any precordial lead. This is not the case (Fig. 4). Step 3 of the algorithm looks for AV dissociation. A careful analysis of the atrial rhythm identifies the presence of P (or possibly F) waves, one before each QRS complex, best visible in lead II (Fig. 5). There is no A–V dissociation. We therefore need to move on to step 4 of the algorithm.

For a wide QRS complex tachycardia with LBBB, arguments in favor of VT are: the presence of an "r wave" > 0.04 s in lead V1 or V2, which is not the case [3]; or the presence of a "QS" in lead V6 or the presence of Josephson's sign, which is not the case. Therefore, according

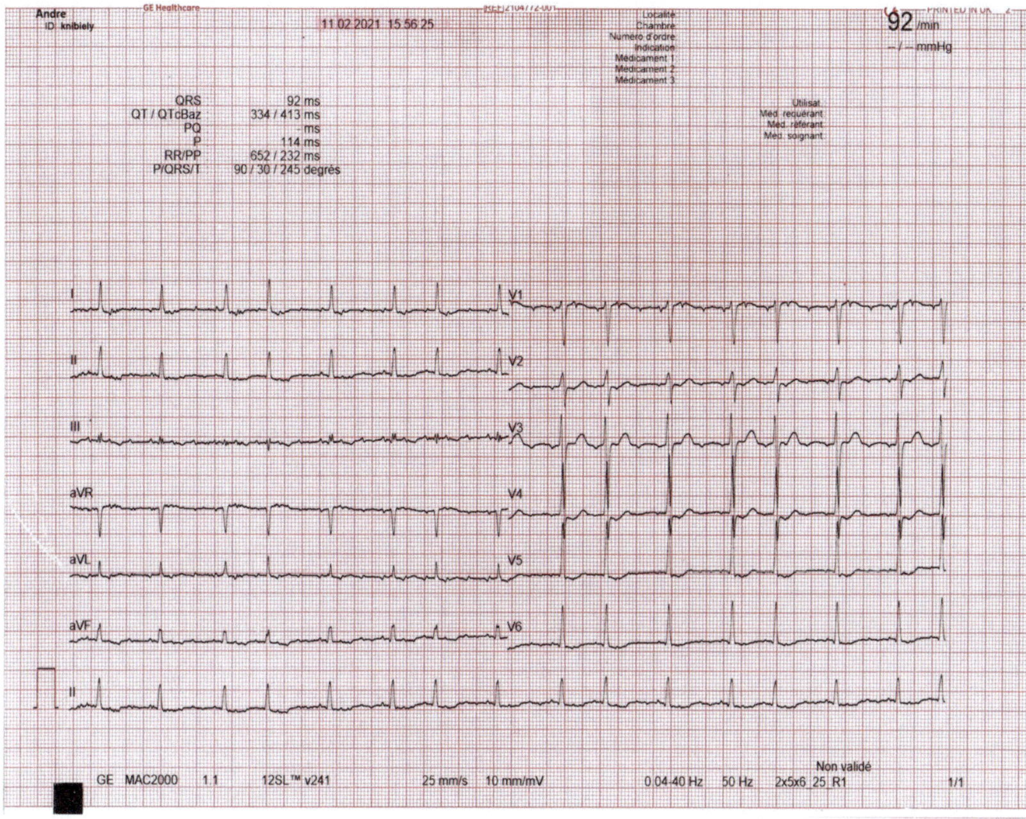

Fig. 2 Twelve-lead ECG recorded 24 h after the first ECG

to the Brugada algorithm, there are no arguments in favor of VT, and the tachycardia is SVT with BBB.

The Vereckei algorithm [4] for the differential diagnosis of wide QRS complex tachycardias also suggests SVT with BBB as the correct answer. The first step of the algorithm looks for A–V dissociation, which is not evaluable on the present ECG. The second step of the algorithm looks for an initial predominant R wave in lead aVR, which, again, is not the case (Fig. 3). The third step "QRS morphology unlike BBB or fascicular block" suggests SVT with BBB, based on the arguments explained above [1].

The Basel algorithm [5] also suggests SVT with BBB as the correct answer. There is no criterion present in favor of a ventricular origin of the wide QRS complex tachycardia: there are no clinical high-risk features (no history of myocardial infarction, no congestive heart failure or LVEF of <35%, and no ICD or CRT device implanted). The other criteria: the time to the first peak in lead II > 40 ms (Fig. 6) and the time to the first peak in lead aVR > 40 ms (Fig. 7) are not present on the ECG from Fig. 1 either. In the Basel algorithm, the diagnosis of ventricular tachycardia can be established if at least two criteria are present, which is not the case for this patient.

Apart from these algorithms, there are two criteria favoring the diagnosis of ventricular tachycardia: 1. for an LBBB QRS morphology, a QRS duration of over 160 ms [6]; 2. a duration of >60 ms from the onset of the QRS to the nadir of the S wave in lead V1 (Fig. 8) [3].

The clinical context of the patient is in favor of Flecainide overdose in the context of acute renal failure (Flecainide is renally excreted), with subsequent QRS enlargement. The patient presented an episode of atrial tachycardia after the catheter

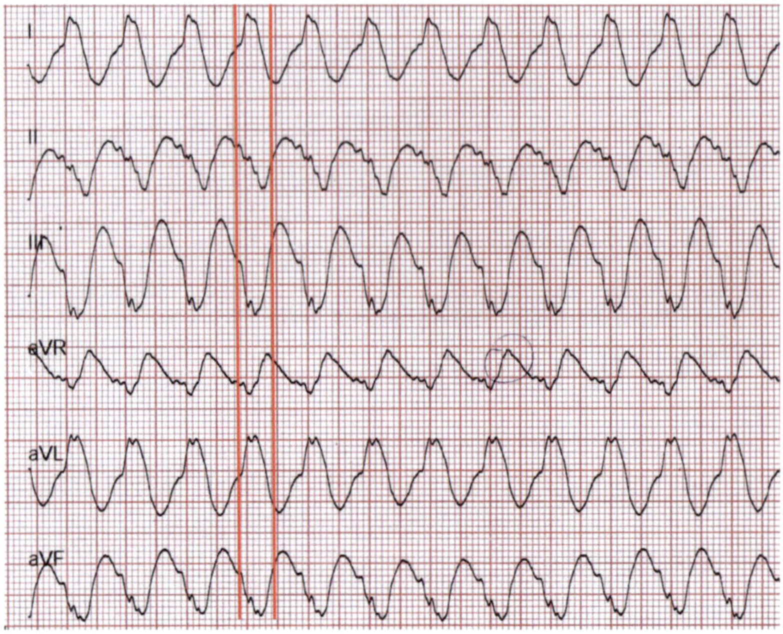

Fig. 3 Limb leads from the ECG presented in Fig. 1 showing the width of the QRS complex of 180 ms

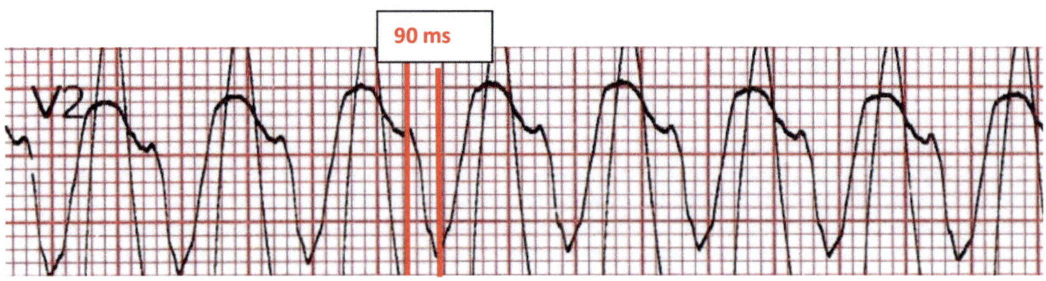

Fig. 4 Detailed analysis of the QRS morphology in lead V2 during the wide QRS complex tachycardia. The RS interval measures 90 ms. This is not diagnostic of ventricular tachycardia (but it does not exclude it either)

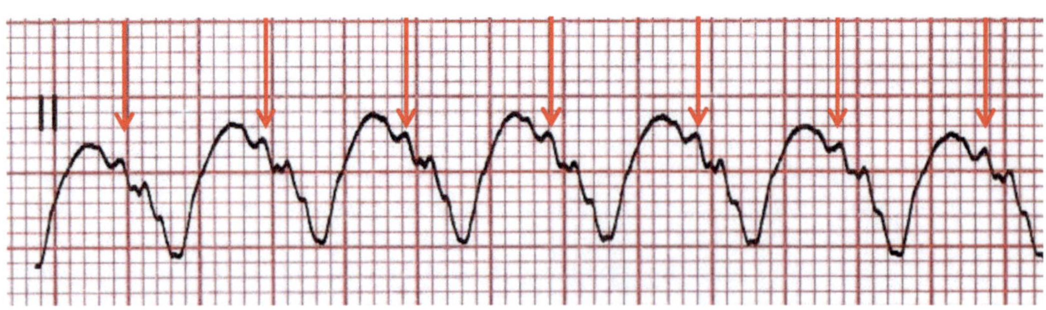

Fig. 5 Detailed analysis of the QRS morphology in lead V2 during the wide QRS complex tachycardia. P (or possibly F) waves are present (red arrows), with one such wave preceding each QRS complex. Therefore, there is no atrioventricular dissociation, and this is not diagnostic of ventricular tachycardia (but it does not exclude it either)

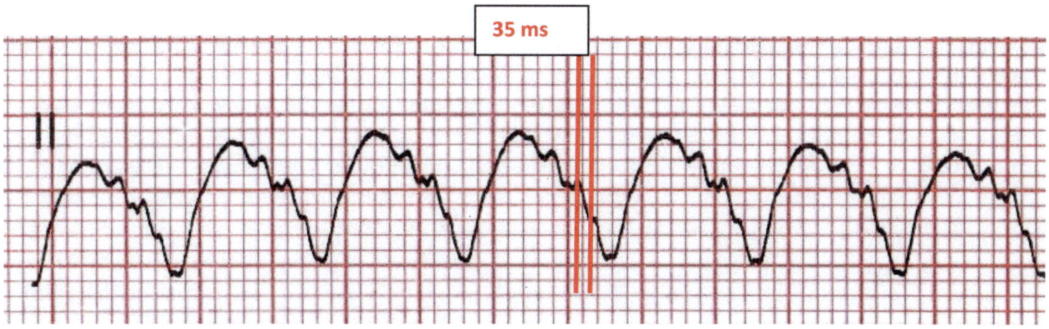

Fig. 6 Lead II from the ECG from Fig. 1 showing the time to the first peak of 35 ms, argument not in favor of ventricular tachycardia (but not excluding it either)

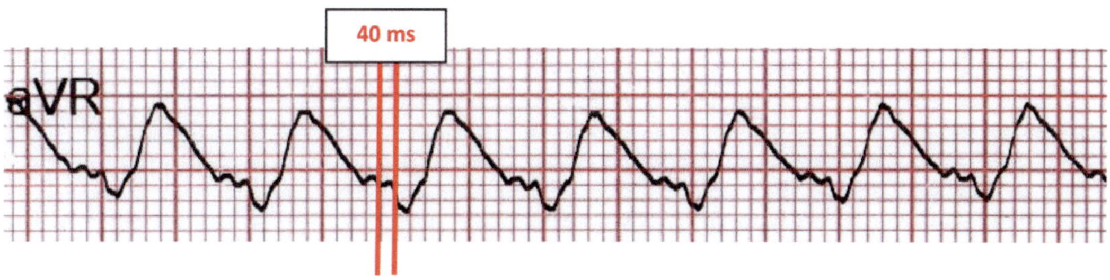

Fig. 7 Lead aVR from the ECG from Fig. 1 showing the time to the first peak of 40 ms, argument not in favor of ventricular tachycardia (but not excluding it either)

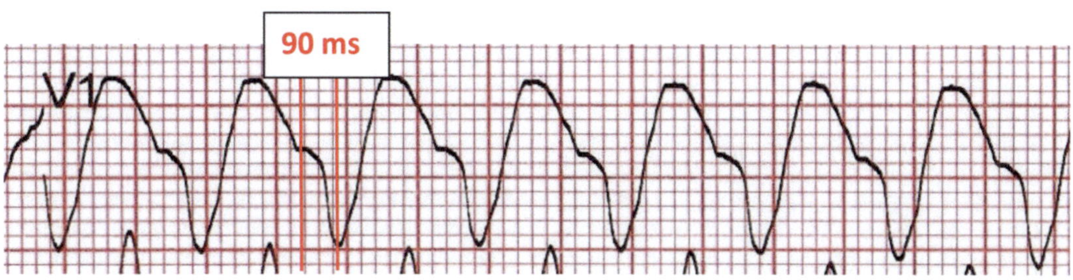

Fig. 8 Lead V1 from the ECG from Fig. 1 showing a duration of >60 ms from the onset of the QRS to the nadir of the S wave, argument in favor of ventricular tachycardia

ablation procedure, as seen in Fig. 2. Flecainide is a class IC antiarrhythmic drug which has as a mechanism of action slowing of conduction. The ECG in Fig. 1 shows atrial tachycardia with 2:1 conduction and functional LBBB.

Flecainide was immediately stopped.

A second catheter ablation procedure was performed, which confirmed the diagnosis of macroreentry atrial tachycardia (counterclockwise peri-mitral) atrial flutter. Ablation of the mitral isthmus converted atrial flutter to sinus rhythm (Fig. 9).

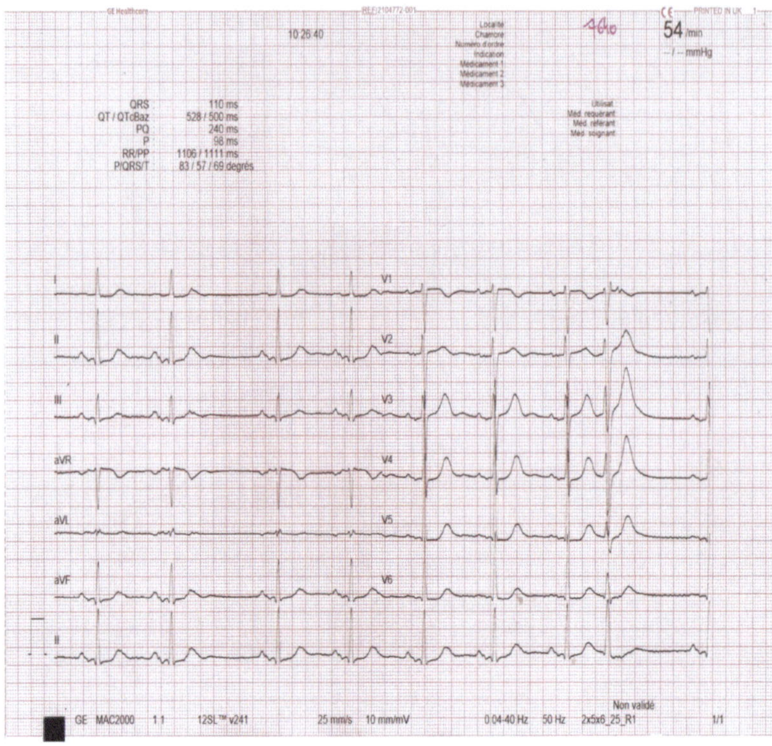

Fig. 9 Twelve-lead ECG after the catheter ablation of the peri-mitral flutter

References

1. Surawicz B, Childers R, Deal BJ, Gettes LS, Bailey JJ, Gorgels A, et al. AHA/ACCF/HRS recommendations for the standardization and interpretation of the electrocardiogram: part III: intraventricular conduction disturbances: a scientific statement from the American Heart Association Electrocardiography and Arrhythmias Committee, Council on Clinical Cardiology; the American College of Cardiology Foundation; and the Heart Rhythm Society. Endorsed by the International Society for Computerized Electrocardiology. J Am Coll Cardiol. 2009;53(11):976–81.
2. Brugada P, Brugada J, Mont L, Smeets J, Andries EW. A new approach to the differential diagnosis of a regular tachycardia with a wide QRS complex. Circulation. 1991;83(5):1649–59.
3. Kindwall KE, Brown J, Josephson ME. Electrocardiographic criteria for ventricular tachycardia in wide complex left bundle branch block morphology tachycardias. Am J Cardiol. 1988;61(15):1279–83.
4. Vereckei A, Duray G, Szenasi G, Altemose GT, Miller JM. Application of a new algorithm in the differential diagnosis of wide QRS complex tachycardia. Eur Heart J. 2007;28(5):589–600.
5. Moccetti F, Yadava M, Latifi Y, Strebel I, Pavlovic N, Knecht S, et al. Simplified integrated clinical and electrocardiographic algorithm for differentiation of wide QRS complex tachycardia: the Basel algorithm. JACC Clin Electrophysiol. 2022;8(7):831–9.
6. Eckardt L, Breithardt G, Kirchhof P. Approach to wide complex tachycardias in patients without structural heart disease. Heart. 2006;92(5):704–11.

ECG 39

Raphael Martins

1 Case Presentation

An 84-year-old male patient with a history of ischemic heart disease treated with triple CABG at the age of 64 years (2004), arterial hypertension, persistent atrial fibrillation, dyslipidemia, and chronic renal failure is admitted to the Cardiology Department for an episode of decompensated heart failure (dyspnea on exertion, nocturnal paroxysmal dyspnea, and peripheral edema) that had progressively worsened over the previous 2 weeks prior to his presentation to the hospital. His ECG recorded at admittance to the Cardiology Department is presented in Fig. 1.

Question: What is the nature of the tachycardia presented in Fig. 1?

(a) Atrial fibrillation and bifascicular block (RBBB and LPFB)
(b) Sinus rhythm with bifascicular block (RBBB and LPFB) and first-degree AV block
(c) Ventricular pre-excitation using a left-sided bypass tract
(d) Accelerated idioventricular rhythm originating from the lateral wall of the LV
(e) Accelerated idioventricular rhythm originating from the septal wall of the LV

R. Martins (✉)
Department of Cardiology, CHU Rennes, Rennes, France
e-mail: raphael.martins@chu-rennes.fr

Hint: A second ECG recorded several minutes later is presented in Fig. 2.

Correct answer: d. Accelerated idioventricular rhythm originating from the lateral wall of the LV.

Explanation: The first ECG shows a regular wide QRS complex rhythm with a heart rate of 92 bpm and RBBB morphology. The width of the QRS complex is 222 ms. The differential diagnosis of this wide QRS complex rhythm includes: accelerated idioventricular rhythm and supraventricular rhythm (atrial fibrillation, atrial flutter, atrial tachycardia, AVNRT, and AVRT) with functional bundle branch block and ventricular pre-excitation.

The morphology of the right bundle branch block of the QRS complex during tachycardia from Fig. 1 might look like a typical one [1]: the QRS duration is of >120 ms; there is an "RsR'" pattern in lead V1; the QRS complex has an "RS" morphology in leads I and aVL and an "rS" morphology in leads V5 and V6; and there is ST segment and T wave modifications opposite to the major deflection of the QRS complex; however, the R-to-S ratio in lead V6 is <1, which is not characteristic of a typical RBBB.

The ECG recorded outside the episode of palpitations can sometimes provide valuable clues

L. Muresan (ed.), *ECG Interpretation of Wide QRS Complex Tachycardia*,
https://doi.org/10.1007/978-3-031-97030-6_40

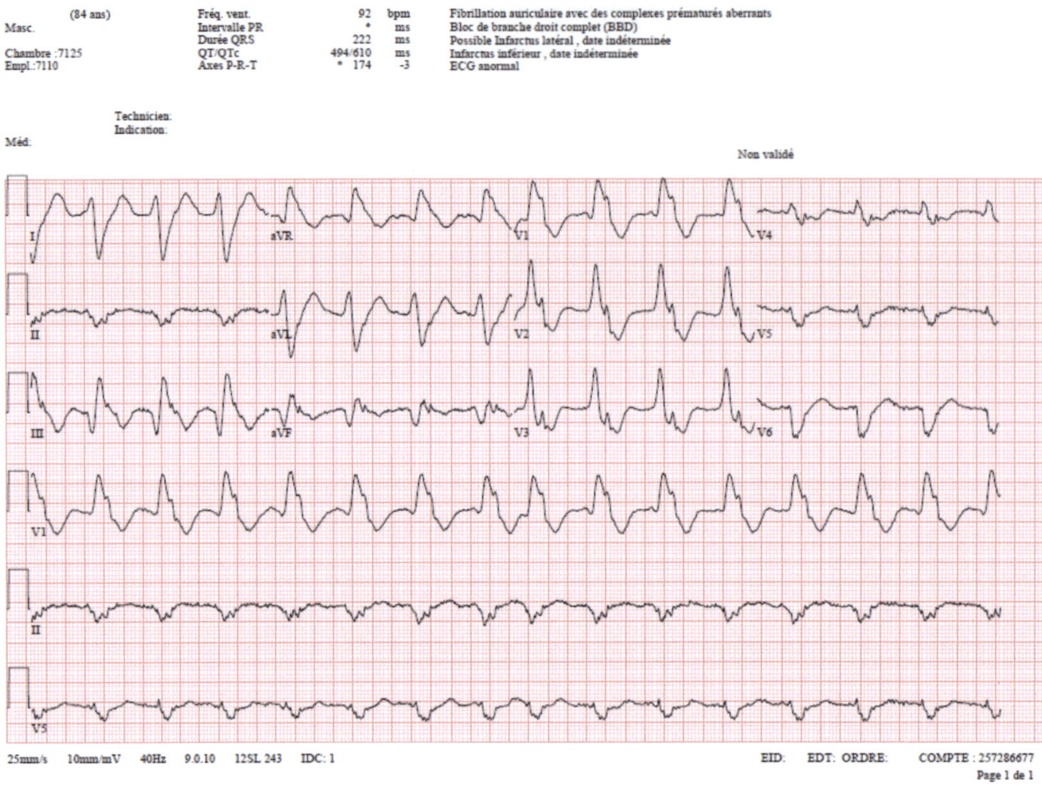

Fig. 1 Twelve-lead ECG recorded at admittance to the Cardiology Department

concerning the most likely and the most unlikely nature of the tachycardia. In the present case, the ECG in Fig. 2 shows atrial fibrillation with a heart rate of 47 bpm, QRS axis at +80°, absence of hypertrophy, negative T waves in leads V4–V6, DII, DIII, and aVF. There are no pathological Q waves in favor of an old myocardial infarction and no elements in favor of ventricular pre-excitation (short PR interval and delta waves). The absence of ventricular pre-excitation on this ECG suggests answer c—"Ventricular pre-excitation using a left-sided bypass tract"—less likely (but not impossible, since transient pre-excitation not recorded on this ECG could still be the case). There is also no RBBB, in favor of a supraventricular rhythm with pre-existing RBBB.

Coming back to the ECG of the wide QRS complex tachycardia, applying the Brugada algorithm [2], it can be seen that: 1. There is no absence of an RS complex in the precordial leads (otherwise said, there are RS complexes in leads V5 and V6). 2. Analysis of the R-to-S interval in any precordial leads finds an interval of more than 100 ms in lead V2 (see Fig. 3). This is an argument in favor of ventricular tachycardia.

Other arguments in favor of VT from the Brugada algorithm, for an RBBB morphology wide QRS complex tachycardia, are the presence of a taller left peak of the QRS complex in lead V1 (the rabbit ear sign) (Fig. 4). Next, in lead V6, an argument in favor of VT is the presence of an "rS" complex. This can also be expressed as a ratio of R/S < 1 in lead V6 (Fig. 5). Therefore, according to the Brugada algorithm, the rhythm on the ECG from Fig. 1 is ventricular in origin.

The Vereckei algorithm [3] for the differential diagnosis of wide QRS complex tachycardias also suggests VT as the correct answer. The first step of the algorithm looks for A–V dissociation, which is not seen on the present ECG (the atrial rhythm is atrial fibrillation, as can be seen on the ECG from Fig. 2). The second step of the algorithm looks for an initial predominant R wave in lead aVR, which is not the case, the morphology

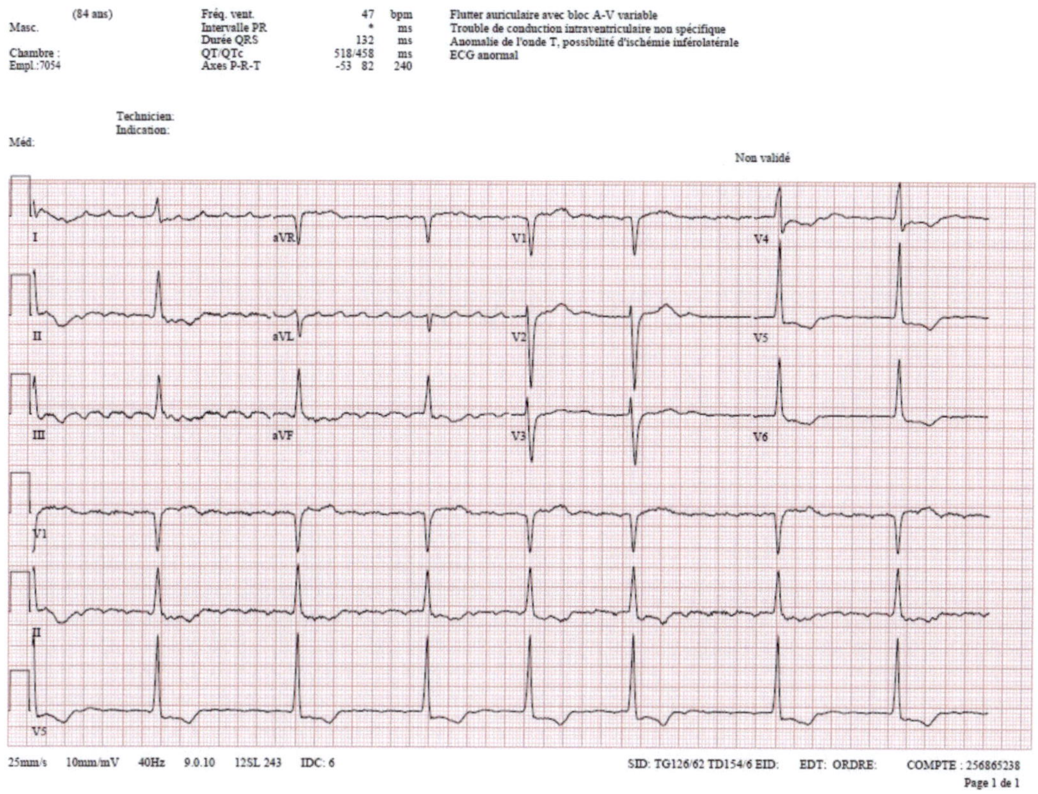

Fig. 2 Twelve-lead ECG recorded several minutes later

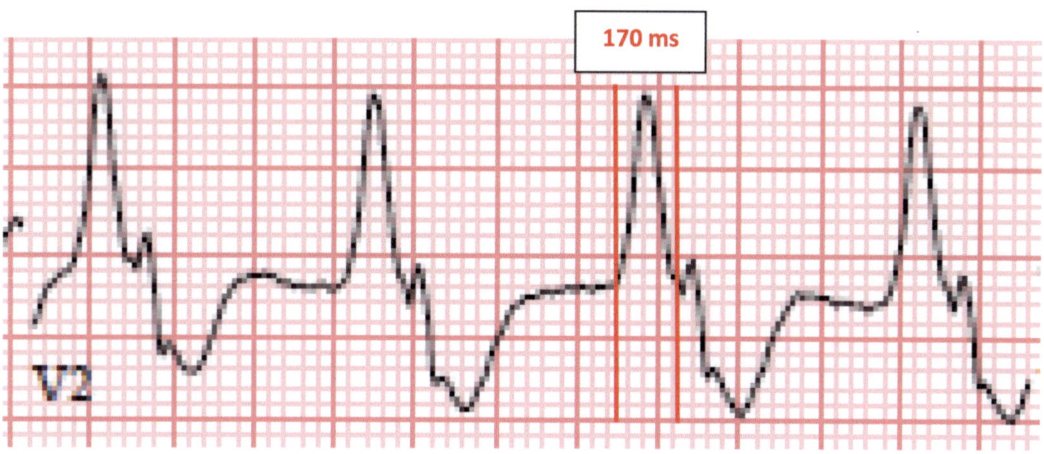

Fig. 3 Lead V3 from the ECG presented in Fig. 1 showing an R-to-S interval of 170 ms, the argument in favor of ventricular tachycardia

being "qR" (Fig. 6). We therefore move to the third step of the algorithm.

The third step "QRS morphology unlike BBB or fascicular block" does not suggest SVT with BBB, based on the arguments explained above (R-to-S ratio < 1 in lead V6). Therefore, based on the Vereckei algorithm, the nature of the tachycardia is also ventricular.

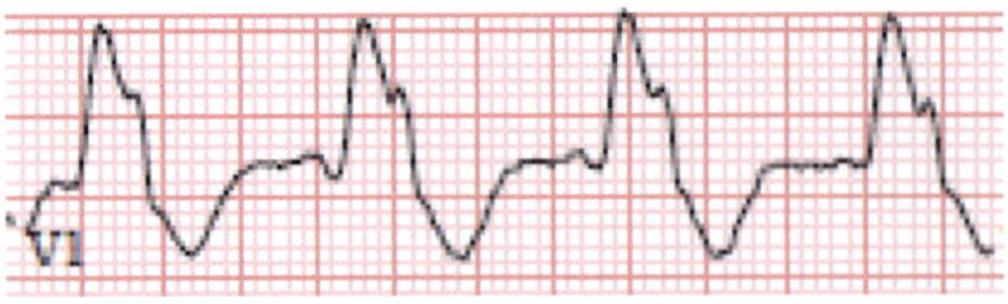

Fig. 4 Lead V1 from the ECG presented in Fig. 1 showing the presence of a taller left peak of the QRS complex in lead V1 (the rabbit ear sign), criterion in favor of ventricular tachycardia

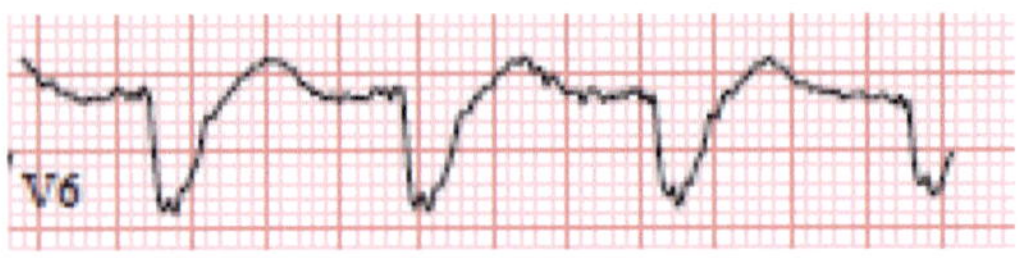

Fig. 5 Lead V6 from the ECG presented in Fig. 1 showing an R-to-S ratio < 1, argument in favor of ventricular tachycardia

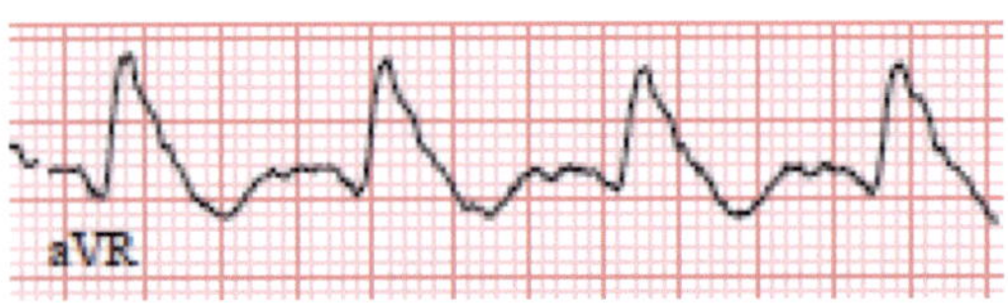

Fig. 6 Lead aVR from the tachycardia presented in Fig. 1, showing an initial R wave, criterion in favor of ventricular tachycardia

Other arguments in favor of ventricular tachycardia are the QRS duration of over 140 ms for a RBBB morphology wide QRS complex tachycardia [4].

Based on all these observations, the rhythm presented in Fig. 1 is accelerated idioventricular rhythm.

The origin of this idioventricular rhythm is in the left ventricle (RBBB morphology) at the level of the lateral wall (predominant S waves in leads I and aVL).

References

1. Surawicz B, Childers R, Deal BJ, Gettes LS, Bailey JJ, Gorgels A, et al. AHA/ACCF/HRS recommendations for the standardization and interpretation of the electrocardiogram: part III: intraventricular conduction disturbances: a scientific statement from the American Heart Association Electrocardiography and Arrhythmias Committee, Council on Clinical Cardiology; the American College of Cardiology Foundation; and the Heart Rhythm Society. Endorsed by the International Society for Computerized Electrocardiology. J Am Coll Cardiol. 2009;53(11):976–81.
2. Brugada P, Brugada J, Mont L, Smeets J, Andries EW. A new approach to the differential diagnosis of a regular tachycardia with a wide QRS complex. Circulation. 1991;83(5):1649–59.
3. Vereckei A, Duray G, Szenasi G, Altemose GT, Miller JM. Application of a new algorithm in the differential diagnosis of wide QRS complex tachycardia. Eur Heart J. 2007;28(5):589–600.
4. Vereckei A, Duray G, Szenasi G, Altemose GT, Miller JM. New algorithm using only lead aVR for differential diagnosis of wide QRS complex tachycardia. Heart Rhythm. 2008;5(1):89–98.

ECG 40

Ronan Le Bouar

1 Case Presentation

A 33-year-old male patient with a history of dextrocardia, L-transposition of the great arteries, ventricular septal defect (VSD), atrial septal defect (ASD), treated with repeated surgical interventions (arterial switch procedure, closure of the VSD and of the ASD, and surgical relief of the subpulmonary obstruction), and paroxysmal atrial fibrillation is admitted to the Cardiology Department for an episode of palpitations accompanied by dyspnea, anxiety, and lightheadedness that had occurred 20 min prior to his presentation to the hospital. His ECG recorded at admittance is presented in Fig. 1.

Question: What is the nature of the tachycardia presented in Fig. 1?

(a) Ventricular tachycardia originating from the RVOT
(b) Ventricular tachycardia originating from the LVOT
(c) Bundle branch re-entry ventricular tachycardia
(d) Antidromic tachycardia using a right-sided bypass tract
(e) Atrial tachycardia with left bundle branch block

Hint: A second ECG recorded after electrical cardioversion is presented in Fig. 2.

Observation: The ECG electrodes were placed over the patient's right anterior thorax because of dextrocardia.

Correct answer: a. Ventricular tachycardia originating from the anterior RVOT.

Explanation: The ECG in Fig. 1 shows a regular wide QRS complex tachycardia with a heart rate of 185 bpm and LBBB morphology. The width of the QRS complex is 140 ms. The QRS axis is at +105°. The differential diagnosis of this regular wide QRS complex tachycardia with LBBB morphology includes: ventricular tachycardia (myocardial-related VT and bundle branch re-entry VT), supraventricular tachycardia (atrial flutter, atrial tachycardia, AVNRT, and AVRT) with functional or pre-existing bundle branch block and antidromic tachycardia (in pre-excitation syndromes).

The ECG from Fig. 2 shows sinus rhythm with a heart rate of 87 bpm, QRS axis at +20°, absence of LV hypertrophy, nonspecific intraventricular conduction delay (QRS duration of

R. Le Bouar (✉)
Department of Cardiology, Emile Muller Hospital, Mulhouse, France
e-mail: LEBOUARR@ghrmsa.fr

L. Muresan (ed.), *ECG Interpretation of Wide QRS Complex Tachycardia*,
https://doi.org/10.1007/978-3-031-97030-6_41

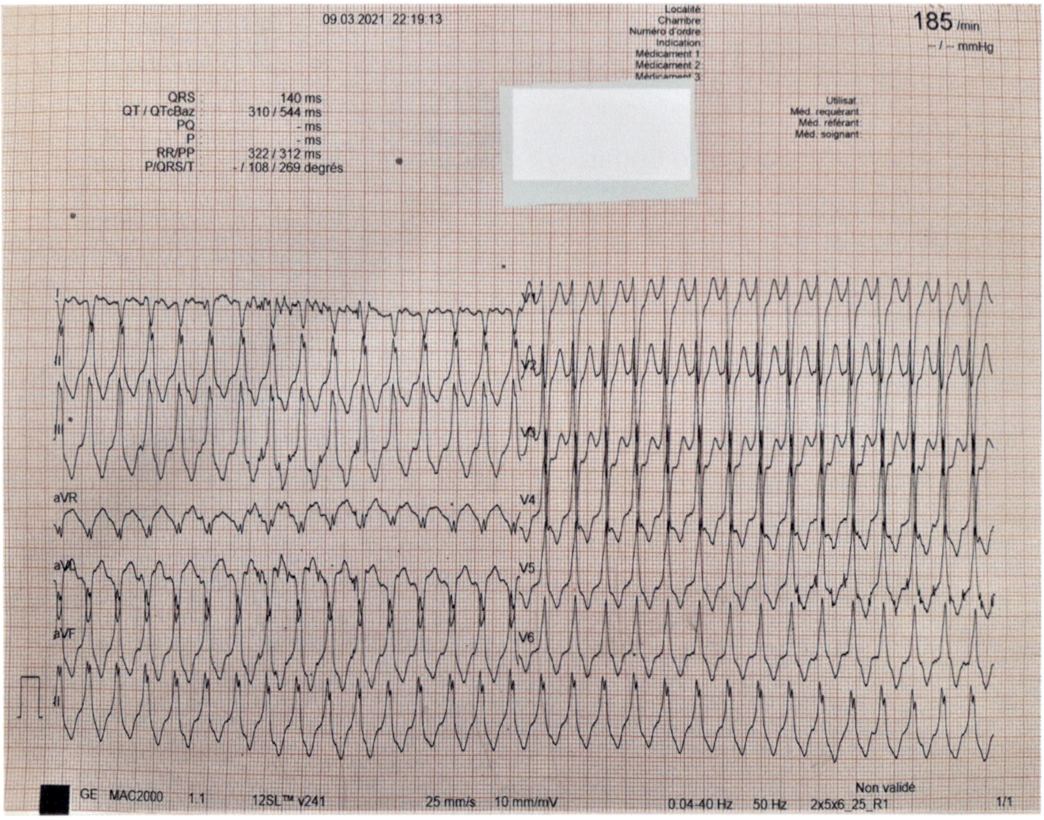

Fig. 1 Twelve-lead ECG recorded at admittance to the Cardiology Department

128 ms), and one isolated PVC (in the beginning of the recording). There are no signs of ventricular pre-excitation (no short PR interval and no delta waves), which makes ventricular pre-excitation unlikely.

The morphology of the left bundle branch block of the QRS complex during tachycardia from Fig. 1 suggests that it might be a typical one [1]: the QRS duration is >120 ms; the QRS is predominantly negative in lead V1, with a "typical" unique R wave in leads V5 and V6; and there is ST segment and T wave modification opposite to the major deflection of the QRS complex: ST segment elevation with positive T waves in leads V1 and V2 and ST segment depression with negative T waves in leads V5 and V6. However, the QRS complex has a "Qr" morphology in lead I and a "QS" morphology in lead aVL, with a precordial transition in lead V4. The r wave in lead V1 is greater than 0.04 ms. All these elements are not in favor of a typical left bundle branch block. This makes SVT with aberrancy unlikely.

Applying the Brugada algorithm [2] to the tachycardia from Fig. 2, it can be seen that there is no absence of an RS complex in the precordial leads (otherwise said, there are rS complexes in leads V1 to V3) (Fig. 3); we therefore move to the second step of the algorithm.

The second step analyzes the absence of an R-to-S interval > 100 ms in any precordial lead. When measured in lead V1, the RS interval is 110 ms (Fig. 4). This is an argument in favor of ventricular tachycardia.

The Vereckei algorithm [3] for the differential diagnosis of wide QRS complex tachycardias also suggests VT as the correct answer. The first step of the algorithm looks for A–V dissociation, which is not seen on the present ECG. The sec-

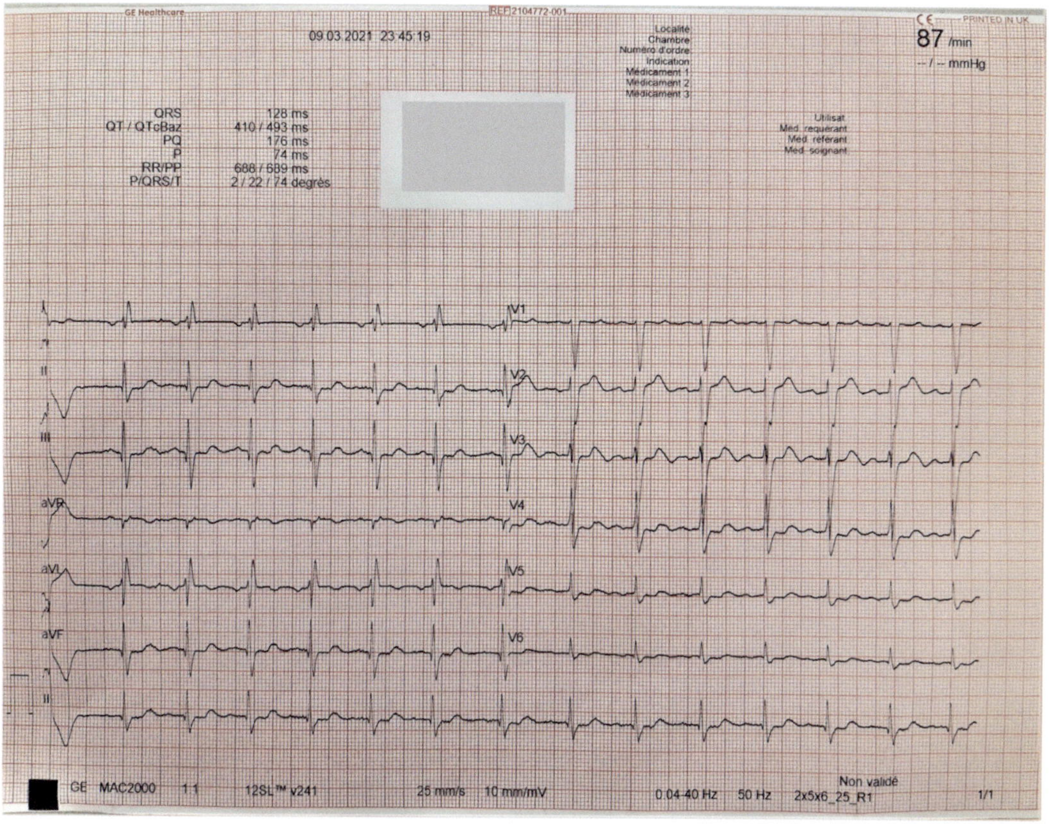

Fig. 2 Twelve-lead ECG recorded after electrical cardioversion

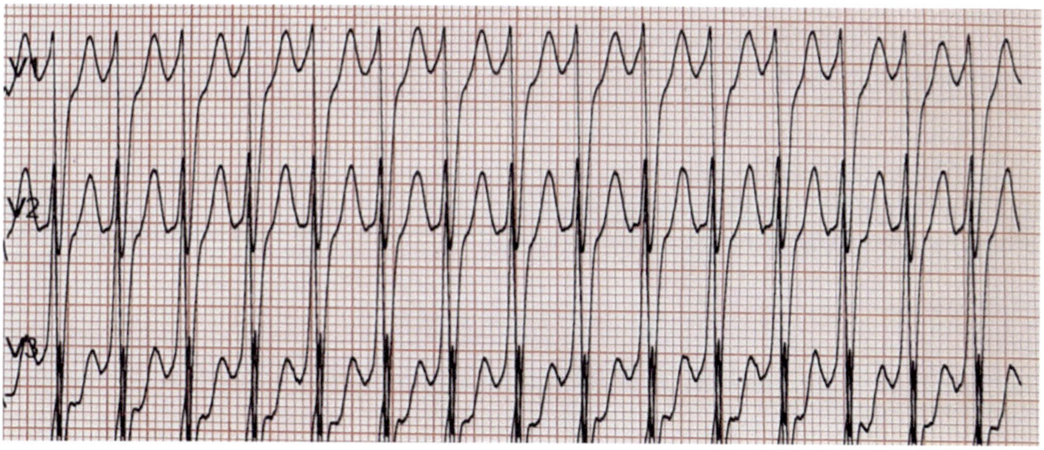

Fig. 3 Leads V1 to V3 from the ECG presented in Fig. 1 demonstrating the presence of RS complexes, argument not in favor of ventricular tachycardia (but not excluding it either)

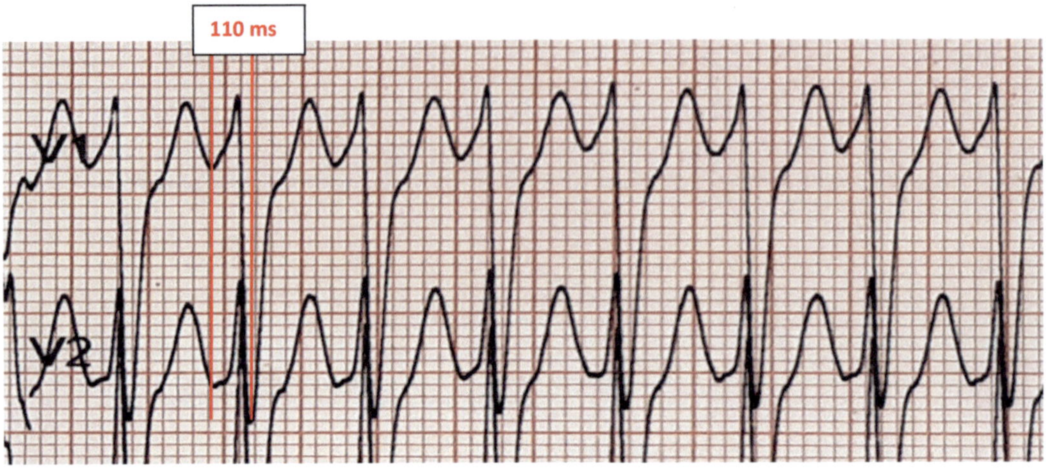

Fig. 4 Lead V1 from the ECG presented in Fig. 1 demonstrating an R-to-S interval of 110 ms, argument in favor of ventricular tachycardia

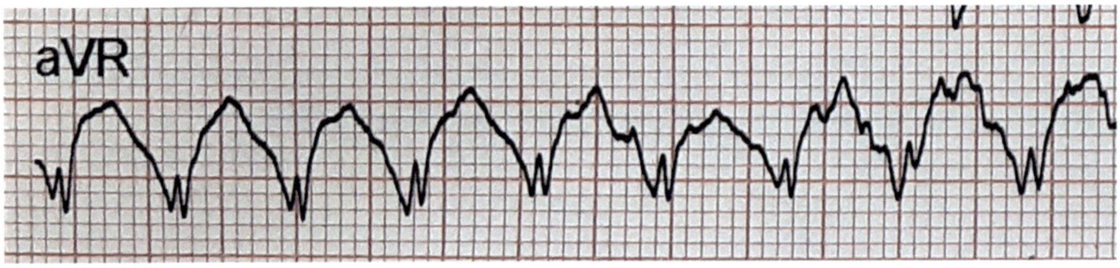

Fig. 5 Lead aVR from the tachycardia presented in Fig. 1, showing the absence of an initial positive tall R wave, criterion not in favor of ventricular tachycardia (but not excluding it either)

ond step of the algorithm looks for an initial predominant R wave in lead aVR, which, again, is not the case (Fig. 5).

The third step "QRS morphology unlike BBB or fascicular block" does not suggest SVT with BBB, based on the arguments presented above: "Qr" morphology in lead I and "QS" in lead aVL, with a precordial transition in lead V4, and the presence of an "r wave" in lead V1 greater than 0.04 ms.

Based on these arguments, the diagnosis of ventricular tachycardia is retained.

The origin of the tachcyardia is the outflow tract region, given its LBBB aspect and inferior axis [4–8]. The precordial transition in lead V3 is in favor of a RVOT origin [4, 7]. This is concordant with the underlying pathology: scar in the RVOT after the surgical relief of the subpulmonary obstruction.

References

1. Surawicz B, Childers R, Deal BJ, Gettes LS, Bailey JJ, Gorgels A, et al. AHA/ACCF/HRS recommendations for the standardization and interpretation of the electrocardiogram: part III: intraventricular conduction disturbances: a scientific statement from the American Heart Association Electrocardiography and Arrhythmias Committee, Council on Clinical Cardiology; the American College of Cardiology Foundation; and the Heart Rhythm Society. Endorsed by the International Society for Computerized Electrocardiology. J Am Coll Cardiol. 2009;53(11):976–81.
2. Brugada P, Brugada J, Mont L, Smeets J, Andries EW. A new approach to the differential diagnosis of a regular tachycardia with a wide QRS complex. Circulation. 1991;83(5):1649–59.
3. Vereckei A, Duray G, Szenasi G, Altemose GT, Miller JM. Application of a new algorithm in the differential diagnosis of wide QRS complex tachycardia. Eur Heart J. 2007;28(5):589–600.
4. Anderson RD, Kumar S, Parameswaran R, Wong G, Voskoboinik A, Sugumar H, et al. Differentiating right-

and left-sided outflow tract ventricular arrhythmias: classical ECG signatures and prediction algorithms. Circ Arrhythm Electrophysiol. 2019;12(6):e007392.
5. Hachiya H, Aonuma K, Yamauchi Y, Harada T, Igawa M, Nogami A, et al. Electrocardiographic characteristics of left ventricular outflow tract tachycardia. Pacing Clin Electrophysiol. 2000;23(11 Pt 2):1930–4.
6. Hoffmayer KS, Bhave PD, Marcus GM, James CA, Tichnell C, Chopra N, et al. An electrocardiographic scoring system for distinguishing right ventricular outflow tract arrhythmias in patients with arrhythmogenic right ventricular cardiomyopathy from idiopathic ventricular tachycardia. Heart Rhythm. 2013;10(4):477–82.
7. Mariani MV, Piro A, Della Rocca DG, Forleo GB, Pothineni NV, Romero J, et al. Electrocardiographic criteria for differentiating left from right idiopathic outflow tract ventricular arrhythmias. Arrhythmia Electrophysiol Rev. 2021;10(1):10–6.
8. Yu M, Liu J, Zhang H, Xia Y, Li X, Fang P. Distinguishing ventricular arrhythmias originating from the posterior right ventricular outflow tract, or near the right coronary cusp or near the his-bundle. Am J Cardiol. 2020;126:37–44.

ECG 41

Crina Muresan

1 Case Presentation

A 70-year-old male patient with a history of recent aortic valve replacement for severe aortic stenosis, tricuspid annuloplasty for severe secondary tricuspid regurgitation (performed 3 days prior), paroxysmal atrial fibrillation, and ischemic stroke is admitted to the Cardiology Department due to repeated episodes of a wide QRS complex rhythm recorded by telemetry in the Post-Surgical Cardiac Surgery Unit. His ECG recorded at admittance to the Cardiology Department is presented in Fig. 1.

Question: What is the nature of the rhythm presented in Fig. 1?

(a) Slow antidromic tachycardia using a left-sided bypass tract
(b) Atrial fibrillation with ventricular pre-excitation
(c) Sinus rhythm with antegrade conduction over the fast and the slow pathway (double-firing) and right bundle branch block
(d) Atrial fibrillation with right bundle branch block
(e) Accelerated idioventricular rhythm originating from the left ventricle

C. Muresan (✉)
Department of Cardiology, Emile Muller Hospital, Mulhouse, France
e-mail: crina.muresan@ghrmsa.fr

Hint: A second ECG recorded several minutes later is presented in Fig. 2.

Correct answer: e. Accelerated idioventricular rhythm originating from the left ventricle.

Explanation: The ECG in Fig. 1 shows a regular wide QRS complex rhythm with a heart rate of 86 bpm and RBBB morphology. The width of the QRS complex is 170 ms. The QRS axis is at +115°. The differential diagnosis of this regular wide QRS complex rhythm with RBBB morphology includes: accelerated idioventricular rhythm, a supraventricular rhythm (atrial fibrillation and sinus rhythm) with functional or pre-existing right bundle branch block, and a supraventricular rhythm with ventricular pre-excitation.

The morphology of the right bundle branch block of the QRS from Fig. 1 is certainly not that of a typical one [1]: the QRS duration is indeed >120 ms, and the QRS complex is positive in lead V1; with the exception of the first QRS complex from the limb leads, the QRS has an "rS" pattern; however, there is a monomorphic R wave in lead V1, a "QS" pattern in lead aVL, and there is a "unique R" pattern in leads V5 and V6, which is not at all compatible with a typical RBBB. This makes answers c and d highly unlikely.

L. Muresan (ed.), *ECG Interpretation of Wide QRS Complex Tachycardia*,
https://doi.org/10.1007/978-3-031-97030-6_42

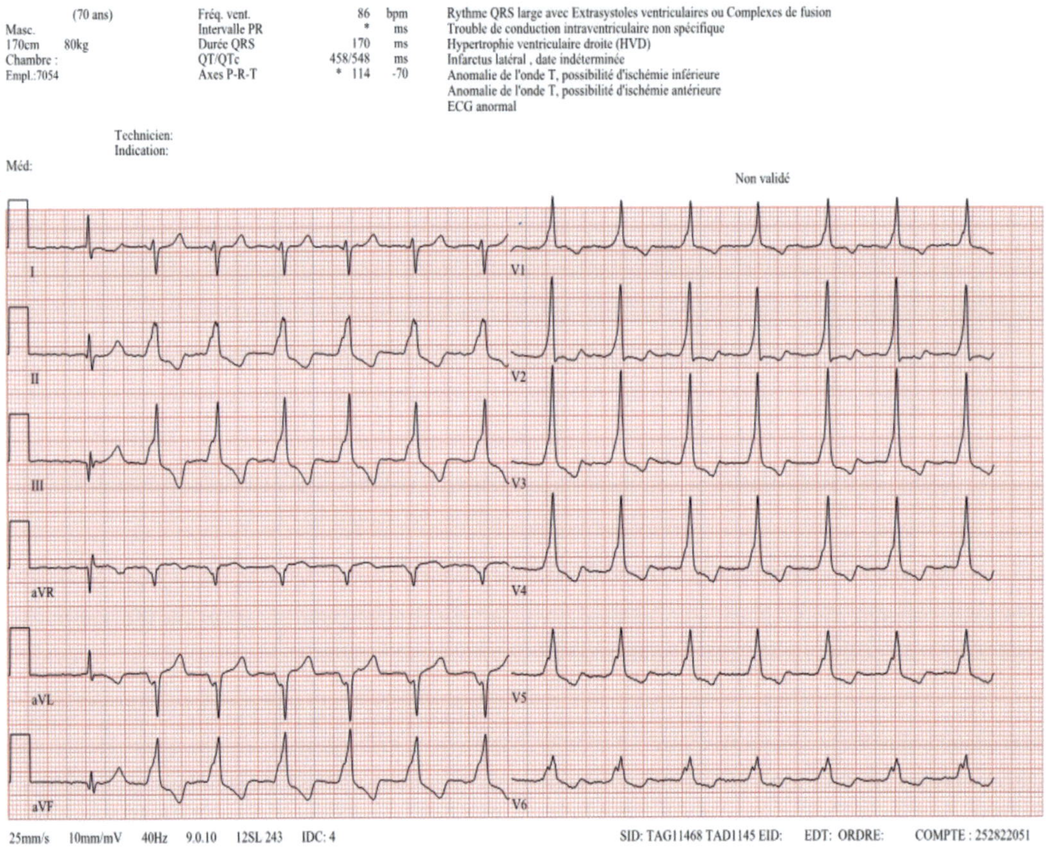

Fig. 1 Twelve-lead ECG recorded at admittance to the Cardiology Department

The ECG from Fig. 2 shows atrial fibrillation with a heart rate of 59 bpm, QRS axis at +30°, absence of LV hypertrophy, and absence of ischemia. There are no signs in favor of ventricular pre-excitation (no delta waves and no wide QRS complexes), which makes answers a and b highly unlikely.

Applying the Brugada algorithm [2] to the tachycardia from Fig. 1, it can be seen that there is an absence of an RS complex in the precordial leads (otherwise said, there are no rS complexes in leads V1 to V6) (Fig. 3). This is a strong argument in favor of a ventricular origin for the rhythm presented in Fig. 1.

The Vereckei algorithm [3] for the differential diagnosis of wide QRS complex tachycardias also suggests ventricular tachycardia as the correct answer. The first step of the algorithm looks for A–V dissociation, which is not seen on the present ECG, since the underlying rhythm is atrial fibrillation (Fig. 2). The second step of the algorithm looks for an initial predominant R wave in lead aVR, which, again, is not the case (Fig. 4).

The third step "QRS morphology unlike BBB or fascicular block" does not suggest SVT with BBB, based on the argument presented above.

Based on these arguments, the diagnosis of a ventricular origin of the rhythm presented in Fig. 1 can be retained. Given the heart rate of 86 bpm, the correct answer is accelerated idioventricular rhythm. Since the QRS complex has a "RBBB" morphology in lead V1, its origin is in the left ventricle.

Accelerated idioventricular rhythm can sometimes be observed post-aortic valve replacement (surgical or percutaneous) [4]. It is usually not associated with hemodynamic compromise, and it is usually transitory [5, 6]. In the absence of clinical and hemodynamic alterations, it does not require specific treatment [7, 8].

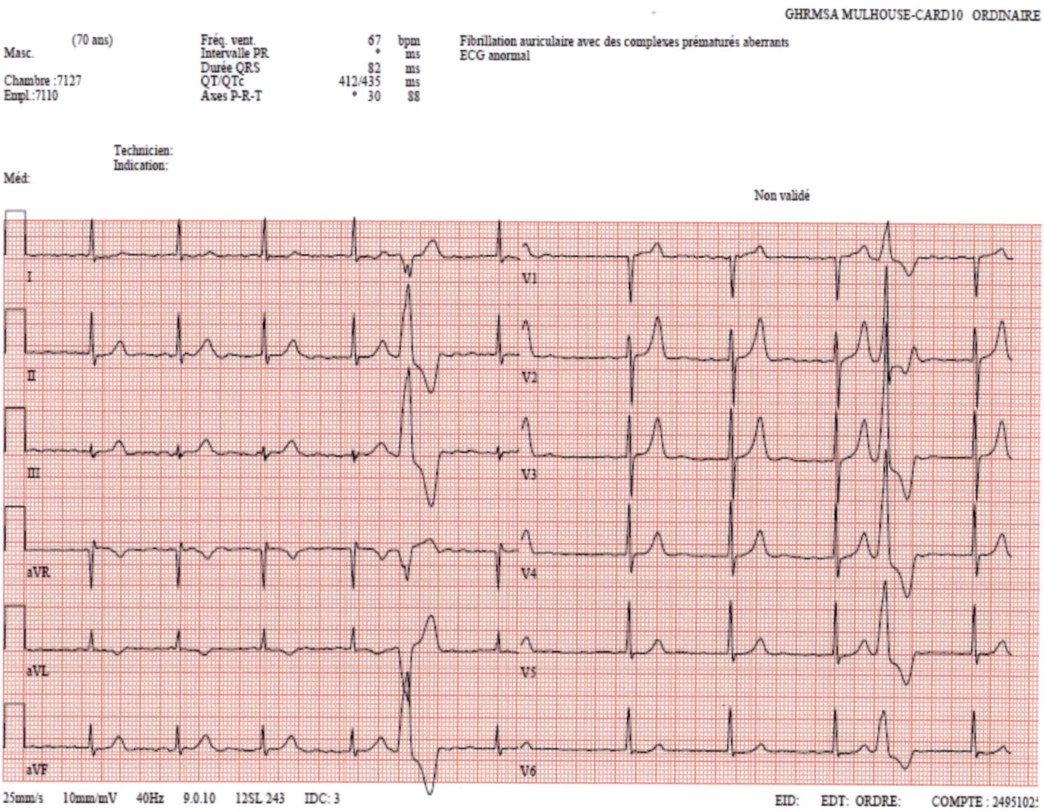

Fig. 2 Twelve-lead ECG recorded after the end of the episode of palpitations

Fig. 3 Precordial leads from the ECG recorded in Fig. 1 showing the absence of RS complexes, argument in favor of ventricular tachycardia

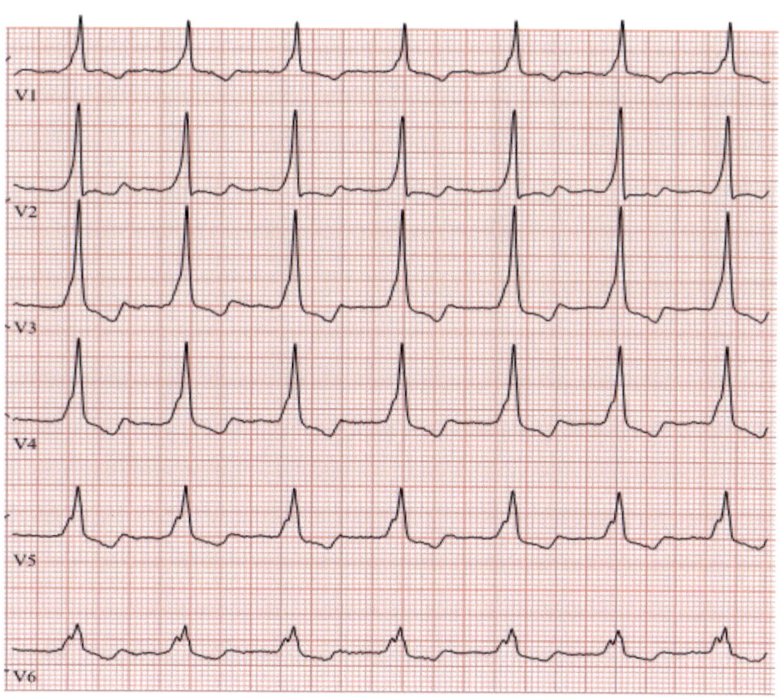

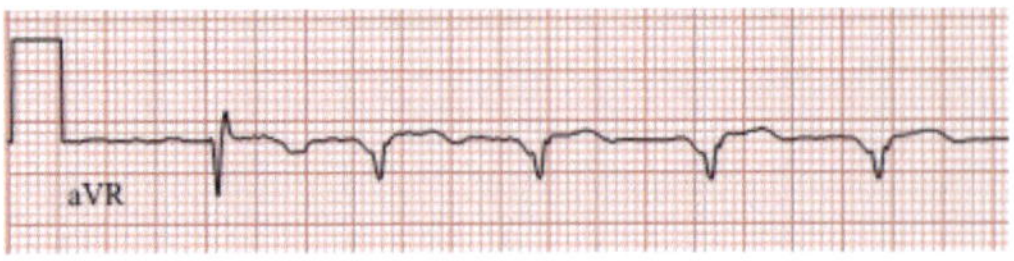

Fig. 4 Lead aVR from the tachycardia presented in Fig. 1, showing the absence of an initial positive tall R wave, criterion not in favor of ventricular tachycardia (but not excluding it either)

References

1. Surawicz B, Childers R, Deal BJ, Gettes LS, Bailey JJ, Gorgels A, et al. AHA/ACCF/HRS recommendations for the standardization and interpretation of the electrocardiogram: part III: intraventricular conduction disturbances: a scientific statement from the American Heart Association Electrocardiography and Arrhythmias Committee, Council on Clinical Cardiology; the American College of Cardiology Foundation; and the Heart Rhythm Society. Endorsed by the International Society for Computerized Electrocardiology. J Am Coll Cardiol. 2009;53(11):976–81.
2. Brugada P, Brugada J, Mont L, Smeets J, Andries EW. A new approach to the differential diagnosis of a regular tachycardia with a wide QRS complex. Circulation. 1991;83(5):1649–59.
3. Vereckei A, Duray G, Szenasi G, Altemose GT, Miller JM. Application of a new algorithm in the differential diagnosis of wide QRS complex tachycardia. Eur Heart J. 2007;28(5):589–600.
4. Morita Y, Endo A, Tanabe K. Accelerated Idioventricular rhythm following transcatheter self-expandable aortic valve implantation. Circ Rep. 2021;3(7):421–2.
5. Gildea TH, Levis JT. ECG diagnosis: accelerated idioventricular rhythm. Perm J. 2018;22:17–173.
6. Jakkoju A, Jakkoju R, Subramaniam PN, Glancy DL. Accelerated idioventricular rhythm. Proceedings. 2018;31(4):506–7.
7. Shirayama T, Nakagawa M. Accelerated idioventricular rhythm. Ryoikibetsu Shokogun Shirizu. 1996;12:458–60.
8. Riera AR, Barros RB, de Sousa FD, Baranchuk A. Accelerated idioventricular rhythm: history and chronology of the main discoveries. Indian Pacing Electrophysiol J. 2010;10(1):40–8.

ECG 42

Jacques Levy

1 Case Presentation

A 76-year-old female patient with a history of severe persistent extrinsic asthma, arterial hypertension, hypothyroidism, and dyslipidemia is admitted to the hospital for aggravated persistent dyspnea that had been going on for 10 days prior to her presentation. She was admitted to the Cardiology Department due to the presence of peripheral edema and increased levels of NT—pro BNP, for suspicion of heart failure. While in the Cardiology Department, she presented an episode of rapid palpitations, accompanied by severe dyspnea and anxiety. Her ECG recorded during the episode of palpitations is presented in Fig. 1.

Question: What is the nature of the tachycardia presented in Fig. 1?

(a) Intrafascicular re-entry ventricular tachycardia (posterior fascicle).
(b) Intrafascicular re-entry ventricular tachycardia (anterior fascicle).
(c) Interfascicular re-entry ventricular tachycardia.
(d) Antidromic tachycardia using a left-sided bypass tract.
(e) Atrial fibrillation with bifascicular block (RBBB + LPFB).

Hint: An ECG recorded several minutes later is presented in Fig. 2.

Correct answer: a. Atrial fibrillation with bifascicular block (RBBB + LPHB)

Explanation: The ECG in Fig. 1 shows an irregular wide QRS complex tachycardia with a heart rate of 165 bpm and RBBB morphology. The width of the QRS complex is 130 ms. The QRS axis is at +100°. The differential diagnosis of this irregular wide QRS complex tachycardia with RBBB morphology includes: ventricular tachycardia (myocardial-related VT and fascicular ventricular tachycardia), supraventricular tachycardia (atrial flutter, atrial tachycardia, AVNRT, and AVRT) with functional or preexisting bundle branch block. Antidromic tachycardia (in pre-excitation syndromes) is usually regular and unlikely present in this case.

The morphology of the right bundle branch block of the QRS complex during tachycardia from Fig. 1 is that of a typical one [1]: the QRS duration is >120 ms; the QRS morphology is "RSR'" in lead V1, and there is an RS pattern in leads I, aVL, V5, and V6. The R-to-S ratio in lead

J. Levy (✉)
Department of Cardiology, Emile Muller Hospital, Mulhouse, France
e-mail: LEVYJ@ghrmsa.fr

L. Muresan (ed.), *ECG Interpretation of Wide QRS Complex Tachycardia*,
https://doi.org/10.1007/978-3-031-97030-6_43

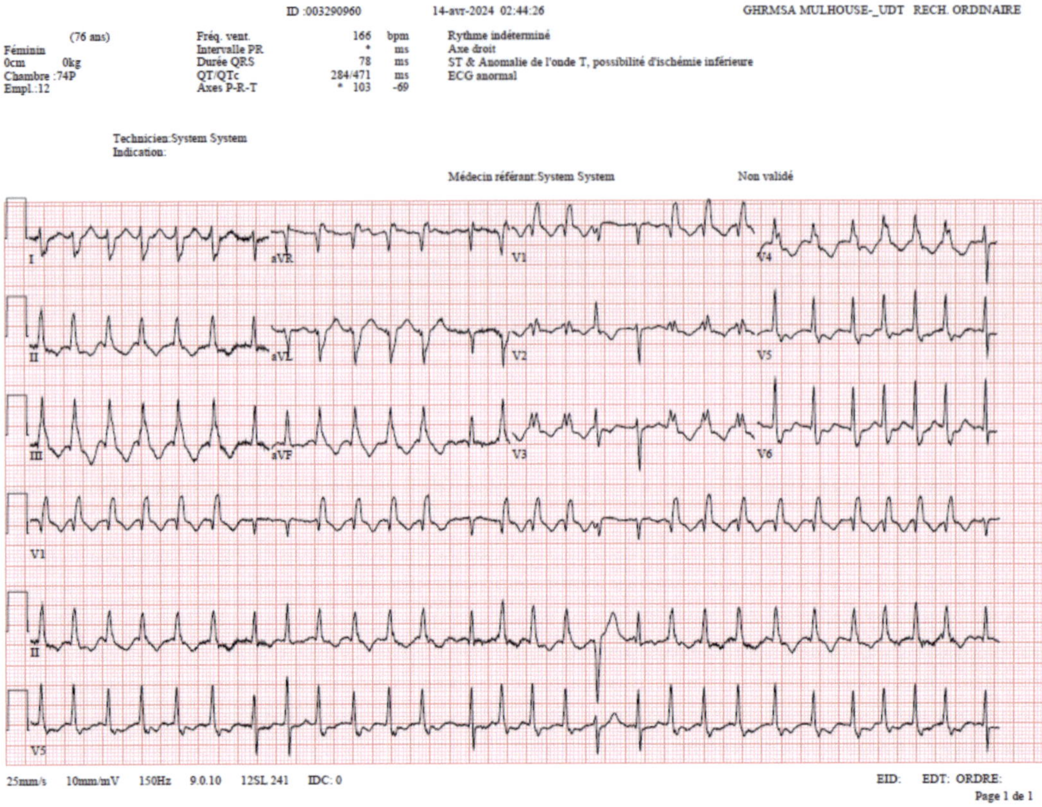

Fig. 1 Twelve-lead ECG recorded at admittance to the Cardiology Department

V6 is <1. Therefore, at this point of the analysis, we cannot say whether this is SVT with RBBB or VT.

The ECG from Fig. 2 shows sinus rhythm with a heart rate of 98 bpm, QRS axis at +70°, absence of LV hypertrophy, and absence of ischemia, with no signs of ventricular pre-excitation (no short PR interval and no delta waves). This makes antidromic tachycardia unlikely.

Applying the Brugada algorithm [2] to the tachycardia from Fig. 2, it can be seen that there is no absence of an RS complex in the precordial leads (otherwise said, there are rS complexes in leads V5 and V6) (Fig. 3); we therefore move to the second step of the algorithm.

The second step analyzes the absence of an R-to-S interval >100 ms in any precordial lead. This is not the case (Fig. 4).

Step 3 of the algorithm looks for A–V dissociation. If we analyze the atrial activity, there are no visible P waves. Therefore, we cannot say if there is AV dissociation. We therefore need to move to step 4 of the algorithm.

For an RBBB morphology wide QRS complex tachycardia, an argument in favor of VT would be the presence of a taller left peak of the QRS complex in lead V1 (the rabbit ear sign) or for biphasic RS or QR complexes, which is not the case. Next, in lead V6, an argument in favor of VT would be the presence of an "rS" complex, which is the case. This can also be expressed as a ratio of R/S < 1 in lead V6. This is also not the case (Fig. 4). Therefore, there are no arguments in favor of VT according to the Brugada algorithm.

The Vereckei algorithm [3] for the differential diagnosis of wide QRS complex tachycardias also finds no arguments in favor of VT. The first step of the algorithm looks for A–V dissociation, which is not seen on the present ECG. The sec-

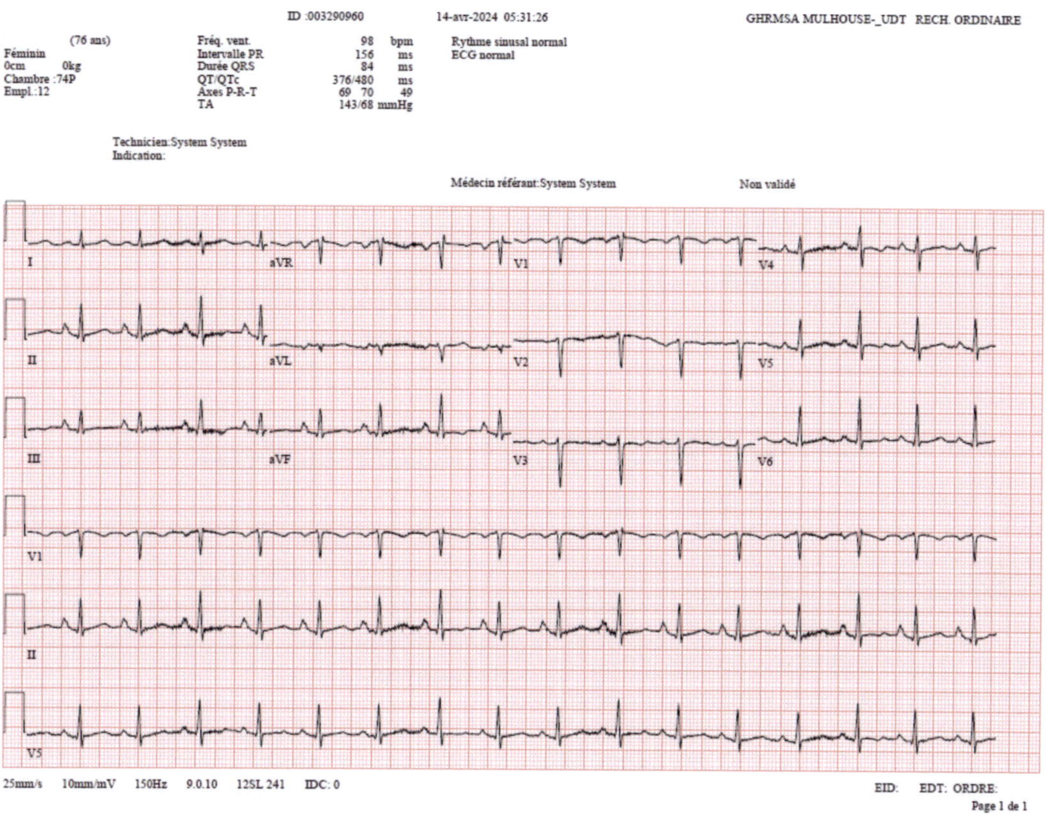

Fig. 2 Twelve-lead ECG recorded after the end of the episode of palpitations

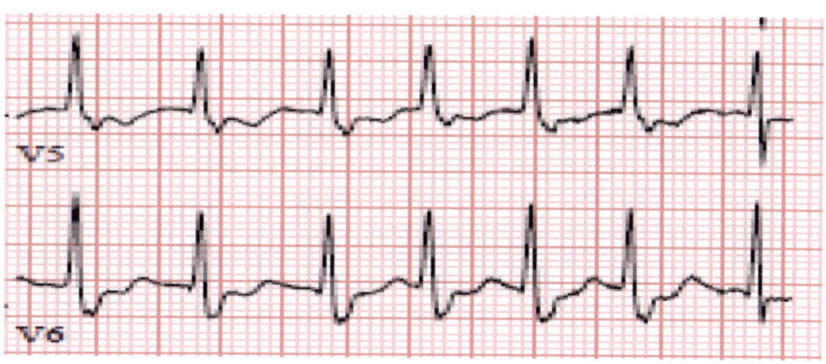

Fig. 3 Leads V5 and V6 from the ECG recorded in Fig. 1 showing the presence of RS complexes, argument not in favor of ventricular tachycardia (but not excluding it either)

ond step of the algorithm looks for an initial predominant R wave in lead aVR, which is not the case (Fig. 5).

The third step "QRS morphology unlike BBB or fascicular block" suggests SVT with RBBB, based on arguments exposed above.

These findings, together with the irregularity of the rhythm, are in favor of SVT with RBBB. A closer inspection of the ECG from Fig. 1 finds the presence of narrow QRS complexes, identical to the ones from the ECG 2. These QRS complexes are present when the preceding RR interval increases; otherwise said, the QRS complexes become large when the RR interval decreases, argument in favor of aberrant conduction. Therefore, this is functional (phase 3) RBBB. No P waves are present, and the rhythm is irregular; this is therefore atrial fibrillation with functional

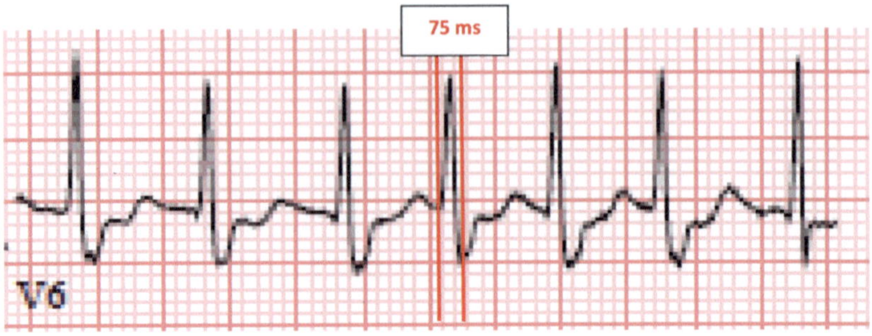

Fig. 4 Lead V6 from the ECG presented in Fig. 1 showing an R-to-S interval of 75 ms, argument not in favor of ventricular tachycardia (but not excluding it either)

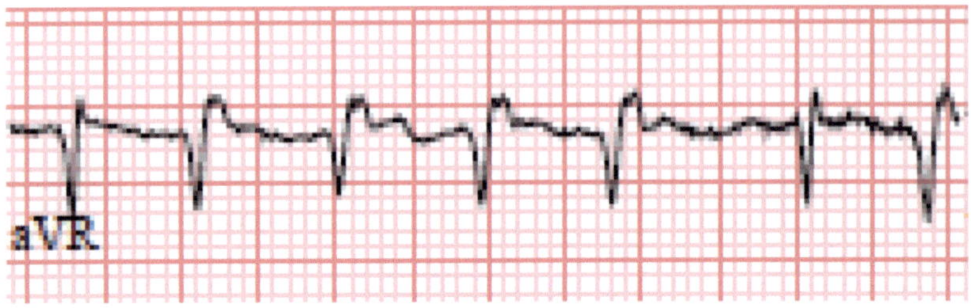

Fig. 5 Lead aVR from the tachycardia presented in Fig. 1, showing the absence of an initial positive tall R wave, criterion not in favor of ventricular tachycardia (but not excluding it either)

RBBB. There is a right axis deviation; therefore, there is associated LPFB. The correct answer is e—"Atrial fibrillation with RBBB and LPFB". The differential diagnosis of this tachycardia includes left posterior fascicular re-entry ventricular tachycardia. However, this type of VT is usually regular, and the "rabbit ear sign" is usually present in lead V1 (which is not the case for the present patient). The narrow QRS complexes should not be mistaken for capture beats during VT, since they represent normal conduction using the His–Purkinje system during atrial fibrillation. The longer RR interval preceding them allows the right bundle and the left posterior fascicle to recover conduction; functional BBB occurs when the RR interval shortens (phase 3 block).

References

1. Surawicz B, Childers R, Deal BJ, Gettes LS, Bailey JJ, Gorgels A, et al. AHA/ACCF/HRS recommendations for the standardization and interpretation of the electrocardiogram: part III: intraventricular conduction disturbances: a scientific statement from the American Heart Association Electrocardiography and Arrhythmias Committee, Council on Clinical Cardiology; the American College of Cardiology Foundation; and the Heart Rhythm Society. Endorsed by the International Society for Computerized Electrocardiology. J Am Coll Cardiol. 2009;53(11):976–81.
2. Brugada P, Brugada J, Mont L, Smeets J, Andries EW. A new approach to the differential diagnosis of a regular tachycardia with a wide QRS complex. Circulation. 1991;83(5):1649–59.
3. Vereckei A, Duray G, Szenasi G, Altemose GT, Miller JM. Application of a new algorithm in the differential diagnosis of wide QRS complex tachycardia. Eur Heart J. 2007;28(5):589–600.

ECG 43

Charline Daval

1 Case Presentation

A 76-year-old male patient with a history of non-ischemic cardiomyopathy with severe systolic dysfunction (LVEF of 15%), implanted with a dual-chamber ICD (Microport Platinum) for the primary prevention of sudden cardiac death, LV apical thrombus treated with oral anticoagulant, and ischemic stroke at the age of 71 years is admitted to the Cardiology Department for an episode of decompensated heart failure, presenting dyspnea on exertion and at rest, bilateral peripheral edema, and signs and symptoms that had progressively worsened during the previous 10 days prior to his presentation to the hospital. His ECG recorded at admittance is presented in Fig. 1.

Question: What is the nature of the tachycardia presented in Fig. 1?

(a) Ventricular tachycardia originating from the superior septal LV wall.
(b) Ventricular tachycardia originating from the superior septal RV wall.
(c) Antidromic tachycardia using a right-sided bypass tract.
(d) Atrial flutter with 2:1 A:V conduction and left bundle branch block.
(e) Supraventricular tachycardia with left bundle branch block.

Hint: A second ECG recorded several minutes later is presented in Fig. 2.

Correct answer: e. Supraventricular tachycardia with left bundle branch block

Explanation: The ECG in Fig. 1 shows a regular wide QRS complex tachycardia with a heart rate of 144 bpm and LBBB morphology. The width of the QRS complex is 144 ms. The QRS axis is at +110°. The differential diagnosis of this regular wide QRS complex tachycardia with LBBB morphology includes: ventricular tachycardia (myocardial-related VT and bundle branch re-entry VT), supraventricular tachycardia (atrial flutter, atrial tachycardia, AVNRT, and AVRT) with functional or pre-existing bundle branch block, and antidromic tachycardia (in pre-excitation syndromes).

There are possible P waves present at the end of each QRS complex, with a 1:1 QRS–P wave relationship (Fig. 3).

The morphology of the left bundle branch block of the QRS complex during tachycardia

C. Daval (✉)
Department of Cardiology, Emile Muller Hospital, Mulhouse, France
e-mail: charline.daval@ghrmsa.fr

L. Muresan (ed.), *ECG Interpretation of Wide QRS Complex Tachycardia*,
https://doi.org/10.1007/978-3-031-97030-6_44

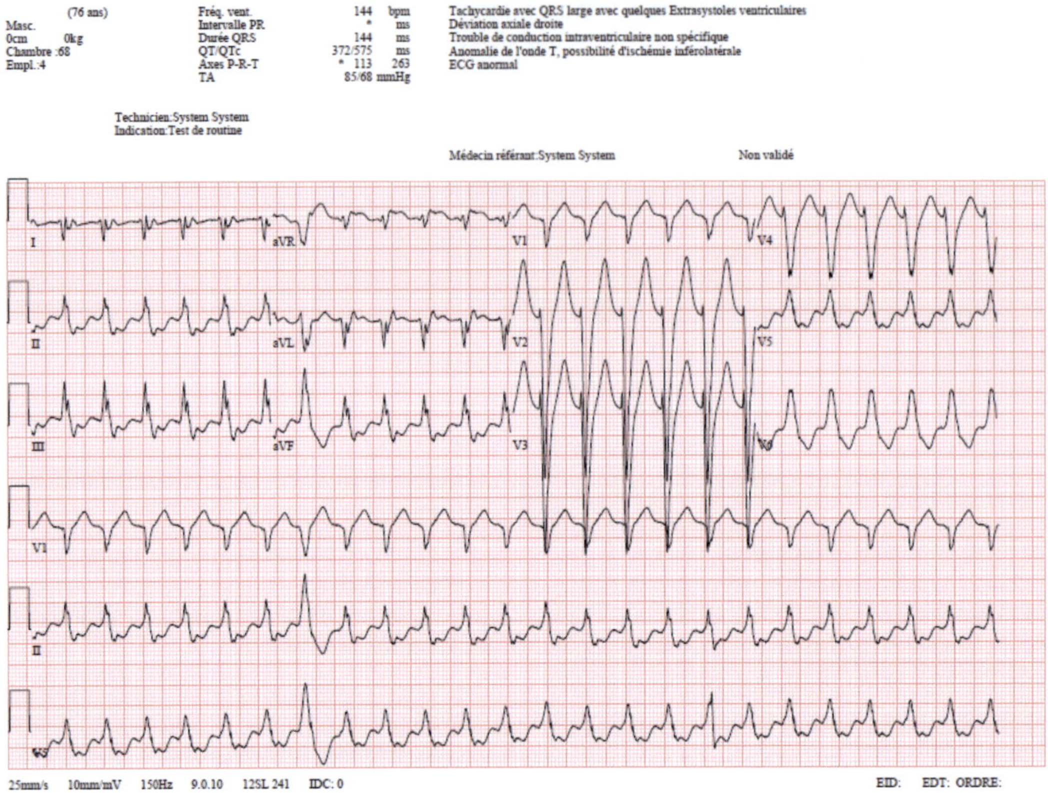

Fig. 1 Twelve-lead ECG recorded at admittance to the Cardiology Department

from Fig. 1 suggests that it might be a typical one [1]: the QRS duration is of >120 ms; there is a "QS" aspect in lead V1, a monomorphic notched R wave in leads V5 and V6; and there is ST segment and T wave modifications opposite to the major deflection of the QRS complex: ST segment elevation with positive T waves in leads V1 to V4. However, the QRS complex has an "rSr'" aspect in leads I and aVL, which is not characteristic of a typical LBBB.

Applying the Brugada algorithm [2] to the tachycardia from Fig. 2, it can be seen that there is no absence of an RS complex in the precordial leads (otherwise said, there are rS complexes in leads V2 to V4) (Fig. 4); we therefore move to the second step of the algorithm.

The second step analyzes the absence of an R-to-S interval >100 ms in any precordial lead. This is not the case (Fig. 5).

Step 3 of the algorithm looks for A–V dissociation. The P to QRS relationship is 1:1. This takes us to step 4 of the algorithm.

For a wide QRS complex tachycardia with LBBB, arguments in favor of VT are: the presence of an "r wave" >0.04 s in lead V1 or V2, which is not the case in the ECG presented in Fig. 1; the presence of a notched S wave in lead V1 or V2, which is also not the case; and the presence of a delayed S nadir >0.06 s in lead V1 or V2, which is also not the case (Fig. 3) [3]. So, according to the Brugada algorithm, there are no arguments in favor of VT.

Another argument in favor of ventricular tachycardia for an LBBB QRS morphology would be a QRS duration of over 160 ms [4], which is also not the case (QRS duration is of 144 ms).

The Vereckei algorithm [5] for the differential diagnosis of wide QRS complex tachycardias also suggests SVT as the correct answer. The first step of the algorithm looks for A–V dissociation, which is not seen on the present ECG. The second step of the algorithm looks for an initial predominant R wave

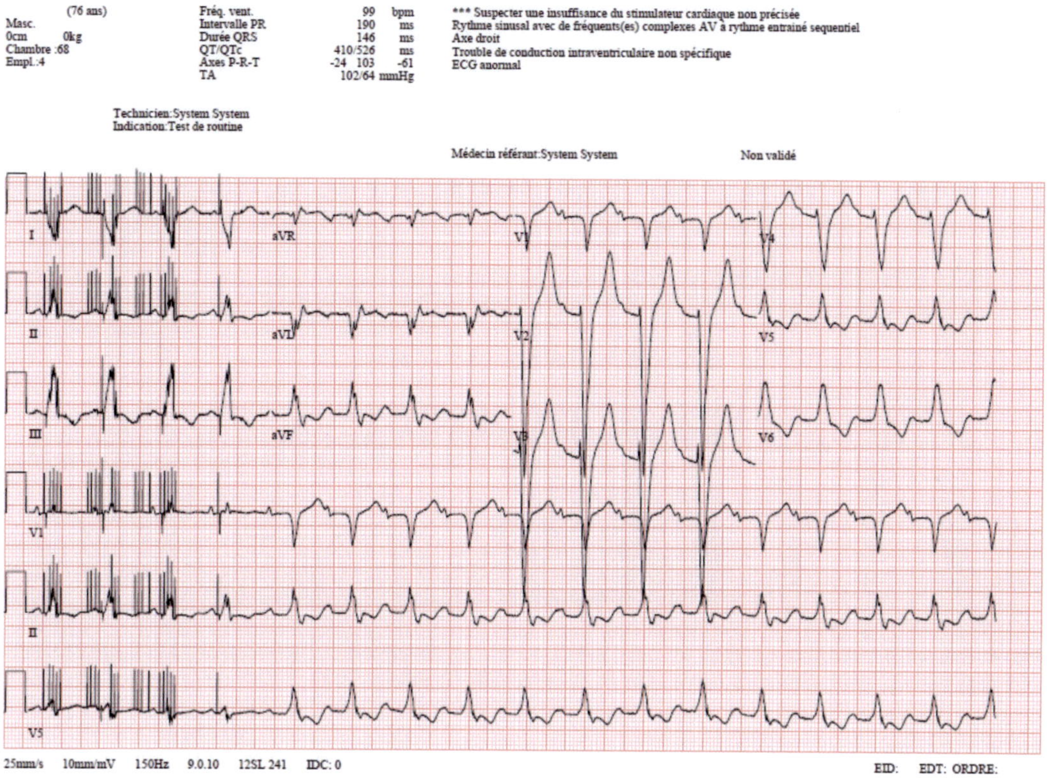

Fig. 2 Twelve-lead ECG recorded after the end of the episode of palpitations

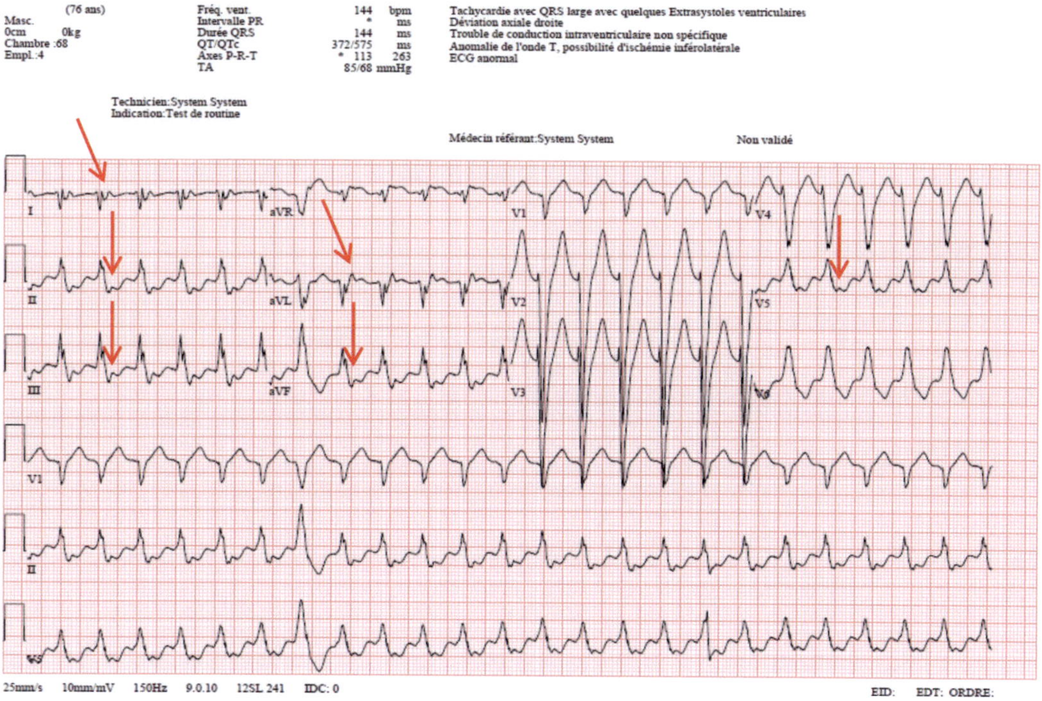

Fig. 3 The same ECG from Fig. 1, with red arrows indicating possible P waves, with a 1:1 P-to-QRS relationship

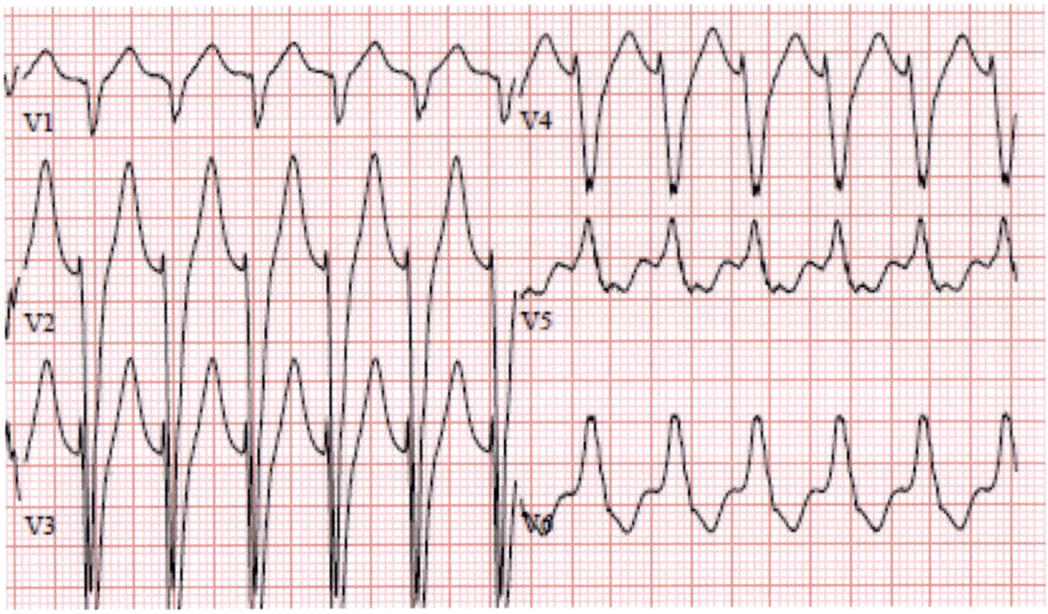

Fig. 4 Precordial leads from the ECG recorded in Fig. 1 showing the presence of RS complexes in leads V2 to V4, argument not in favor of ventricular tachycardia (but not excluding it either)

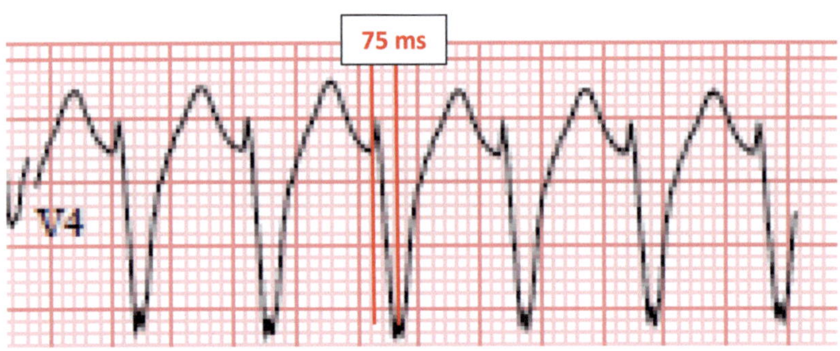

Fig. 5 Lead V6 from the ECG presented in Fig. 1 showing an R-to-S interval of 75 ms, argument not in favor of ventricular tachycardia (but not excluding it either)

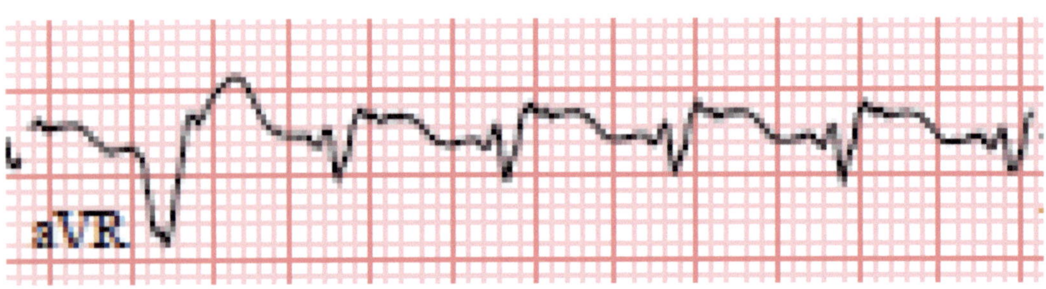

Fig. 6 Lead aVR from the tachycardia presented in Fig. 1, showing the absence of an initial positive tall R wave, criterion not in favor of ventricular tachycardia (but not excluding it either)

in lead aVR, which, again, is not the case (Fig. 6).

The third step "QRS morphology unlike BBB or fascicular block" does not suggest SVT with BBB, given the presence of an "rSr'" aspect in leads I and aVL, which is not characteristic of a typical LBBB. The fourth step of the algorithm analyzes the vi/vt index. This index compares the

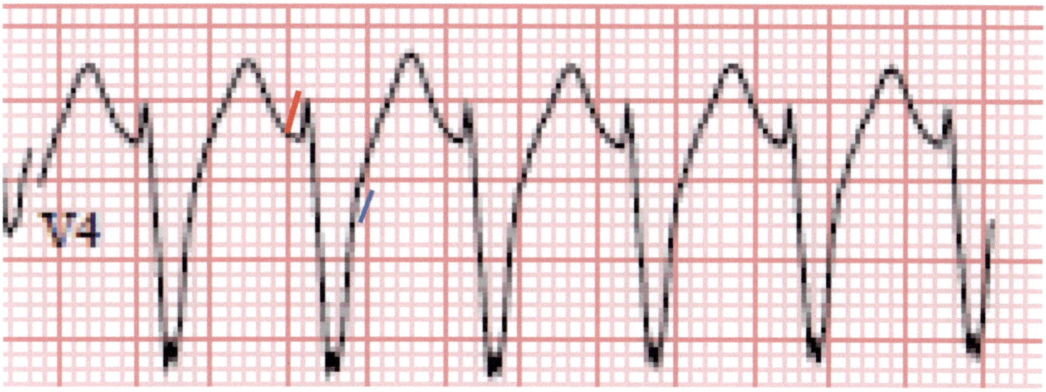

Fig. 7 The vi/vt index from the Vereckei algorithm in lead V1. The ratio of the initial 40 ms and the last 40 ms of the QRS complex is 2 mV vs 1.5 mV; therefore, 2/1.5 = 1.33, which is >1. This is in favor of a supraventricular tachycardia

amplitude of the first 40 ms of a QRS complex to the amplitude of the last 40 ms of the QRS complex in a lead where the QRS has both an R and an S wave, such as lead V4. In the present case, this is illustrated in Fig. 7.

The ECG from Fig. 2 shows in the first part of the tracing (leads I, II, and III) sinus rhythm with paced QRS complexes, followed by sinus rhythm with spontaneous QRS complexes with a heart rate of 99 bpm, QRS axis at +100°, first-degree AV block best seen in lead V1 (despite the automatic measure of the PR interval of 190 ms, the PR interval is of more than 200 ms), and most importantly, LBBB, with a QRS morphology that is identical to the morphology of the QRS complex from the wide QRS complex tachycardia presented in Fig. 1. There are no signs of ventricular pre-excitation (no short PR interval and no delta waves). This is a strong argument in favor of a supraventricular origin for the tachycardia from Fig. 1, with LBBB. Antidromic tachycardia is highly unlikely.

Based on all these arguments, the diagnosis is supraventricular tachycardia with LBBB.

Answer d—"Atrial flutter with 2:1 A:V conduction and left bundle branch block"—is not correct since there is no 2:1 A:V conduction during the tachycardia.

References

1. Surawicz B, Childers R, Deal BJ, Gettes LS, Bailey JJ, Gorgels A, et al. AHA/ACCF/HRS recommendations for the standardization and interpretation of the electrocardiogram: part III: intraventricular conduction disturbances: a scientific statement from the American Heart Association Electrocardiography and Arrhythmias Committee, Council on Clinical Cardiology; the American College of Cardiology Foundation; and the Heart Rhythm Society. Endorsed by the International Society for Computerized Electrocardiology. J Am Coll Cardiol. 2009;53(11):976–81.
2. Brugada P, Brugada J, Mont L, Smeets J, Andries EW. A new approach to the differential diagnosis of a regular tachycardia with a wide QRS complex. Circulation. 1991;83(5):1649–59.
3. Kindwall KE, Brown J, Josephson ME. Electrocardiographic criteria for ventricular tachycardia in wide complex left bundle branch block morphology tachycardias. Am J Cardiol. 1988;61(15):1279–83.
4. Eckardt L, Breithardt G, Kirchhof P. Approach to wide complex tachycardias in patients without structural heart disease. Heart. 2006;92(5):704–11.
5. Vereckei A, Duray G, Szenasi G, Altemose GT, Miller JM. Application of a new algorithm in the differential diagnosis of wide QRS complex tachycardia. Eur Heart J. 2007;28(5):589–600.

ECG 44

Serban Schiau

1 Case Presentation

A 43-year-old male patient with a history of remote inferior myocardial infarction treated with PTCA and stent implantation at the level of his right coronary artery at the age of 34 years and ischemic cardiomyopathy with moderate LV dysfunction (LVEF of 44%) is admitted to the Cardiology Department for an episode of palpitations accompanied by chest pain, dyspnea, anxiety, and lightheadedness that had started 40 min prior to his presentation to the hospital. His ECG recorded at admittance to the Cardiology Department is presented in Fig. 1.

Question: What is the nature of the tachycardia presented in Fig. 1?

(a) Ventricular tachycardia originating from the inferior septal LV wall.
(b) Ventricular tachycardia originating from the inferior lateral RV wall.
(c) Ventricular tachycardia originating from the inferior septal RV wall.
(d) Antidromic tachycardia using a right-sided bypass tract.
(e) Atrial tachycardia with left bundle branch block.

S. Schiau (✉)
Department of Cardiology, Emile Muller Hospital, Mulhouse, France
e-mail: serban.schiau@ghrmsa.fr

Hint: A second ECG recorded during the end of the episode of palpitations is presented in Fig. 2.

Correct answer: a. Ventricular tachycardia originating from the inferior septal LV wall

Explanation: The ECG in Fig. 1 shows a regular wide QRS complex tachycardia with a heart rate of 145 bpm and LBBB morphology. The width of the QRS complex is 160 ms. The QRS axis is at −30°. The differential diagnosis of this regular wide QRS complex tachycardia with LBBB morphology includes: ventricular tachycardia (myocardial-related VT and bundle branch re-entry VT), supraventricular tachycardia (atrial flutter, atrial tachycardia, AVNRT, and AVRT) with functional or pre-existing bundle branch block, and antidromic tachycardia (in pre-excitation syndromes).

The ECG in Fig. 2 shows the end of the tachycardia and conversion to sinus rhythm. The heart rate during the sinus rhythm is 79 bpm; the QRS axis is at +30°; and there are deep Q waves in leads II, III, and aVF, compatible with the necrosis of the inferior LV wall. The QRS complex is narrow; there is no bundle branch block; and there are no signs of ventricular pre-excitation (no short PR interval and no delta waves).

L. Muresan (ed.), *ECG Interpretation of Wide QRS Complex Tachycardia*,
https://doi.org/10.1007/978-3-031-97030-6_45

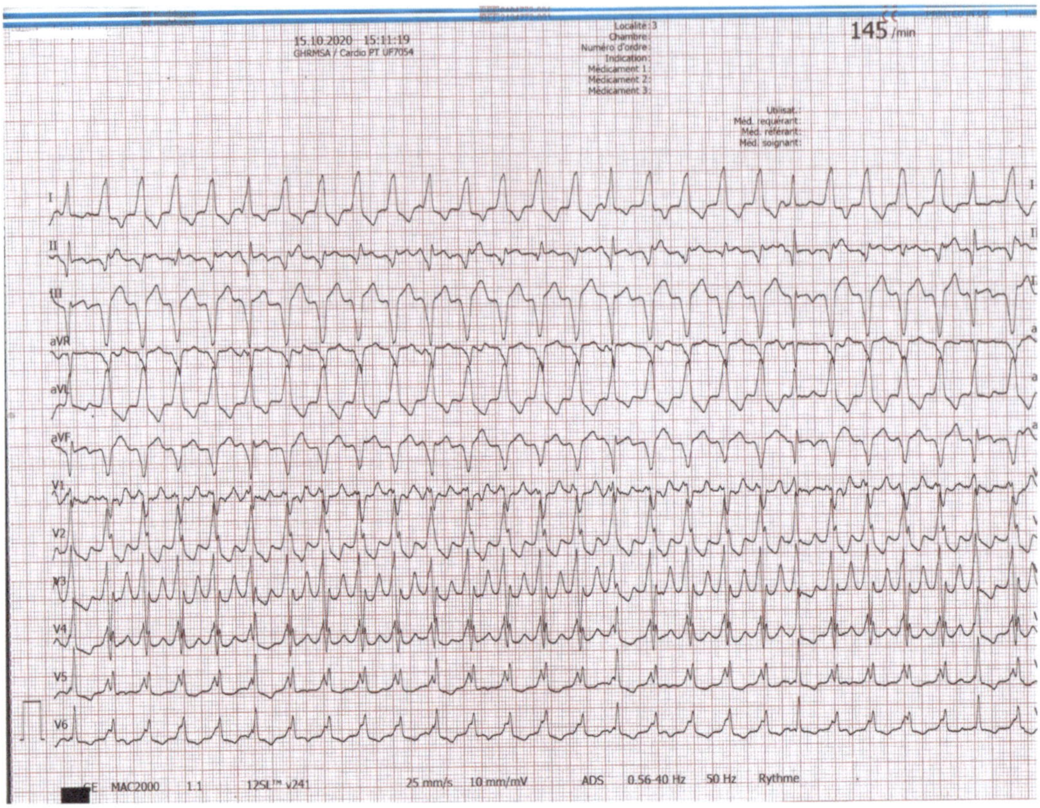

Fig. 1 Twelve-lead ECG recorded at admittance to the Cardiology Department

Therefore, answer d—Antidromic tachycardia"— is unlikely.

The morphology of the left bundle branch block of the QRS complex during tachycardia from Fig. 1 suggests that it might be a typical one [1]: the QRS duration is >120 ms; there is a monomorphic R wave in leads I, aVL, V5, and V6; and there is ST segment and T wave modification opposite to the major deflection of the QRS complex: ST segment elevation with positive T waves in lead V1 and negative in V5 and V6. However, the transition of the QRS complex in the precordial leads takes place in lead V2, which is unusual for a typical LBBB. Also, the presence of an r wave >0.04 s in lead V1 is not in favor of a typical LBBB [2]. Therefore, answer e—"Atrial tachycardia with left bundle branch block"—is unlikely.

Applying the Brugada algorithm [3] to the tachycardia from Fig. 2, it can be seen that: 1. There is no absence of an RS complex in the precordial leads (otherwise said, there are rS complexes in leads V1 and V3; we therefore move to the second step of the algorithm: 2. This step analyzes the absence of an R-to-S interval >100 ms in any precordial lead. The R-to-S interval in lead V3 is 120 ms (Fig. 3), criterion in favor of ventricular tachycardia.

The Vereckei algorithm [4] for the differential diagnosis of wide QRS complex tachycardias also suggests VT as the correct answer. The first step of the algorithm looks for A–V dissociation, which is indeed seen on the present ECG. This is best seen in leads V5 and V6 (Fig. 4).

Another argument from the Vereckei algorithm in favor of ventricular tachycardia is the vi/vt index. This index compares the amplitude of the first 40 ms of a QRS complex to the amplitude of the last 40 ms of the QRS complex in a lead where the QRS has both an R and an S wave. In the present case, this is illustrated in Fig. 5.

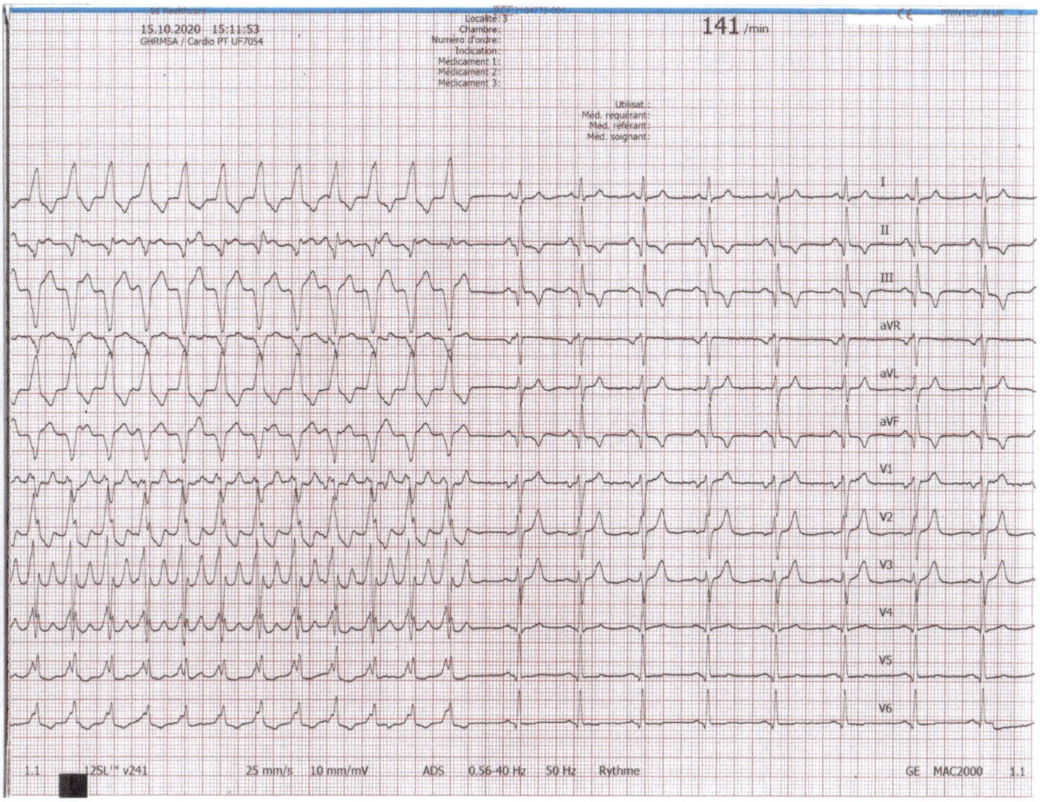

Fig. 2 Twelve-lead ECG recorded during the end of the episode of palpitations

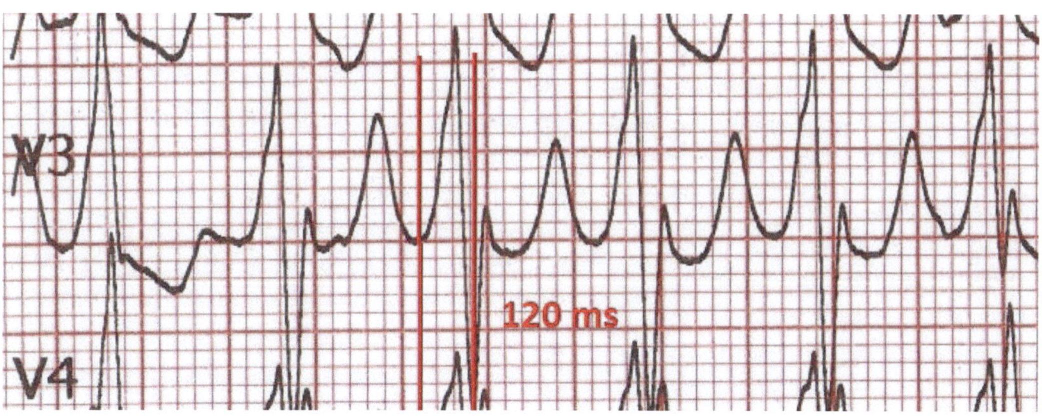

Fig. 3 Lead V3 from the ECG presented in Fig. 1 showing an R-to-S interval of 120 ms, argument in favor of ventricular tachycardia

Another argument in favor of VT is the presence of **c**apture beats (*) and fusion beats (Fig. 6). A–V dissociation is also pointed out in this figure.

Based on these arguments, the diagnosis of ventricular tachycardia was established.

The origin of the VT is at the level of the LV (aspect of LBBB with rapid transition in the pre-

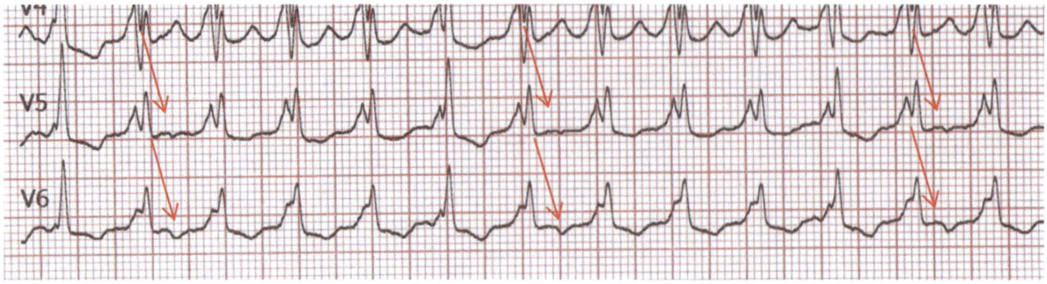

Fig. 4 Leads V5 and V6 demonstrating A–V dissociation (red arrows point to the P waves)

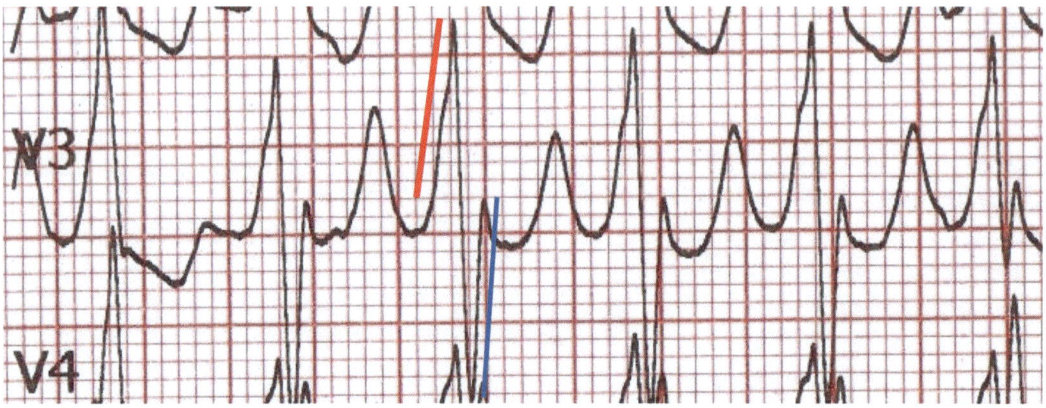

Fig. 5 The vi/vt index from the Vereckei algorithm in lead V3. The ratio of the initial 40 ms and the last 40 ms of the QRS complex is 10 mV vs 12 mV; therefore, 10/11.5 = 0.87, which is <1. This is in favor of ventricular tachycardia

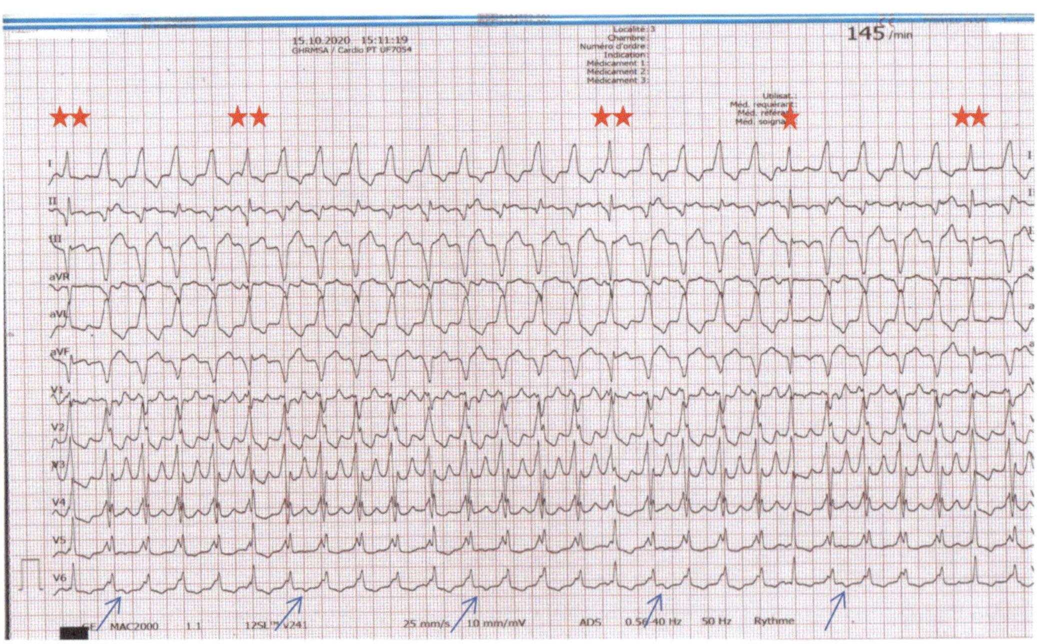

Fig. 6 The same ECG from Fig. 1 recorded at admittance to the Cardiology Department showing capture beats (*) and fusion beats (**), favoring the diagnosis of ventricular tachycardia. Of note, the aspect of the QRS complex is not that of a typical LBBB, with the transition of the QRS complex in precordial leads in V2, another argument in favor of VT. A–V dissociation is also observed, with blue arrows pointing to P waves

cordial leads), at the inferior LV wall (negative QRS complexes in leads II, III, and aVF), and septal wall (positive QRS in leads I and aVL).

The patient underwent an electrophysiological study with successful catheter ablation of his ventricular tachycardia.

References

1. Surawicz B, Childers R, Deal BJ, Gettes LS, Bailey JJ, Gorgels A, et al. AHA/ACCF/HRS recommendations for the standardization and interpretation of the electrocardiogram: part III: intraventricular conduction disturbances: a scientific statement from the American Heart Association Electrocardiography and Arrhythmias Committee, Council on Clinical Cardiology; the American College of Cardiology Foundation; and the Heart Rhythm Society. Endorsed by the International Society for Computerized Electrocardiology. J Am Coll Cardiol. 2009;53(11):976–81.
2. Eckardt L, Breithardt G, Kirchhof P. Approach to wide complex tachycardias in patients without structural heart disease. Heart. 2006;92(5):704–11.
3. Brugada P, Brugada J, Mont L, Smeets J, Andries EW. A new approach to the differential diagnosis of a regular tachycardia with a wide QRS complex. Circulation. 1991;83(5):1649–59.
4. Vereckei A, Duray G, Szenasi G, Altemose GT, Miller JM. Application of a new algorithm in the differential diagnosis of wide QRS complex tachycardia. Eur Heart J. 2007;28(5):589–600.

ECG 45

Lucien Diene

1 Case Presentation

A 56-year-old male patient with a history of MINOCA at the age of 40 years, with cardiac MRI-confirmed subendocardial necrosis of the inferior LV wall, with near-normal LVEF (LVEF of 53%) was admitted to the Cardiology Department for an episode of palpitations accompanied by chest pain, dyspnea, and anxiety that had occurred 45 min prior to his presentation to the hospital. His ECG recorded at admittance to the Cardiology Department is presented in Fig. 1.

Question: What is the nature of the tachycardia presented in Fig. 1?

(a) Ventricular tachycardia originating from the inferior septal LV wall.
(b) Ventricular tachycardia originating from the inferior septal RV wall.
(c) Antidromic tachycardia using a left-sided bypass tract.
(d) Antidromic tachycardia using a right-sided bypass tract.
(e) Atrial tachycardia with 1:1 atrioventricular conduction with right bundle branch block.

L. Diene (✉)
Department of Cardiology, Clinique Le Noirmont, Le Noirmont, Switzerland

Hint: A second ECG recorded several minutes later is presented in Fig. 2.

Correct answer: a. Ventricular tachycardia originating from the inferior septal LV wall.

Explanation: The ECG in Fig. 1 shows a regular wide QRS complex tachycardia with a heart rate of 191 bpm and RBBB morphology. The width of the QRS complex is 190 ms (Fig. 3).

The QRS axis is at −70°. The differential diagnosis of this regular wide QRS complex tachycardia with LBBB morphology includes: ventricular tachycardia (myocardial-related VT, bundle branch re-entry VT, and fascicular VT), supraventricular tachycardia (atrial flutter, atrial tachycardia, AVNRT, and AVRT) with functional or pre-existing bundle branch block, and antidromic tachycardia (in pre-excitation syndromes).

The ECG in Fig. 2 shows sinus rhythm with a heart rate of 70 bpm, QRS axis at +50°, right atrial enlargement, absence of LV hypertrophy, absence of ischemia, and one nonconducted PAC. The QRS complexes are narrow. There are no signs of ventricular pre-excitation (no short PR interval and no delta waves). Therefore, answer c—"Antidromic tachycardia using a left-sided bypass tract"—and answer d—"Antidromic

L. Muresan (ed.), *ECG Interpretation of Wide QRS Complex Tachycardia*,
https://doi.org/10.1007/978-3-031-97030-6_46

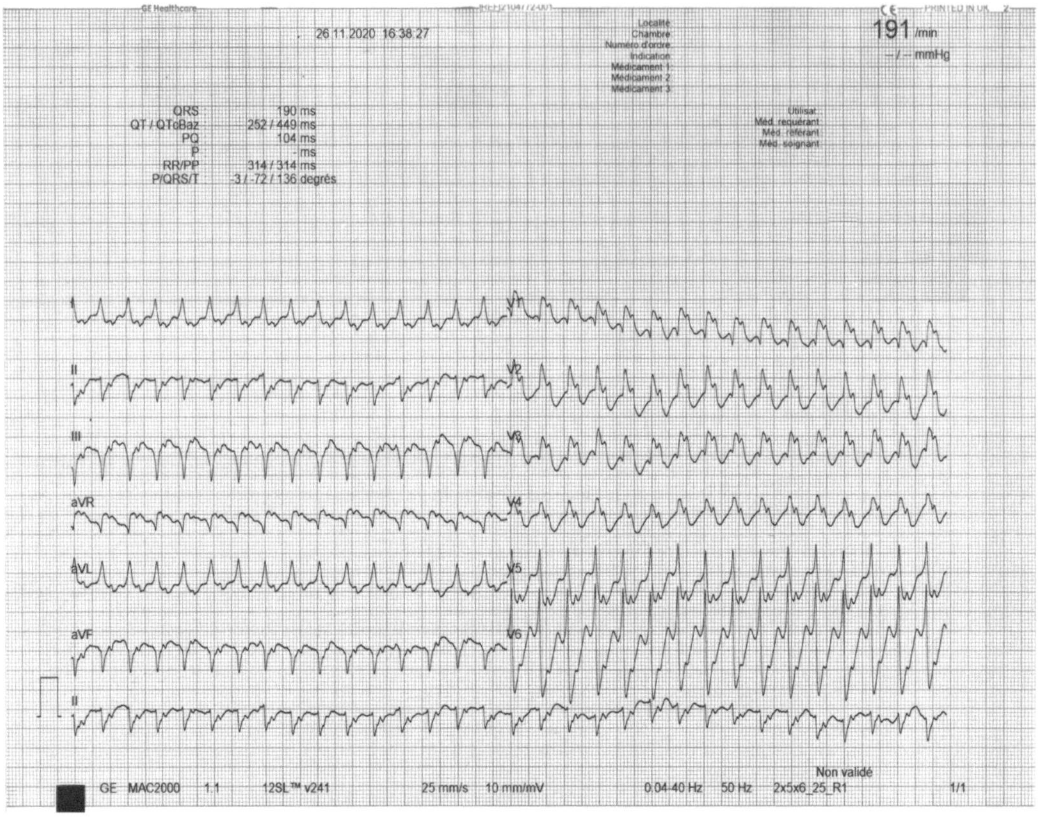

Fig. 1 Twelve-lead ECG recorded at admittance to the Cardiology Department

tachycardia using a right-sided bypass tract"—are unlikely.

The morphology of the right bundle branch block of the QRS complex during tachycardia from Fig. 1 is not that of a typical one [1]: the QRS duration is indeed >120 ms, but there is a "qR" pattern in lead V1, and there are no S waves in leads I and aVL. Therefore, answer e—"Atrial tachycardia with 1:1 atrioventricular conduction with right bundle branch block"—is unlikely.

Applying the Brugada algorithm [2] to the tachycardia from Fig. 1, it can be seen that: 1. There is no absence of an RS complex in the precordial leads (otherwise said, there are rS complexes in leads V5 and V6); we therefore move to the second step of the algorithm: 2. This step analyzes the absence of an R-to-S interval >100 ms in any precordial lead. This measures exactly 100 ms (Fig. 4). Therefore, according to the Brugada algorithm, the correct diagnosis is ventricular tachycardia.

Another argument from the Brugada algorithm for an RBBB morphology wide QRS complex tachycardia in favor of VT is the presence of a taller left peak of the QRS complex in lead V1 (the rabbit ear sign) or for biphasic RS or QR complexes, which is actually the case (qR morphology) (Fig. 5).

The Vereckei algorithm [3] for the differential diagnosis of wide QRS complex tachycardias also suggests VT as the correct answer. The first step of the algorithm looks for A–V dissociation, which is not the case. A close analysis of the ECG identifies P waves, best seen in lead I, with a 1:1 relationship to the QRS complexes (Fig. 6).

The second step of the algorithm looks for an initial predominant R wave in lead aVR, which, again, is not the case (Fig. 7).

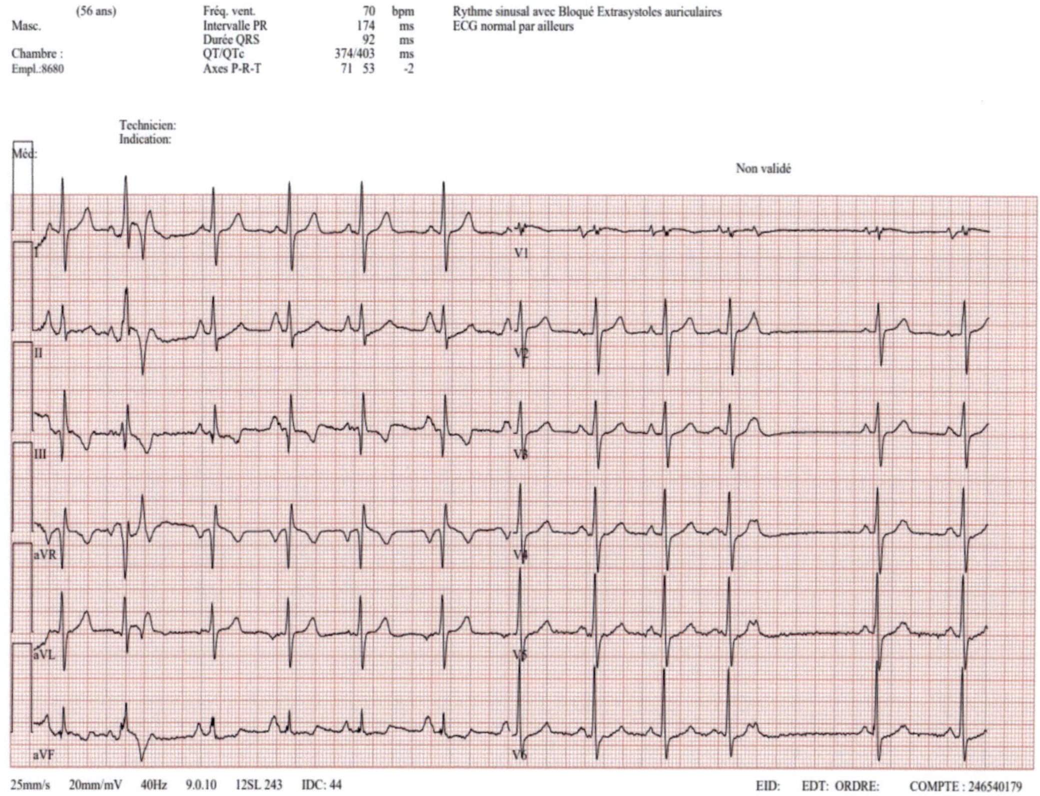

Fig. 2 Twelve-lead ECG recorded after the end of the episode of palpitations

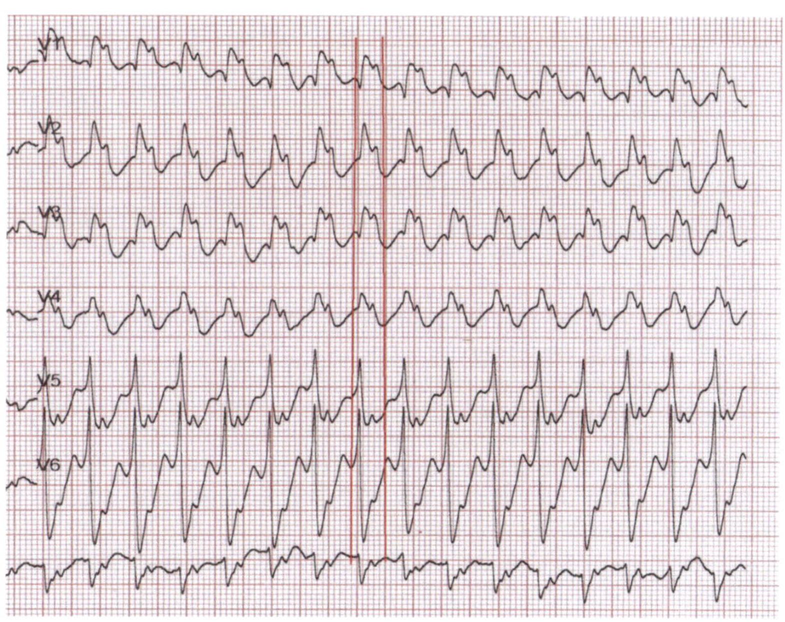

Fig. 3 Precordial leads from the ECG presented in Fig. 1 showing the delineation of the QRS complex

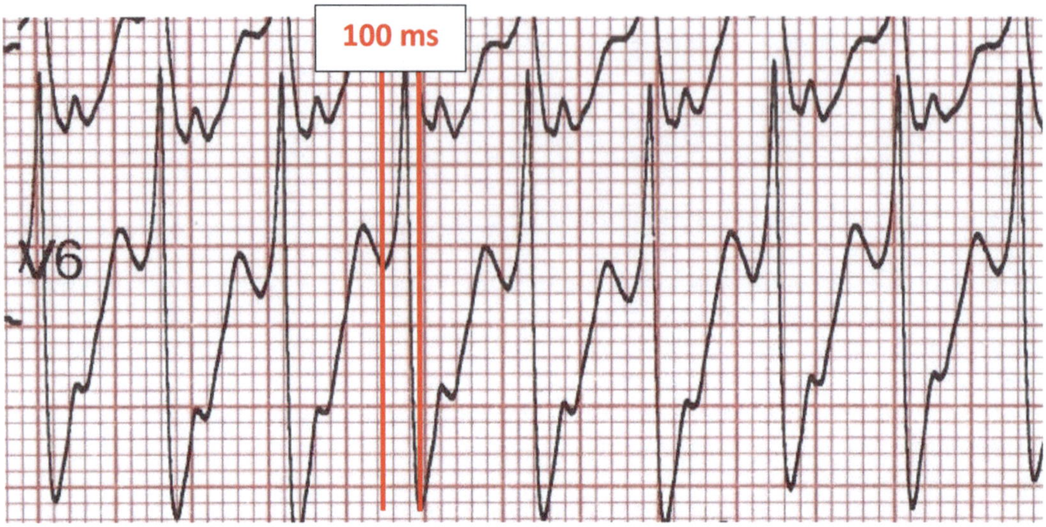

Fig. 4 Lead V6 from the ECG from Fig. 1 showing an R-to-S interval of 100 ms, argument in favor of ventricular tachycardia

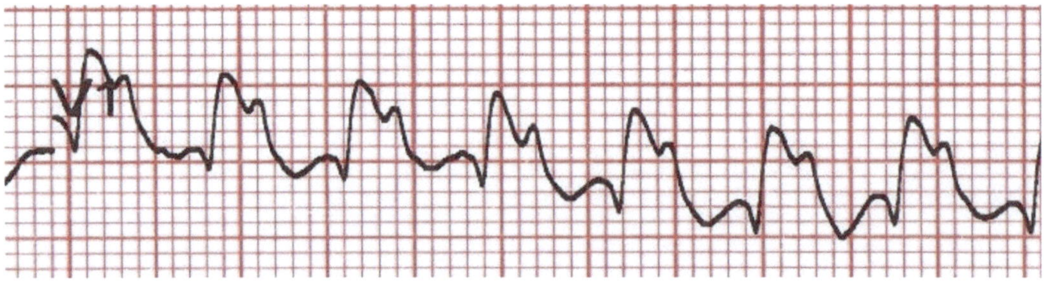

Fig. 5 Lead V1 from the ECG from Fig. 1 showing a "qR" pattern, the argument in favor of ventricular tachycardia

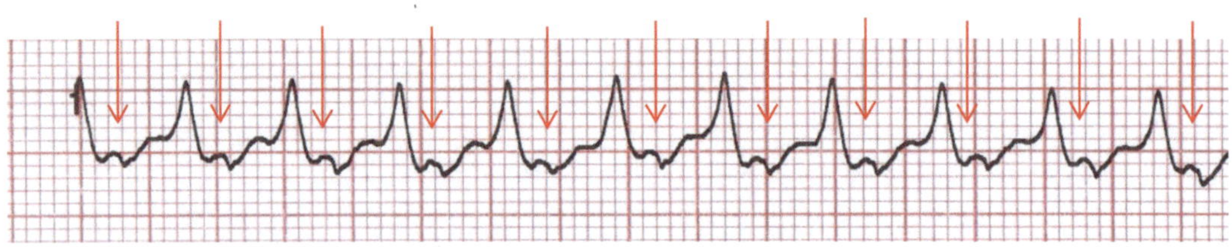

Fig. 6 Lead I from the ECG from Fig. 1 showing the presence of P waves (red arrows) with a 1:1 relationship with the QRS complexes (see text for further explanation)

The third step "QRS morphology unlike BBB or fascicular block" does not suggest SVT with BBB, given the presence of q waves in lead V1 and the absence of S waves in leads I and aVL [1]. Therefore, according to the Vereckei algorithm, the diagnosis of ventricular tachycardia can be established.

Another argument in favor of ventricular tachycardia for an LBBB QRS morphology would be a QRS duration of over 160 ms [4], which is also the case.

Based on these arguments, the diagnosis of ventricular tachycardia was retained.

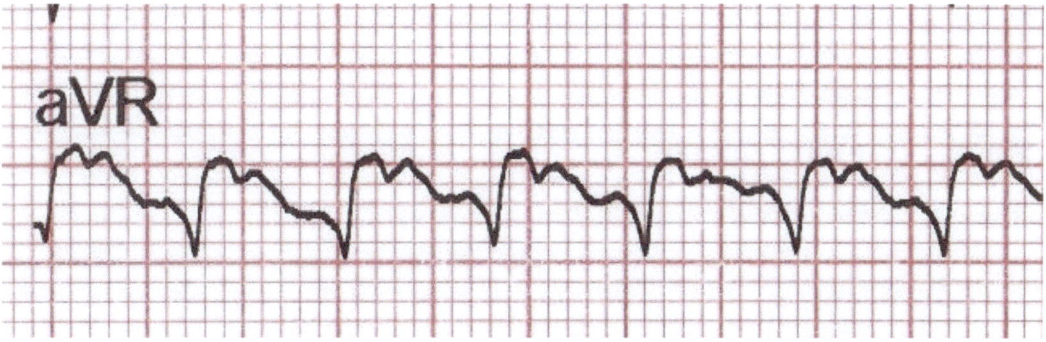

Fig. 7 Lead aVR from the ECG from Fig. 1 showing a "QR" pattern, argument not in favor of ventricular tachycardia (but not excluding it either)

The origin of the VT is the inferior septal LV wall (negative QRS complexes in leads II, III, and aVF, positive in leads I and aVL, and an RBBB morphology).

The patient underwent an electrophysiological study which confirmed the diagnosis and a subsequent catheter ablation procedure.

References

1. Surawicz B, Childers R, Deal BJ, Gettes LS, Bailey JJ, Gorgels A, et al. AHA/ACCF/HRS recommendations for the standardization and interpretation of the electrocardiogram: part III: intraventricular conduction disturbances: a scientific statement from the American Heart Association Electrocardiography and Arrhythmias Committee, Council on Clinical Cardiology; the American College of Cardiology Foundation; and the Heart Rhythm Society. Endorsed by the International Society for Computerized Electrocardiology. J Am Coll Cardiol. 2009;53(11):976–81.
2. Brugada P, Brugada J, Mont L, Smeets J, Andries EW. A new approach to the differential diagnosis of a regular tachycardia with a wide QRS complex. Circulation. 1991;83(5):1649–59.
3. Vereckei A, Duray G, Szenasi G, Altemose GT, Miller JM. Application of a new algorithm in the differential diagnosis of wide QRS complex tachycardia. Eur Heart J. 2007;28(5):589–600.
4. Eckardt L, Breithardt G, Kirchhof P. Approach to wide complex tachycardias in patients without structural heart disease. Heart. 2006;92(5):704–11.

ECG 46

Gabriel Gusetu

1 Case Presentation

A 71-year-old male patient with a history of persistent atrial fibrillation, tachycardia-induced cardiomyopathy with severe systolic dysfunction (LVEF of 25%), external electrical cardioversion with conversion to sinus rhythm, with LVEF of 47% demonstrated by transthoracic echocardiography 2 months later, catheter ablation of atrial fibrillation (pulmonary veins isolation) ischemic stroke, ischemic cardiomyopathy (severe stenosis of the left main coronary artery treated with stent implantation), LVEF of 25%, sustained monomorphic ventricular tachycardia, and implanted with a dual-chamber Biotronik Acticor 7 VR-T ICD is admitted to the Cardiology Department for an episode of palpitations accompanied by dyspnea at rest. His ECG recorded at admittance is presented in Fig. 1.

Question: What is the nature of the tachycardia presented in Fig. 1?

(a) Ventricular tachycardia originating from the inferior septal LV wall.
(b) Ventricular tachycardia originating from the inferior septal RV wall.
(c) Bundle branch re-entry ventricular tachycardia.
(d) Antidromic tachycardia using a right-sided bypass tract.
(e) Atrial tachycardia with 1:1 atrioventricular conduction and left bundle branch block.

Hint: A second ECG recorded after carotid sinus massage is presented in Fig. 2.

Correct answer: e. Atrial tachycardia with 1:1 atrioventricular conduction and left bundle branch block

Explanation: The ECG in Fig. 1 shows a regular wide QRS complex tachycardia with a heart rate of 105 bpm and LBBB morphology. The width of the QRS complex is 162 ms. The QRS axis is at −90°. The differential diagnosis of this regular wide QRS complex tachycardia with LBBB morphology includes: ventricular tachycardia (myocardial-related VT and bundle branch re-entry VT), supraventricular tachycardia (atrial flutter, atrial tachycardia, AVNRT, and AVRT) with functional or pre-existing left bundle branch block, and antidromic tachycardia (in pre-excitation syndromes).

The morphology of the left bundle branch block of the QRS complex during tachycardia

G. Gusetu (✉)
Department of Cardiology, Emile Muller Hospital, Mulhouse, France

L. Muresan (ed.), *ECG Interpretation of Wide QRS Complex Tachycardia*,
https://doi.org/10.1007/978-3-031-97030-6_47

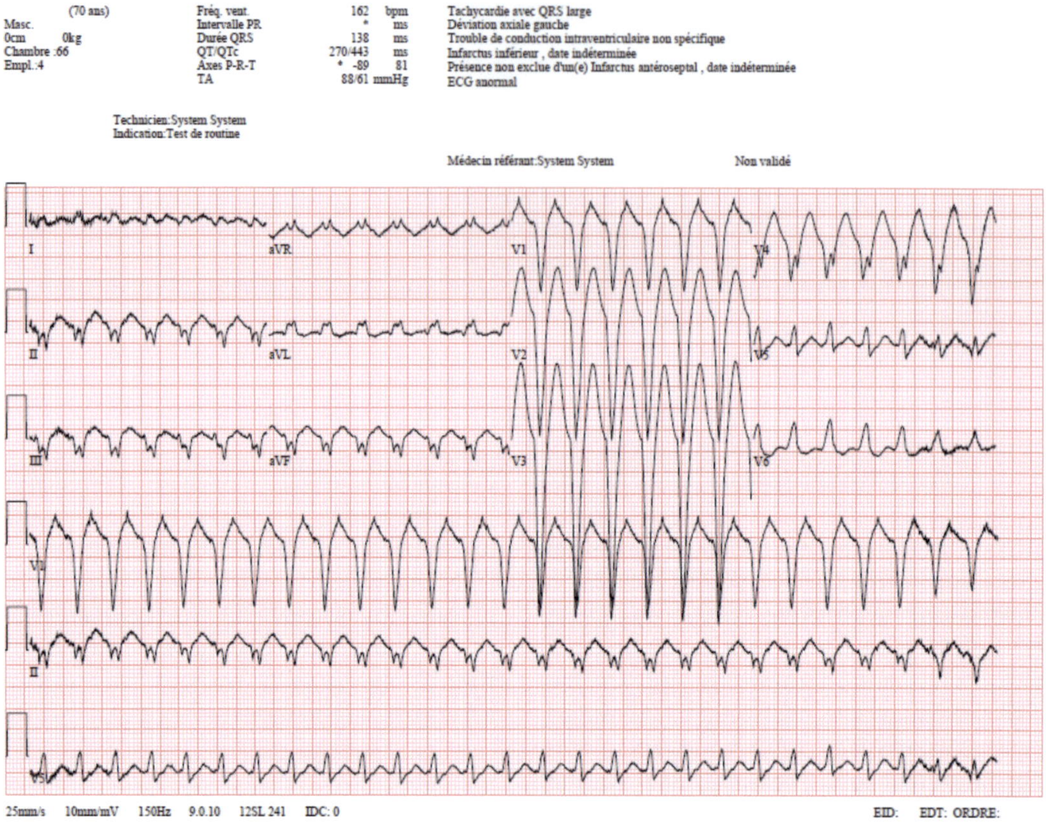

Fig. 1 Twelve-lead ECG recorded at admittance to the Cardiology Department

from Fig. 1 might be compatible with a typical one: the QRS duration is of >120 ms; there is a monomorphic notched R wave in leads I and aVL and a monomorphic R wave in lead V6; and there is ST segment and T wave modification opposite to the major deflection of the QRS complex: ST segment elevation with positive T waves in leads V1 to V5. This is an argument in favor of an SVT with LBBB. However, given the patient's personal history of ischemic cardiomyopathy and ventricular tachycardia, this might also be ventricular tachycardia originating from the septal LV wall. So, at this stage of the analysis, the answer to the question is not yet established.

Applying the Brugada algorithm [1] to the tachycardia from Fig. 1, it can be seen that: 1. There is no absence of an RS complex in the precordial leads (otherwise said, there are rS complexes in leads V5 and V6) (Fig. 3); we therefore move to the second step of the algorithm.

The second step analyzes the absence of an R-to-S interval >100 ms in any precordial lead. This is not the case (Fig. 4).

Step 3 of the algorithm looks for A–V dissociation. This is not obvious. We therefore need to move to step 4 of the algorithm.

For a wide QRS complex tachycardia with LBBB, arguments in favor of VT are: the presence of an "r wave" >0.04 s in lead V1 or V2, which is not the case; the presence of a notched S wave in lead V1 or V2, which is also not the case; and the presence of a delayed S nadir >0.06 s in lead V1 or V2, which is also not the case [2] (Fig. 5).

Therefore, according to the Brugada algorithm, there are no arguments in favor of ventric-

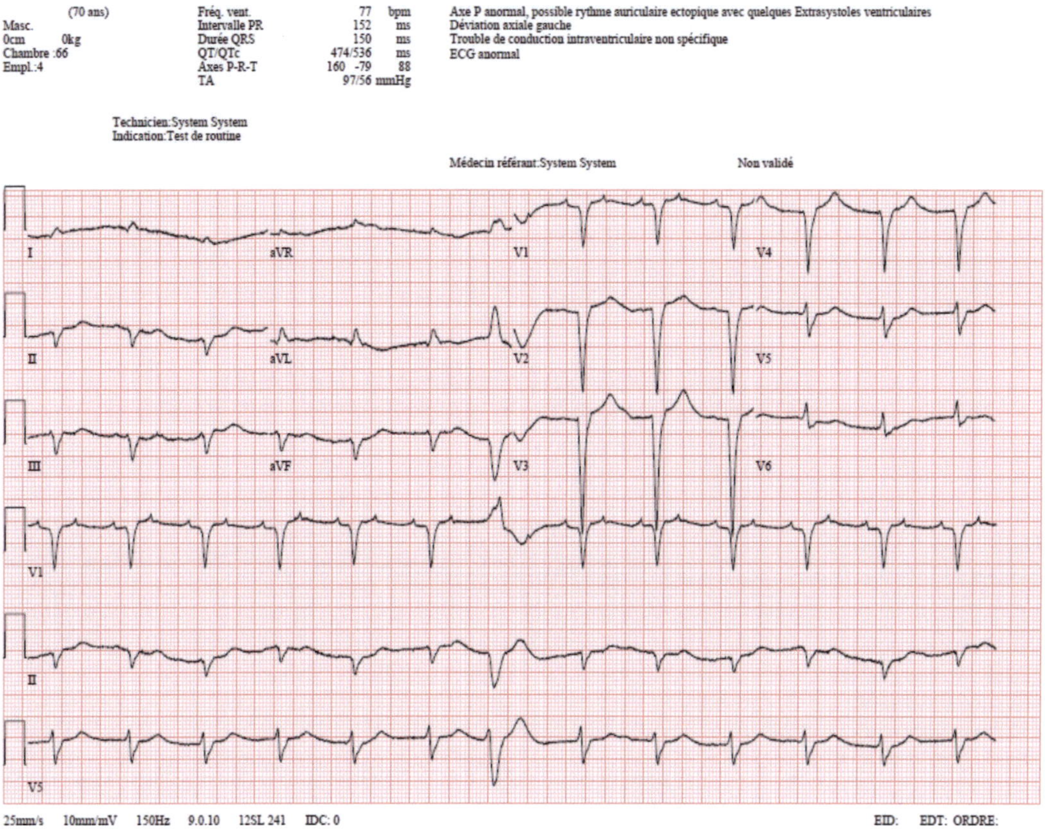

Fig. 2 Twelve-lead ECG recorded after the end of the episode of palpitations

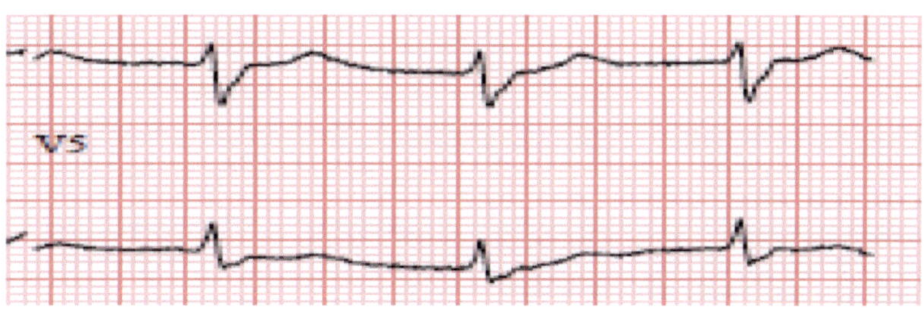

Fig. 3 Leads V5 and V6 from the ECG from Fig. 1 showing the presence of RS complexes, argument not in favor of ventricular tachycardia (but not excluding it either)

ular tachycardia, and this is therefore supraventricular tachycardia with LBBB, which is correct.

Another argument in favor of ventricular tachycardia for a LBBB QRS morphology would be a QRS duration of over 160 ms [3], which is also not the case (QRS duration of 118 ms).

The Vereckei algorithm [4] for the differential diagnosis of wide QRS complex tachycardias also suggests SVT as the correct answer. The first step of the algorithm looks for A–V dissociation, which is not seen on the present ECG. The second step of the algorithm looks for an initial predominant R wave in lead aVR, which, again, is not the case (Fig. 6).

The third step "QRS morphology unlike BBB or fascicular block" actually suggests SVT with LBBB, due to the reasons explained above.

The nature of the tachycardia becomes obvious after looking at the ECG from Fig. 2. This

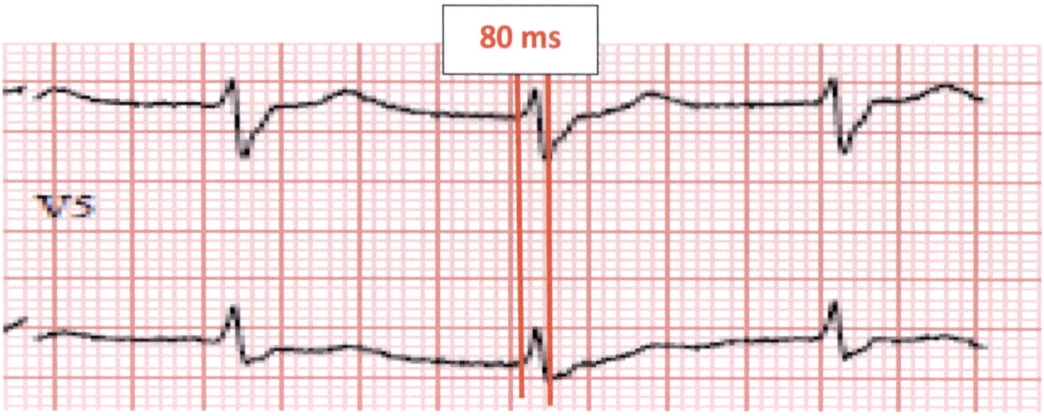

Fig. 4 Lead V5 from the ECG from Fig. 1 showing an R-to-S interval of 80 ms, argument not in favor of ventricular tachycardia (but not excluding it either)

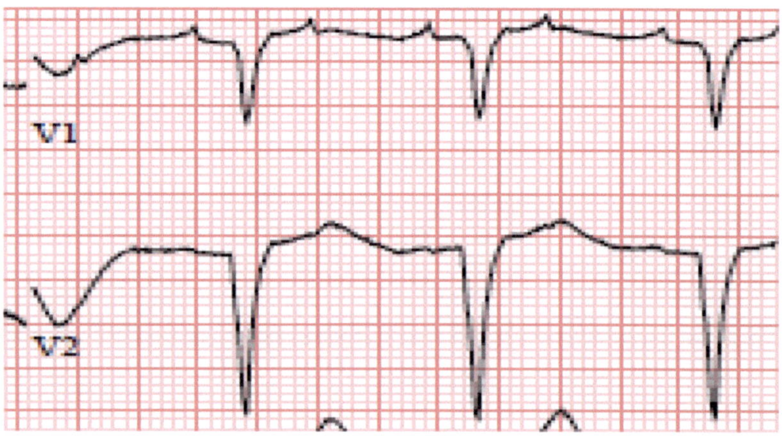

Fig. 5 Leads V1 and V2 from the ECG from Fig. 1 showing the absence of an "r wave" > 0.04 s; the absence of a notched S wave in lead V1 or V2; and the absence of a delayed S nadir >0.06 s

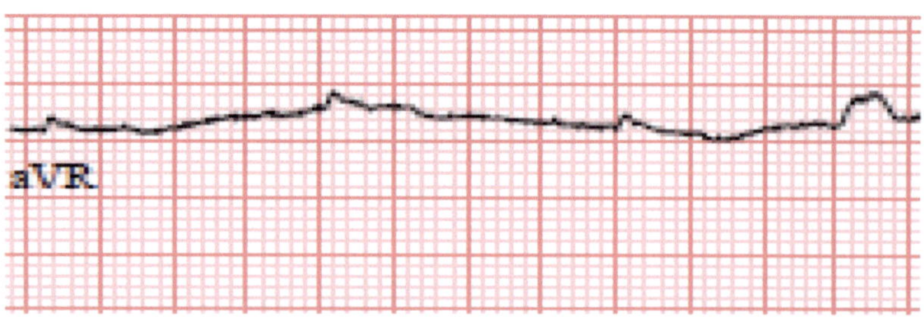

Fig. 6 Lead aVR from the ECG from Fig. 1 showing the absence of a tall initial R wave, argument not in favor of ventricular tachycardia (but not excluding it either)

shows a regular rhythm with a heart rate of about 80 bpm, with a QRS axis at −80° and incomplete LBBB (QRS duration of 118 ms). Analysis of lead V1 shows the presence of P waves, with 2:1 atrioventricular conduction (Fig. 7).

The patient underwent electrical cardioversion. The ECG post-cardioversion is presented in Fig. 8.

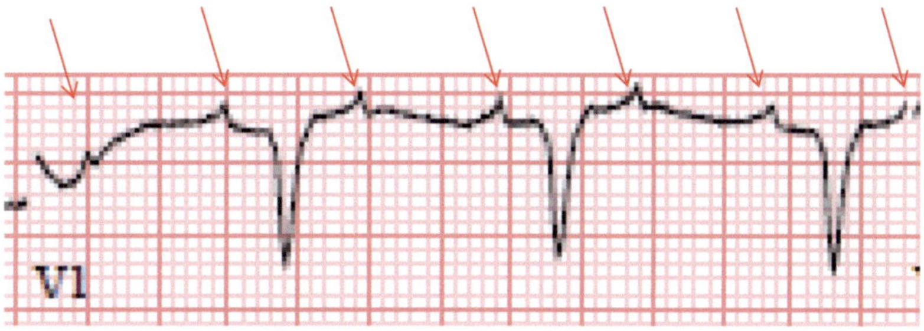

Fig. 7 Lead V1 demonstrating atrial tachycardia with 2:1 atrioventricular conduction (red arrows point to the P waves)

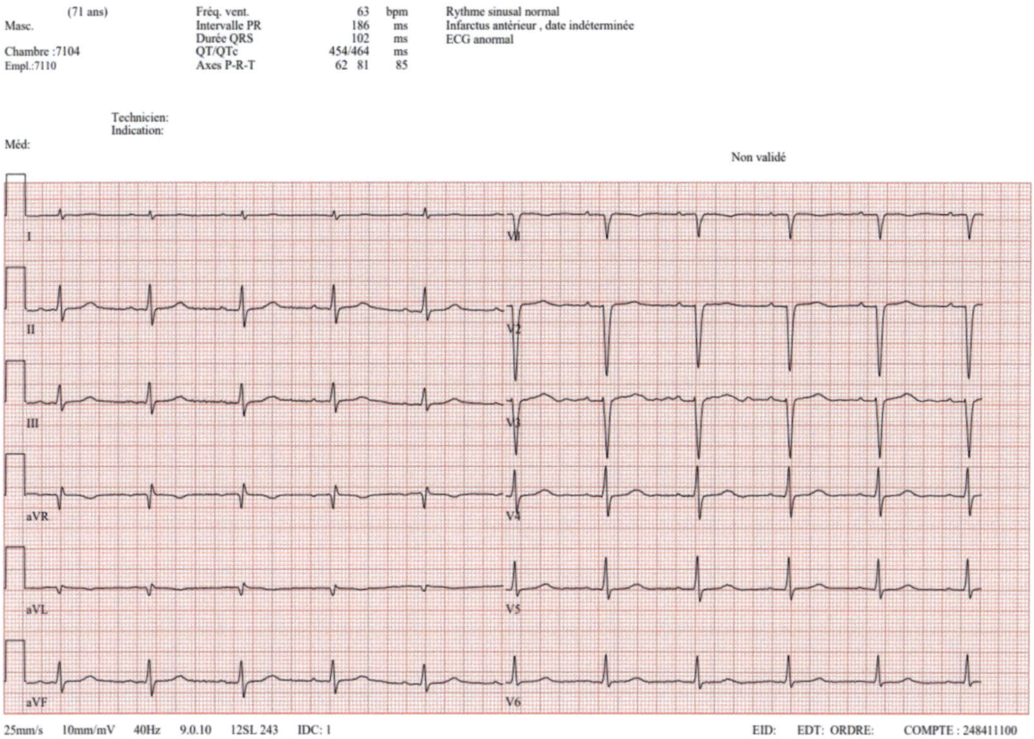

Fig. 8 ECG recorded after external electrical cardioversion

References

1. Brugada P, Brugada J, Mont L, Smeets J, Andries EW. A new approach to the differential diagnosis of a regular tachycardia with a wide QRS complex. Circulation. 1991;83(5):1649–59.
2. Kindwall KE, Brown J, Josephson ME. Electrocardiographic criteria for ventricular tachycardia in wide complex left bundle branch block morphology tachycardias. Am J Cardiol. 1988;61(15):1279–83.
3. Eckardt L, Breithardt G, Kirchhof P. Approach to wide complex tachycardias in patients without structural heart disease. Heart. 2006;92(5):704–11.
4. Vereckei A, Duray G, Szenasi G, Altemose GT, Miller JM. Application of a new algorithm in the differential diagnosis of wide QRS complex tachycardia. Eur Heart J. 2007;28(5):589–600.

ECG 47

Gabriel Cismaru

1 Case Presentation

A 73-year-old male patient with a history of MINOCA (2000), with a confirmed small area of subendocardial necrosis by cardiac MRI, with LVEF of 50% is admitted to the Cardiology Department for an episode of palpitations accompanied by dyspnea, anxiety, and lightheadedness that had occurred 20 min prior to his presentation to the hospital. His ECG recorded at the arrival to the Cardiology Department is presented in Fig. 1.

Question: What is the nature of the tachycardia presented in Fig. 1?

(a) Ventricular tachycardia originating from the inferior lateral LV wall.
(b) Ventricular tachycardia originating from the anterior LV wall.
(c) Ventricular tachycardia originating from the anterior septal LV wall.
(d) Antidromic tachycardia using a left-sided bypass tract.
(e) AVNRT with right bundle branch block.

Hint: A second ECG recorded in the Cardiology Department after electrical cardioversion is presented in Fig. 2.

G. Cismaru (✉)
Department of Cardiology, Rehabilitation Hospital, Cluj-Napoca, Romania

Correct answer: b. Ventricular tachycardia originating from the anterior lateral LV wall

Explanation: The ECG in Fig. 1 shows a regular wide QRS complex tachycardia with a heart rate of 129 bpm and RBBB morphology. The width of the QRS complex is 180 ms (the automatic measurement of 152 ms is inaccurate). The QRS axis is at +140°. The differential diagnosis of this regular wide QRS complex tachycardia with RBBB morphology includes: ventricular tachycardia (myocardial-related VT and bundle branch re-entry VT), supraventricular tachycardia (atrial flutter, atrial tachycardia, AVNRT, and AVRT) with functional or pre-existing bundle branch block, and antidromic tachycardia (in pre-excitation syndromes).

The morphology of the right bundle branch block of the QRS complex during tachycardia from Fig. 1 is not that of a typical one: the QRS duration is indeed >120 ms; the QRS morphology is "notched R wave" in lead V1, and there is an RS pattern in leads I and aVL. However, the QRS complex has a "QS" morphology in V6, element that is not in favor of a typical right bundle branch block. This makes SVT with RBBB highly unlikely.

The ECG from Fig. 2 shows sinus rhythm with a heart rate of 49 bpm, QRS axis at 0°, absence of LV hypertrophy, and absence of

L. Muresan (ed.), *ECG Interpretation of Wide QRS Complex Tachycardia*,
https://doi.org/10.1007/978-3-031-97030-6_48

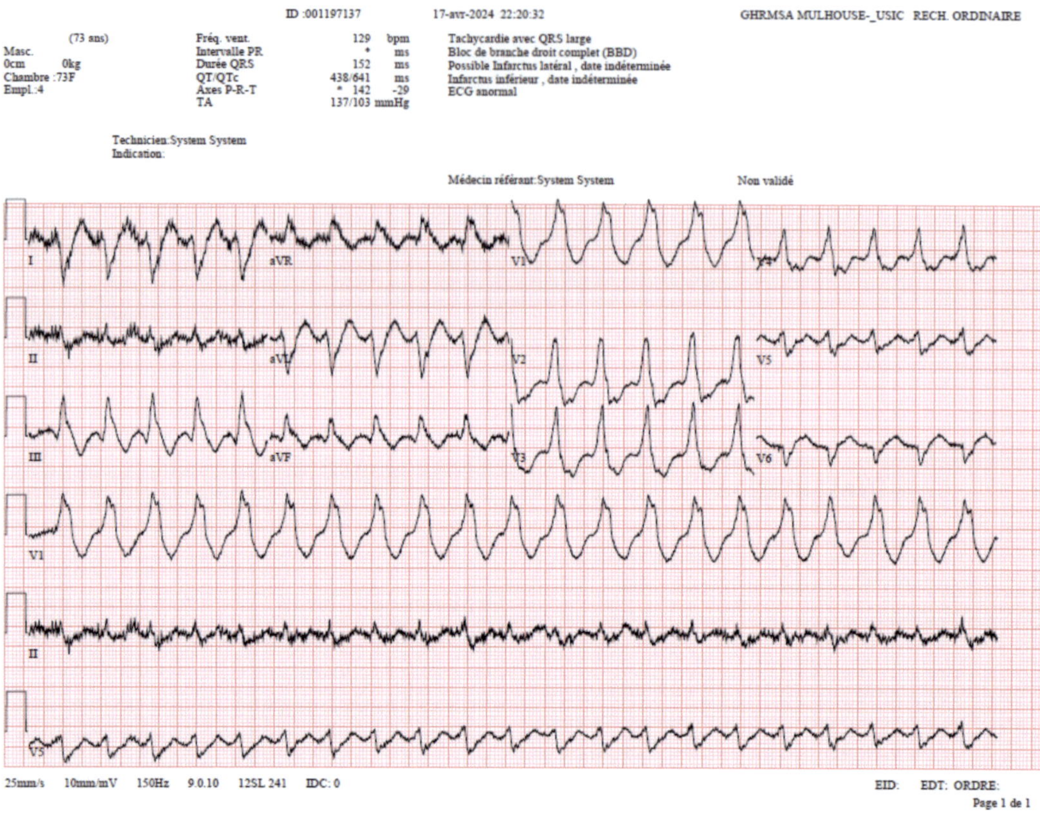

Fig. 1 Twelve-lead ECG recorded at admittance to the Cardiology Department

ischemia, with no signs of ventricular pre-excitation (no short PR interval and no delta waves). This makes antidromic tachycardia unlikely.

Applying the Brugada algorithm [1] to the tachycardia from Fig. 2, it can be seen that: 1. There is no absence of an RS complex in the precordial leads (otherwise said, there are rS complexes in leads V4 and V5); we therefore move to the second step of the algorithm: 2. This step analyzes the absence of an R-to-S interval > 100 ms in any precordial lead. The RS interval in lead V4 is 160 ms, criterion in favor of ventricular tachycardia (Fig. 3).

Another element from the Brugada algorithm in favor of VT is the "rabbit ear" sign, clearly visible in lead V1 (Fig. 4), and the R-to-S ratio < 1 in lead V6.

The Vereckei algorithm [2] for the differential diagnosis of wide QRS complex tachycardias also suggests VT as the correct answer. The first step of the algorithm looks for A–V dissociation, which is not seen on the present ECG. The second step of the algorithm looks for an initial predominant R wave in lead aVR, which is not the case, the QRS complex having a "qR" morphology (Fig. 5).

The third step of the algorithm "QRS morphology unlike BBB or fascicular block" does not suggest SVT with RBBB, based on the arguments exposed above. The fourth step of the algorithm analyzes the vi/vt index. This index compares the amplitude of the first 40 ms of a QRS complex to the amplitude of the last 40 ms of the QRS complex in a lead where the QRS has both an R and an S wave. In the present case, this is illustrated in Fig. 6.

Another argument in favor of ventricular tachycardia for this wide QRS complex tachycardia with RBBB morphology is the QRS duration >140 ms.

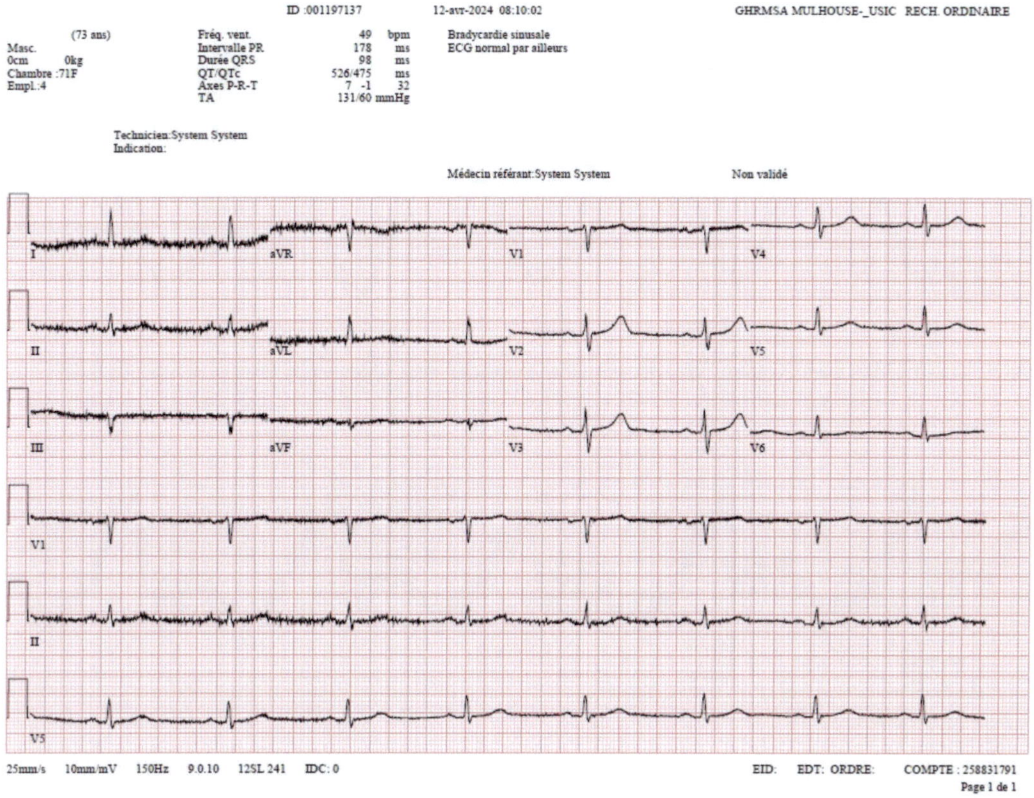

Fig. 2 Twelve-lead ECG recorded after electrical cardioversion

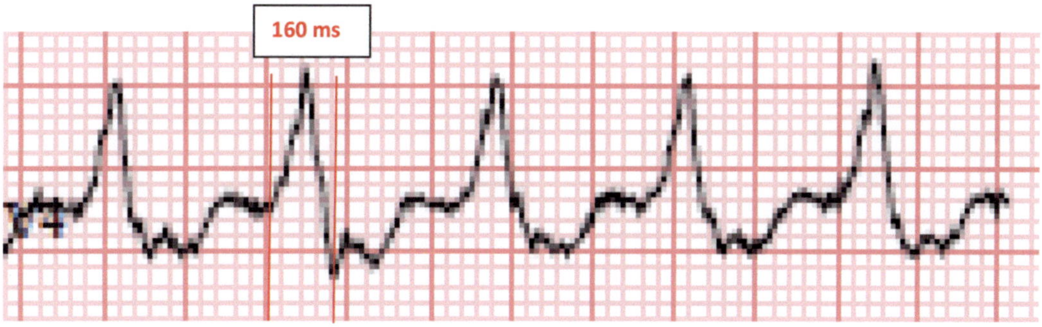

Fig. 3 Lead V4 from the ECG from Fig. 1 showing the presence of an R-to-S interval of 160 ms, argument in favor of ventricular tachycardia

The diagnosis is therefore ventricular tachycardia. Its origin is at the level of the left ventricle (RBBB morphology), anterior wall (positive QRS complexes in leads II, III, and aVF), and at the level of the lateral wall (negative QRS complex in leads I and aVL).

The patient underwent an electrophysiological study which confirmed the ventricular nature of the tachycardia, with a subsequent catheter ablation procedure (epicardial and endocardial approaches).

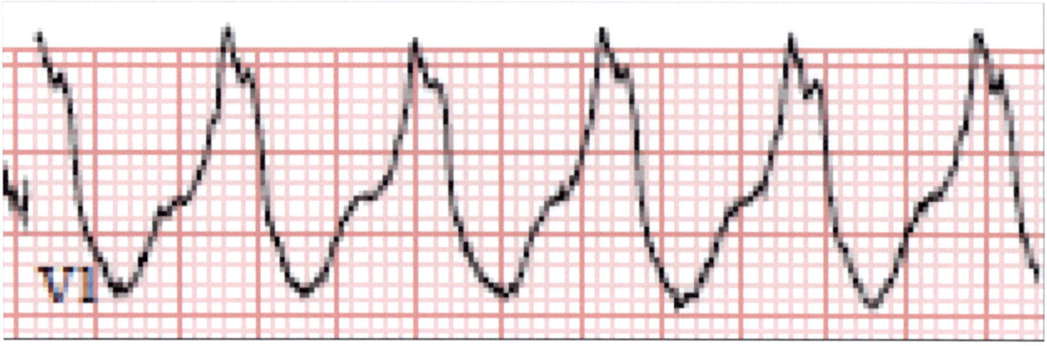

Fig. 4 Lead V1 from the ECG from Fig. 1 showing the "rabbit ear" sign, argument in favor of ventricular tachycardia

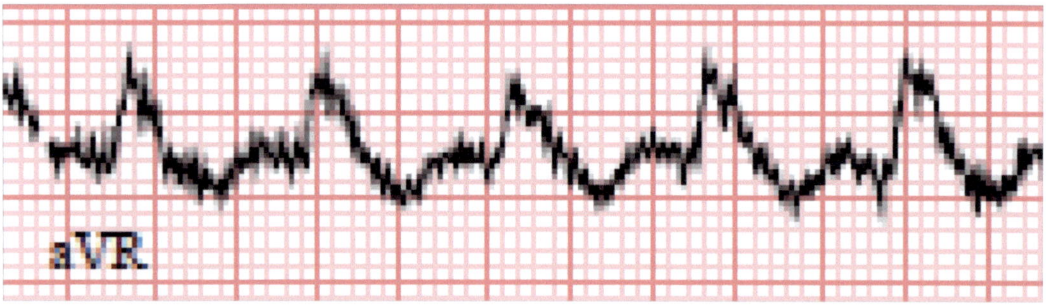

Fig. 5 Lead aVR from the ECG from Fig. 1 showing the presence of a "qR" morphology, argument not in favor of ventricular tachycardia (but not excluding it either)

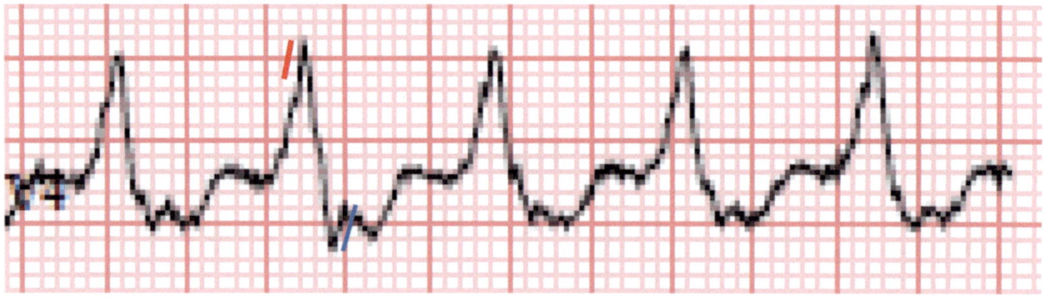

Fig. 6 The vi/vt index from the Vereckei algorithm in lead V1. The ratio of the initial 40 ms and the last 40 ms of the QRS complex is 3 mV vs 3.5 mV; therefore, 3/3.5 = 0.85, which is <1. This is in favor of ventricular tachycardia

References

1. Brugada P, Brugada J, Mont L, Smeets J, Andries EW. A new approach to the differential diagnosis of a regular tachycardia with a wide QRS complex. Circulation. 1991;83(5):1649–59.
2. Eckardt L, Breithardt G, Kirchhof P. Approach to wide complex tachycardias in patients without structural heart disease. Heart. 2006;92(5):704–11.
3. Vereckei A, Duray G, Szenasi G, Altemose GT, Miller JM. Application of a new algorithm in the differential diagnosis of wide QRS complex tachycardia. Eur Heart J. 2007;28(5):589–600.

ECG 48

Radu Rosu

1 Case Presentation

A 41-year-old female patient with no significant past medical history is admitted to the Cardiology Department for a first episode of palpitations accompanied by dyspnea, anxiety, and lightheadedness that had started 30 min prior to her presentation to the hospital. Her ECG recorded at the arrival to the Cardiology Department is presented in Fig. 1.

Question: What is the nature of the tachycardia presented in Fig. 1?

(a) AVNRT with left bundle branch block.
(b) ORT using a left-sided bypass tract and left bundle branch block.
(c) Ventricular tachycardia originating from the moderator band (right ventricle).
(d) Upper septal fascicular ventricular tachycardia (left ventricle).
(e) Left posterior fascicular ventricular tachycardia (left ventricle).

Hint: A second ECG recorded several minutes later is presented in Fig. 2.

R. Rosu (✉)
Rehabilitation Hospital, Department of Cardiology, Cluj-Napoca, Romania

Correct answer: c. Ventricular tachycardia originating from the moderator band (right ventricle).

Explanation: The ECG in Fig. 1 shows a regular wide QRS complex tachycardia with a heart rate of 165 bpm and LBBB morphology. The width of the QRS complex is 120 ms, as measured in lead V2. The QRS axis is at −60°. The differential diagnosis of this regular wide QRS complex tachycardia with LBBB morphology includes: ventricular tachycardia (myocardial-related VT and fascicular VT), supraventricular tachycardia (atrial flutter, atrial tachycardia, AVNRT, and AVRT) with functional or pre-existing bundle branch block, and antidromic tachycardia (in pre-excitation syndromes).

The morphology of the left bundle branch block of the QRS complex during tachycardia from Fig. 1 might be that of a typical one [1]: the QRS duration is of 120 ms; there is a monomorphic notched R wave in leads I and aVL; there is an "RSr'" aspect in lead V6; and there is ST segment and T wave modification opposite to the major deflection of the QRS complex: ST segment elevation with positive T waves in leads V1 to V4. So, at this point of the analysis, SVT with LBBB is a possible answer.

Applying the Brugada algorithm [2] to the tachycardia from Fig. 1, it can be seen that: 1.

L. Muresan (ed.), *ECG Interpretation of Wide QRS Complex Tachycardia*,
https://doi.org/10.1007/978-3-031-97030-6_49

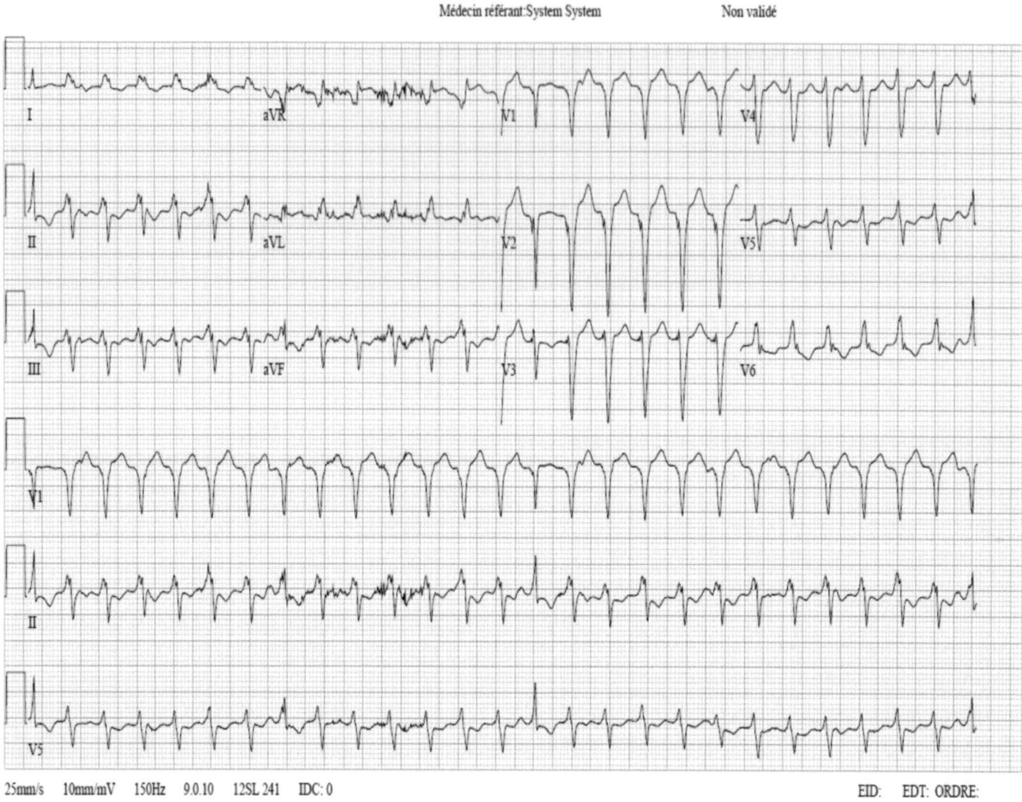

Fig. 1 Twelve-lead ECG recorded at admittance to the Cardiology Department

There is no absence of an RS complex in the precordial leads (otherwise said, there are RS complexes in leads V3 to V5); we therefore move to the second step of the algorithm: 2. This step analyzes the absence of an R-to-S interval > 100 ms in any precordial lead. This is not the case (Fig. 3).

Step 3 of the algorithm looks for A–V dissociation. This is not very obvious at a first glance; however, at a closer look, P waves can be identified, especially in lead V1, and A–V dissociation is present (Fig. 4).

So, according to the Brugada algorithm, the tachycardia from Fig. 1 is ventricular tachycardia.

The Vereckei algorithm [3] for the differential diagnosis of wide QRS complex tachycardias also suggests VT as the correct answer. The first step of the algorithm looks for A–V dissociation, which is seen on the present ECG (Fig. 4).

Based on these arguments, the diagnosis of ventricular tachycardia was retained.

Another argument in favor of ventricular tachycardia is the presence of fusion beats (starred QRS complexes in Fig. 5).

The origin of the tachycardia is close to the His–Purkinje system, explaining the relatively narrow duration of the QRS complex and its morphology, closely similar to a normal QRS, due to the septal origin of the tachycardia.

Re-entry in the posterior fascicle of the left bundle branch is one of the common etiologies of VT in patients with structurally normal hearts. However, the aspect on the 12-lead ECG is different than the VT from Fig. 1: the tachycardia has an RBBB morphology [4–8]. For the upper septal variant of fascicular VT, even though it has an LBBB morphology, the QRS complexes have a tall R wave in leads II, III, and aVF [9], which is not the case of this patient. The 12-lead morphol-

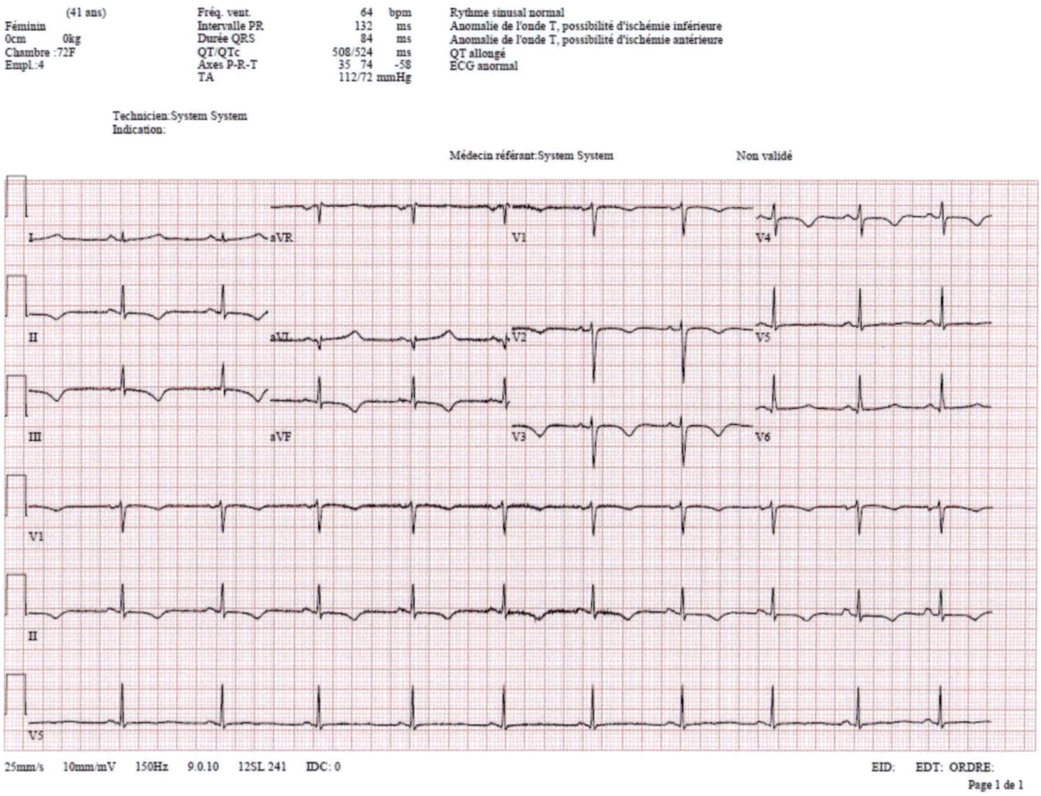

Fig. 2 Twelve-lead ECG recorded after the end of the episode of palpitations

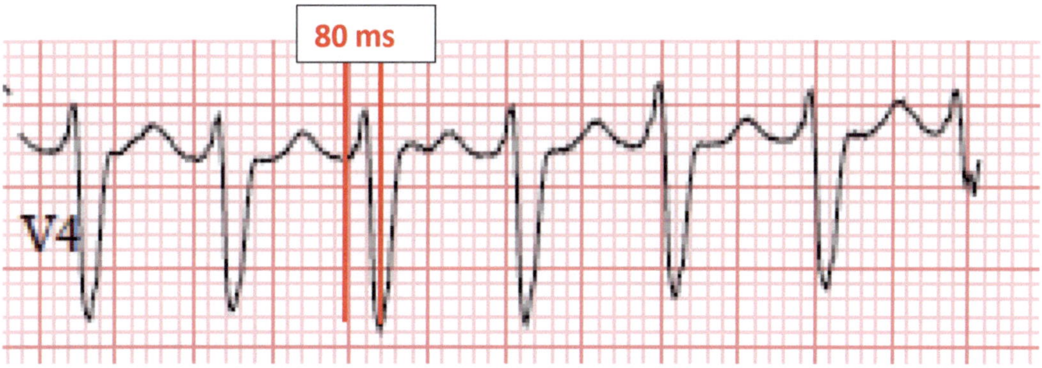

Fig. 3 Lead V4 from the ECG from Fig. 1, showing an R-to-S interval of 80 ms, criterion not in favor of ventricular tachycardia (but not excluding it either)

ogy is compatible with an origin in the right ventricle (LBBB morphology, with a late transition) at the level of the moderator band [10].

The patient underwent an electrophysiological study which confirmed the diagnosis and the origin of VT.

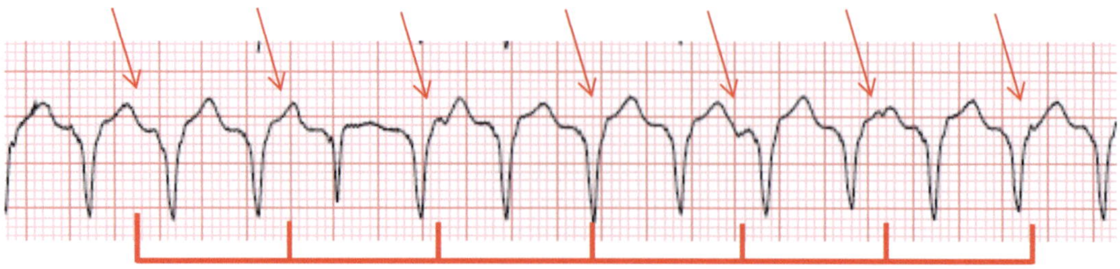

Fig. 4 Limb leads and leads V1 to V3 from the ECG from Fig. 1. Red arrows point to P waves, with A–V dissociation

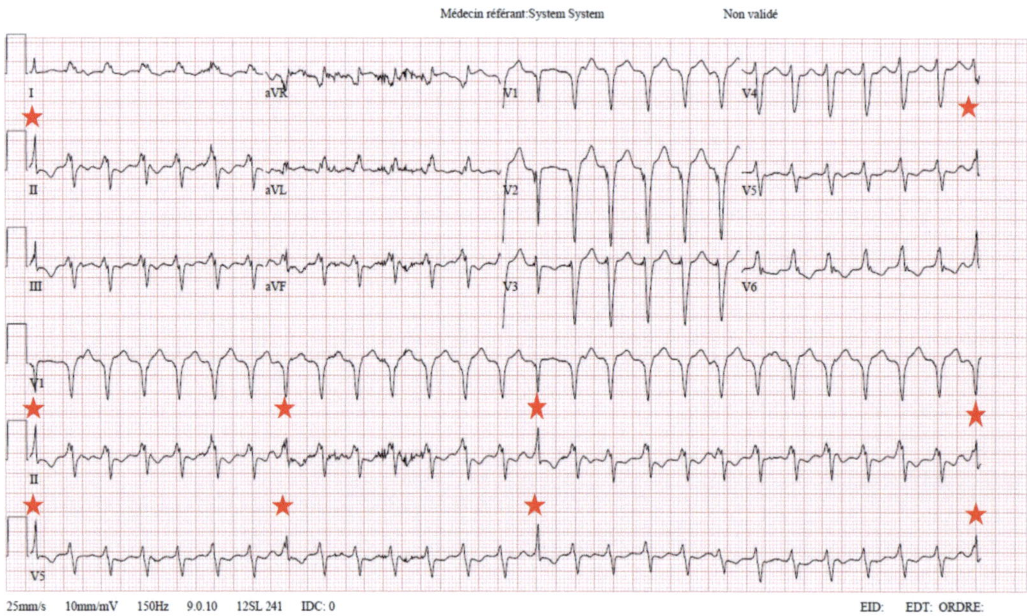

Fig. 5 ECG from Fig. 1 showing the wide QRS complex tachycardia. Red stars indicate beats with a fused morphology between the QRS complex during the wide QRS complex tachycardia and the QRS morphology during sinus rhythm, which can be seen in the ECG from Fig. 2. These are fusion beats, a strong argument in favor of ventricular tachycardia

References

1. Surawicz B, Childers R, Deal BJ, Gettes LS, Bailey JJ, Gorgels A, et al. AHA/ACCF/HRS recommendations for the standardization and interpretation of the electrocardiogram: part III: intraventricular conduction disturbances: a scientific statement from the American Heart Association Electrocardiography and Arrhythmias Committee, Council on Clinical Cardiology; the American College of Cardiology Foundation; and the Heart Rhythm Society. Endorsed by the International Society for Computerized Electrocardiology. J Am Coll Cardiol. 2009;53(11):976–81.
2. Brugada P, Brugada J, Mont L, Smeets J, Andries EW. A new approach to the differential diagnosis of a regular tachycardia with a wide QRS complex. Circulation. 1991;83(5):1649–59.
3. Vereckei A, Duray G, Szenasi G, Altemose GT, Miller JM. Application of a new algorithm in the differential diagnosis of wide QRS complex tachycardia. Eur Heart J. 2007;28(5):589–600.
4. Alahmad Y, Asaad NA, Arafa SO, Ahmad Khan SH, Mahmoud A. Idiopathic fascicular left ventricular tachycardia. Heart Views. 2017;18(3):83–7.
5. Andrade FR, Eslami M, Elias J, Kinoshita O, Nakazato Y, Marcus FI, et al. Diagnostic clues from the surface ECG to identify idiopathic (fascicular) ventricular tachycardia: correlation with electrophysiologic findings. J Cardiovasc Electrophysiol. 1996;7(1):2–8.

6. Magalhaes S, Goncalves H, Primo J, Sa AP, Silva P, Rosas R, et al. Fascicular ventricular tachycardia: experience with radiofrequency ablation. Rev Port Cardiol. 2006;25(5):485–97.
7. Creta A, Chow AW, Sporton S, Finlay M, Papageorgiou N, Honarbakhsh S, et al. Catheter ablation for fascicular ventricular tachycardia: a systematic review. Int J Cardiol. 2019;276:136–48.
8. Geller L, Szilagyi S, Solymossy K, Srej M, Zima E, Tahin T, et al. Ablation of idiopathic fascicular ventricular tachycardia. Orv Hetil. 2009;150(31):1463–9.
9. Nair GM, Thomas V, Stoyanov N, Nery PB, Sadek MM, Green MS. Upper septal transformation of verapamil-sensitive idiopathic left ventricular tachycardia during catheter ablation: wolf in sheep's clothing? HeartRhythm Case Rep. 2016;2(1):101–6.
10. Jiang D, Lv J, Han B, Yang X, Zhao L, Yi Y, et al. Electrocardiographic characteristics and catheter ablation of ventricular arrhythmias originating from the moderator band in children. Front Pediatr. 2022;10:740230.

ECG 49

Mihai Puiu

1 Case Presentation

A 54-year-old male patient with a history of arterial hypertension, ischemic cardiomyopathy (chronic total occlusion of the middle segment of the LAD, CX, and RCA) treated with a CABG procedure (left internal mammary artery – LAD), and with moderate systolic dysfunction (LVEF of 42%) is admitted to the Cardiology Department for an episode of palpitations accompanied by dyspnea, anxiety, and lightheadedness that had started 30 min prior to his presentation to the hospital. His ECG recorded at admittance to the Cardiology Department is shown in Fig. 1.

Question: What is the nature of the tachycardia presented in Fig. 1?

(a) AVNRT with right bundle branch block.
(b) Typical atrial flutter with right bundle branch block.
(c) Antidromic tachycardia using a left-sided bypass tract.
(d) Ventricular tachycardia originating from the inferior LV wall.
(e) Ventricular tachycardia originating from the inferior RV wall.

M. Puiu (✉)
Department of Cardiology, Rehabilitation Hospital, Cluj-Napoca, Romania

Hint: A second ECG recorded several minutes later is presented in Fig. 2.

Correct answer: d. Ventricular tachycardia originating from the inferior wall of the LV.

Explanation: The ECG in Fig. 1 shows a regular wide QRS complex tachycardia with a heart rate of 186 bpm and RBBB morphology. The width of the QRS complex is 144 ms. The QRS axis is at −120° (extreme or "north-west" axis deviation). The differential diagnosis of this regular wide QRS complex tachycardia with RBBB morphology includes: ventricular tachycardia (myocardial-related VT, bundle branch re-entry VT, and fascicular VT), supraventricular tachycardia (atrial flutter, atrial tachycardia, AVNRT, and AVRT) with functional or pre-existing right bundle branch block, and antidromic tachycardia (in pre-excitation syndromes).

The morphology of the left bundle branch block of the QRS complex during tachycardia from Fig. 1 suggests that it might be a typical one: the QRS duration is of >120 ms; the QRS complex has a "RSR'" morphology in lead V1, an "Rs" pattern in leads I and aVL; and there is ST segment and T wave modification opposite to the major deflection of the QRS complex: ST segment elevation with negative T waves in leads

L. Muresan (ed.), *ECG Interpretation of Wide QRS Complex Tachycardia*,
https://doi.org/10.1007/978-3-031-97030-6_50

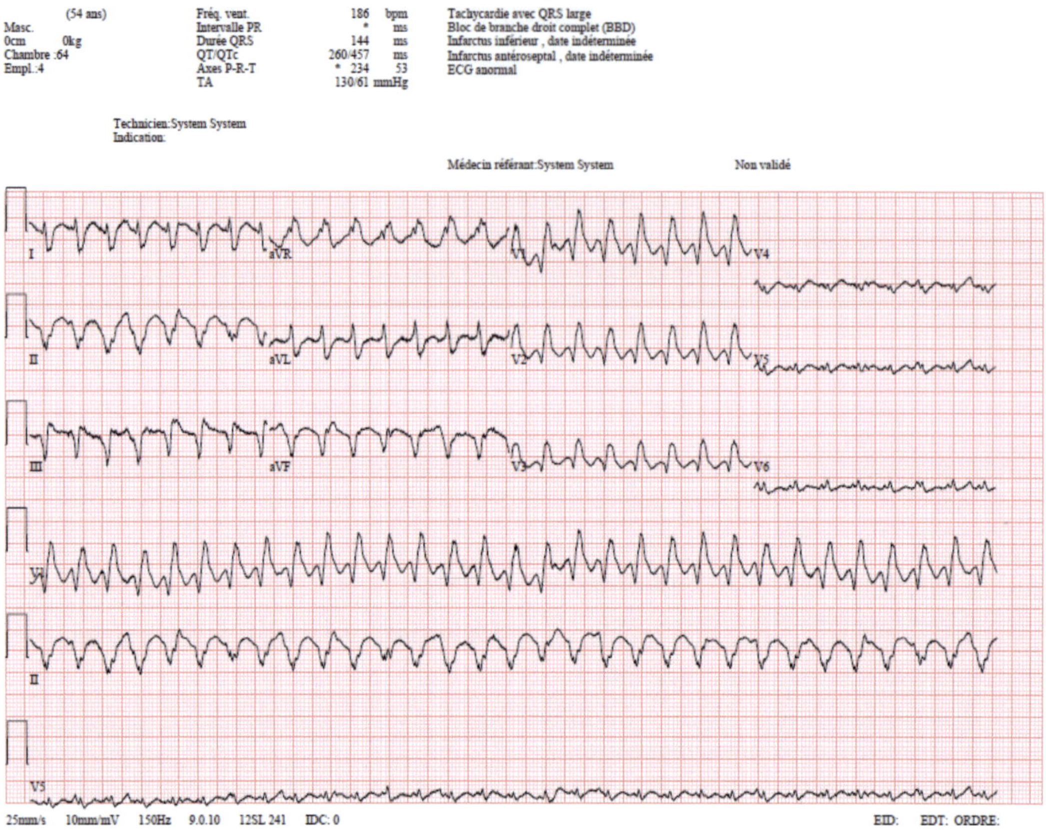

Fig. 1 Twelve-lead ECG recorded at admittance to the Cardiology Department

V1 to V3. However, what is peculiar is that the QRS complex has an RSR'S′ aspect in lead V6, which is not characteristic of a typical RBBB, which should have an "RS" aspect. This makes SVT with RBBB less likely.

The ECG from Fig. 2 shows sinus rhythm with a heart rate of 57 bpm, with a QRS axis at −10°, absence of LVH, necrosis at the level of the inferior LV wall, and no signs of ventricular preexcitation (no short PR interval and no delta waves). This makes answer c—"Antidromic tachycardia using a left-sided bypass tract"—less likely.

Applying the Brugada algorithm (1) to the tachycardia from Fig. 2, it can be seen that: 1. There is an absence of an RS complex in the precordial leads. The QRS complex has an RSR' morphology from V1 to V3 and an RSR'S′ morphology from V4 to V6 (Fig. 3). So, according to the Brugada algorithm, the tachycardia from Fig. 1 is ventricular in origin.

The Vereckei algorithm (2) for the differential diagnosis of wide QRS complex tachycardias also suggests VT as the correct answer. The first step of the algorithm looks for A–V dissociation, which is not seen on the present ECG. The second step of the algorithm looks for an initial predominant R wave in lead aVR, which is actually the case (Fig. 4).

Another argument in favor of VT is the extreme or "north-west" axis deviation, which is not a common finding for SVT with BBB (3).

The origin of the ventricular tachycardia is in the left ventricle (RBBB aspect), at the level of the inferior wall ("QS" morphology in leads II, III, and aVF).

The patient underwent an ICD implantation and a catheter ablation procedure of the ventricualr tachycardia.

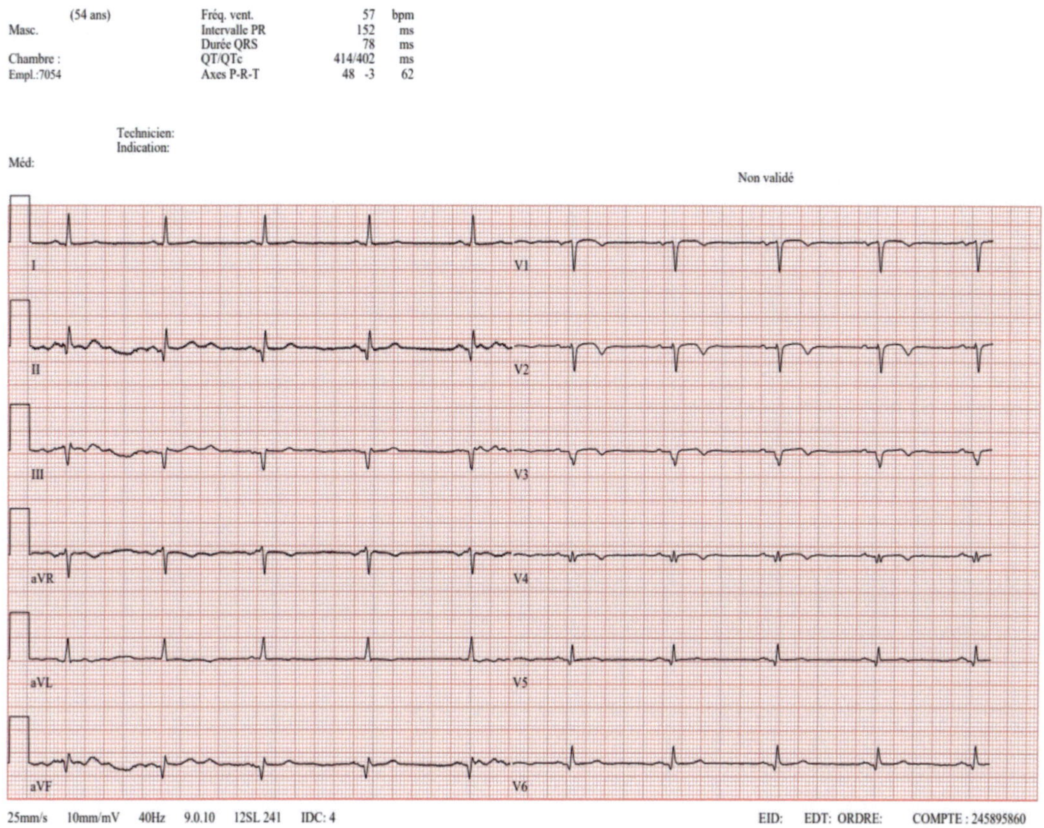

Fig. 2 Twelve-lead ECG recorded after the end of the episode of palpitations

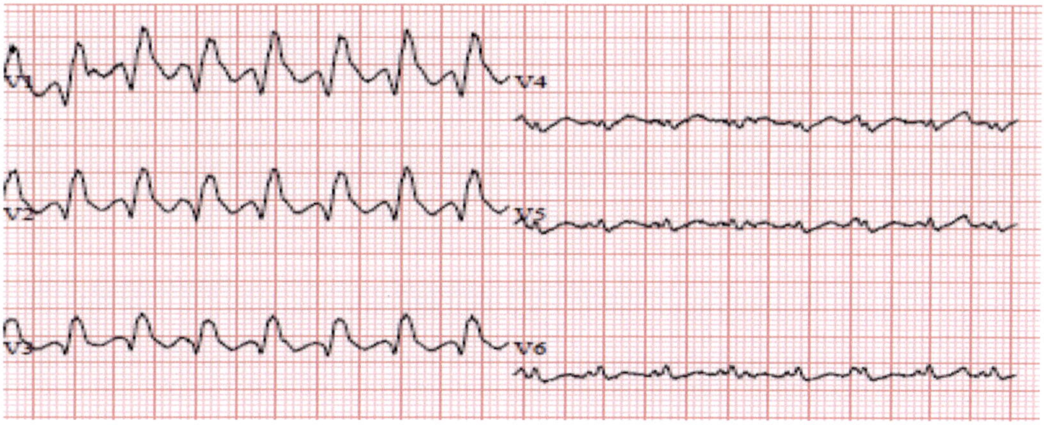

Fig. 3 Precordial leads from the ECG from Fig. 1 recorded during the wide QRS complex tachycardia showing the absence of an "RS complex", argument in favor of ventricular tachycardia

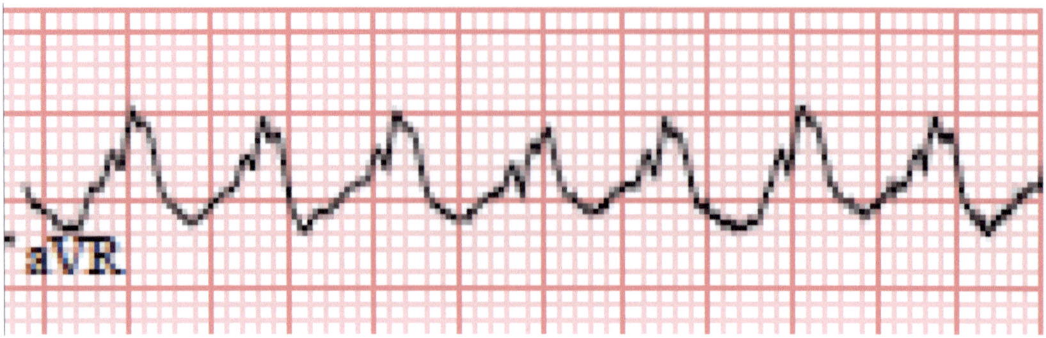

Fig. 4 Lead aVR from the ECG from Fig. 1 recorded during the wide QRS complex tachycardia showing the presence of an initial tall R wave in lead aVR, argument in favor of ventricular tachycardia

References

1. Brugada P, Brugada J, Mont L, Smeets J, Andries EW. A new approach to the differential diagnosis of a regular tachycardia with a wide QRS complex. Circulation. 1991;83(5):1649–59.
2. Vereckei A, Duray G, Szenasi G, Altemose GT, Miller JM. Application of a new algorithm in the differential diagnosis of wide QRS complex tachycardia. Eur Heart J. 2007;28(5):589–600.
3. Wellens HJ, Bar FW, Lie KI. The value of the electrocardiogram in the differential diagnosis of a tachycardia with a widened QRS complex. Am J Med. 1978;64(1):27–33.

ECG 50

Stefan-Lucian Popa

1 Case Presentation

A 41-year-old male patient with no significant past medical history presents to the Emergency Department for repeated episodes of palpitations accompanied by anxiety that had started the same morning of his presentation to the hospital. His ECG recorded during one such episode in the Cardiology Department after transfer from the Emergency Department is presented in Fig. 1.

Question: What is the nature of the tachycardia presented in Fig. 1?

(a) Ventricular tachycardia originating from the anterior septal LV wall.
(b) Ventricular tachycardia originating from the anterior septal RV wall.
(c) Lest posterior fascicular ventricular tachycardia.
(d) Antidromic tachycardia using a left-sided bypass tract.
(e) Atrial tachycardia with right bundle branch block.

Hint: A second ECG recorded several minutes later is presented in Fig. 2.

S.-L. Popa (✉)
Department of Internal Medicine, Second Medical Clinic, Cluj-Napoca, Romania
e-mail: popa.stefan@umfcluj.ro

Correct answer: e. Atrial tachycardia with right bundle branch block

Explanation: The ECG in Fig. 1 shows a regular wide QRS complex tachycardia with a heart rate of 195 bpm and RBBB morphology. The width of the QRS complex is 135 ms (despite the erroneous automatic interpretation of 96 ms). The QRS axis is at +100°. The differential diagnosis of this regular wide QRS complex tachycardia with RBBB morphology includes: ventricular tachycardia (myocardial-related VT and fascicular VT), supraventricular tachycardia (atrial flutter, atrial tachycardia, AVNRT, and AVRT) with functional or pre-existing right bundle branch block, and antidromic tachycardia (in pre-excitation syndromes).

The morphology of the right bundle branch block of the QRS complex during tachycardia from Fig. 1 is that of a typical one: the QRS duration is >120 ms; the QRS complex has an "RSR" pattern in lead V1; there is an "RS" pattern in leads I, aVL, V5, and V6; and there is ST segment and T wave modification opposite to the major deflection of the QRS complex: ST segment depression with negative T waves in leads V1 to V3. So, at this point of the analysis, we cannot say whether this is VT or SVT with RBBB.

L. Muresan (ed.), *ECG Interpretation of Wide QRS Complex Tachycardia*,
https://doi.org/10.1007/978-3-031-97030-6_51

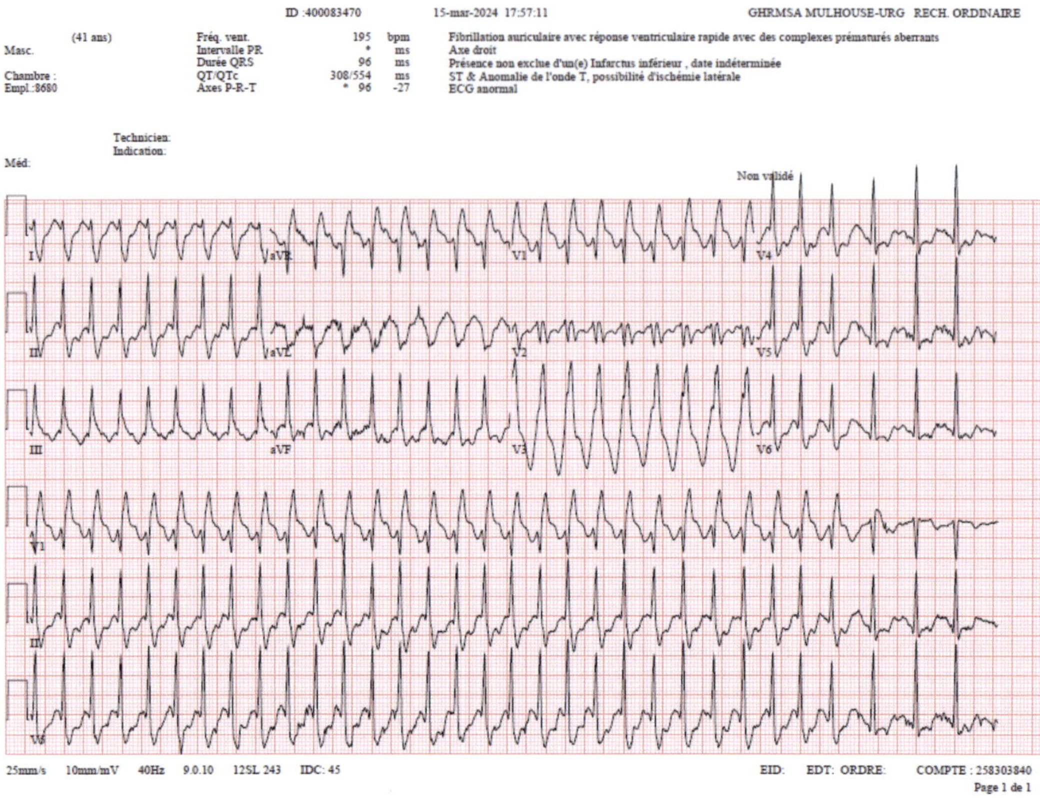

Fig. 1 Twelve-lead ECG recorded at admittance to the Cardiology Department

At a first glance, the ECG from Fig. 2 shows sinus rhythm with a heart rate of 114 bpm, QRS axis at +80°, absence of LVH, and absence of ischemia. Importantly, there are no signs of ventricular pre-excitation (no short PR interval and no delta waves), which makes the diagnosis of antidromic tachycardia for the wide QRS complex tachycardia from Fig. 1 unlikely.

Applying the Brugada algorithm [1] to the tachycardia from Fig. 2, it can be seen that there is no absence of an RS complex in the precordial leads (otherwise said, there are rS complexes in leads V4 to V6) (Fig. 3); we therefore move to the second step of the algorithm.

This step analyzes the absence of an R-to-S interval >100 ms in any precordial lead. This is not the case (Fig. 4).

Step 3 of the algorithm looks for A–V dissociation. P waves are visible on the ECG during tachycardia, best seen in lead aVF, but there seem to be 1:1 atrioventricular (or perhaps ventriculo-atrial) conduction (Fig. 5). So, there probably is no A–V dissociation. We therefore need to move to step 4 of the algorithm.

For an RBBB morphology wide QRS complex tachycardia, an argument in favor of VT would be the presence of a taller left peak of the QRS complex in lead V1 (the rabbit ear sign) or for biphasic RS or QR complexes, which is not the case. Next, in lead V6, an argument in favor of VT would be the presence of an "rS" complex, which is also not the case. This can also be expressed as a ratio of R/S < 1 in lead V6 (Fig. 6). Therefore, according to the Brugada algorithm, there are no arguments in favor of ventricular tachycardia, and therefore, this is probably SVT with RBBB.

The Vereckei algorithm [2] for the differential diagnosis of wide QRS complex tachycardias also suggests SVT as the correct answer. The first step of the algorithm looks for A–V dissociation, which is not seen on the present ECG. The second

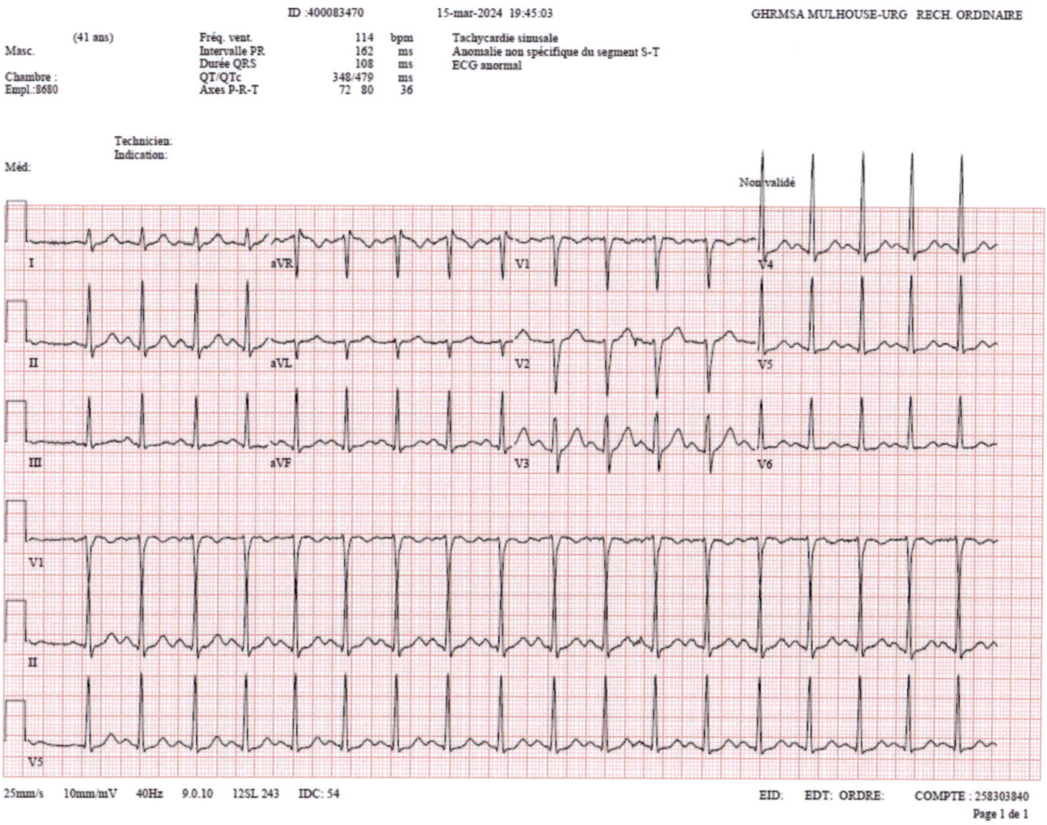

Fig. 2 Twelve-lead ECG recorded after the end of the episode of palpitations

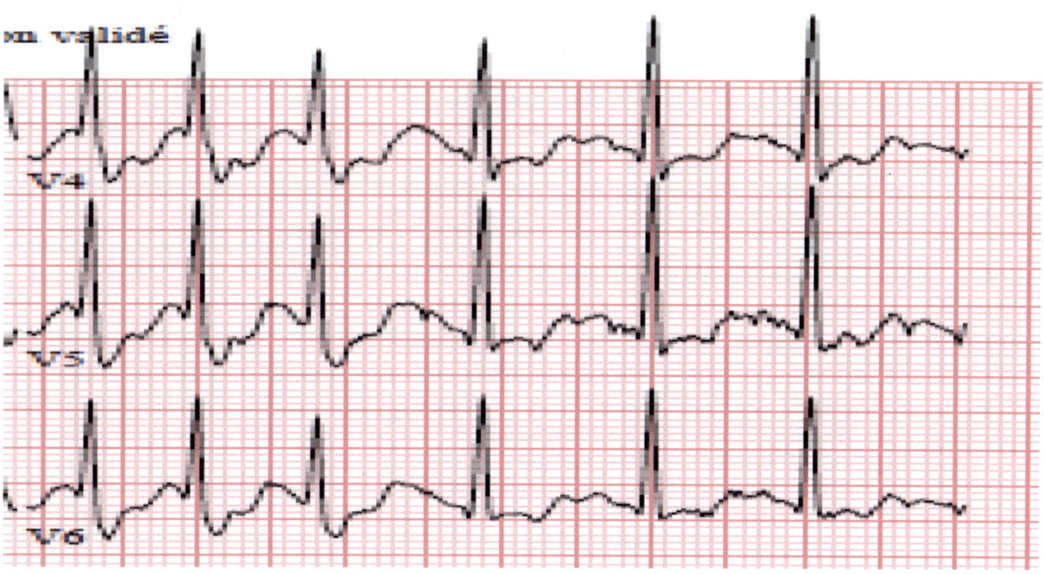

Fig. 3 Leads V4 to V6 from the ECG from Fig. 1 showing the presence of RS complexes, argument not in favor of ventricular tachycardia (but not excluding it either)

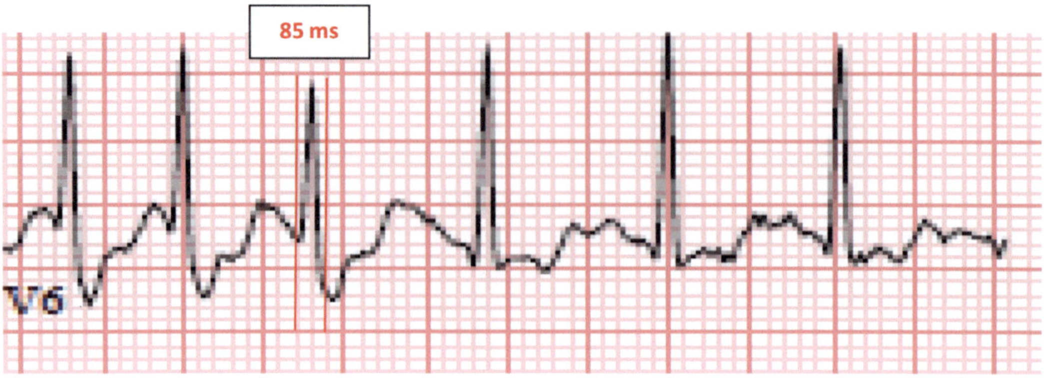

Fig. 4 Lead V4 from the ECG from Fig. 1 showing the presence of an R-to-S interval of 85 ms, argument not in favor of ventricular tachycardia (but not excluding it either)

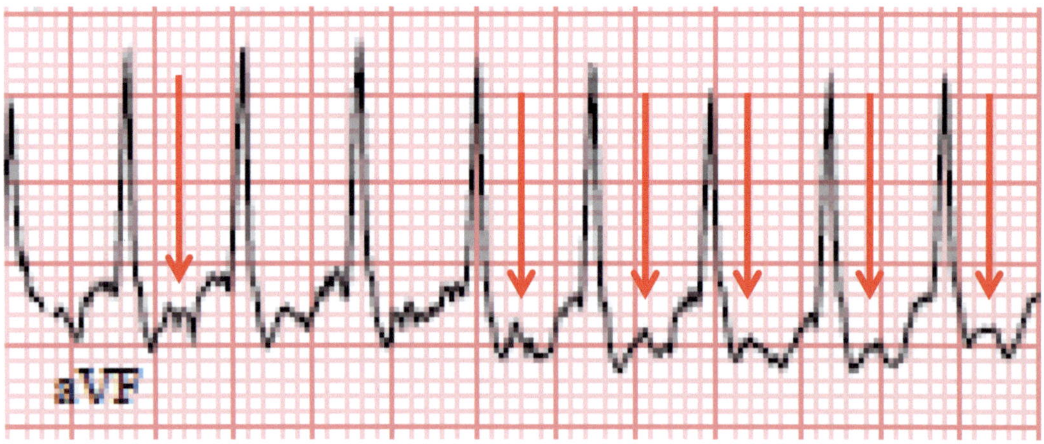

Fig. 5 Lead aVF demonstrating the presence of P waves, with a 1:1 atrioventricular (or ventriculo-atrial) conduction. There is no A–V dissociation

step of the algorithm looks for an initial predominant R wave in lead aVR, which, again, is not the case (Fig. 7).

The third step "QRS morphology unlike BBB or fascicular block" suggests SVT with RBBB, based on the arguments explained above.

Concerning the nature of the SVT, a closer re-examination of the ECG from Fig. 2 identifies two different morphologies of the P wave: the first P wave recorded in leads I, II, III, V1, and V5 is different from the other P waves that follow it. It is positive but more flattened in leads II, III, and V5 compared to the rest of the P waves (Fig. 8). We do not see the previous QRS complex, but the RR interval containing this P wave is clearly longer than the next ones. Otherwise said, the heart rate accelerates following the first P wave of the second morphology. This is actually compatible with the first P wave being sinus in origin and the second P wave corresponding to an atrial tachycardia focus.

This hypothesis was confirmed by an electrophysiological study. The patient underwent catheter ablation of an automatic focus situated in the right atrial appendage.

The wide QRS complex tachycardia is therefore an automatic atrial tachycardia with functional right bundle branch block.

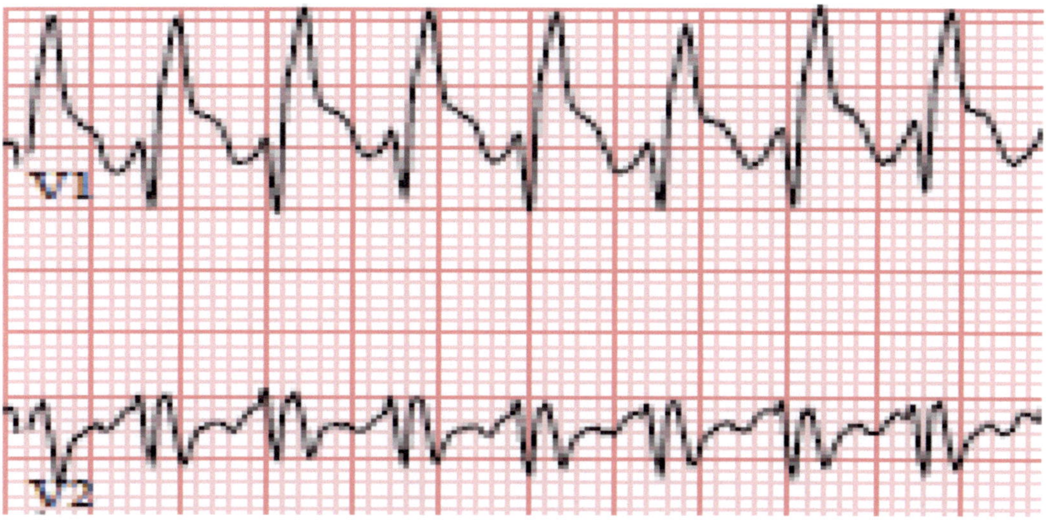

Fig. 6 Leads V4 to V6 from the ECG from Fig. 1 showing the presence of RS complexes, argument not in favor of ventricular tachycardia (but not excluding it either)

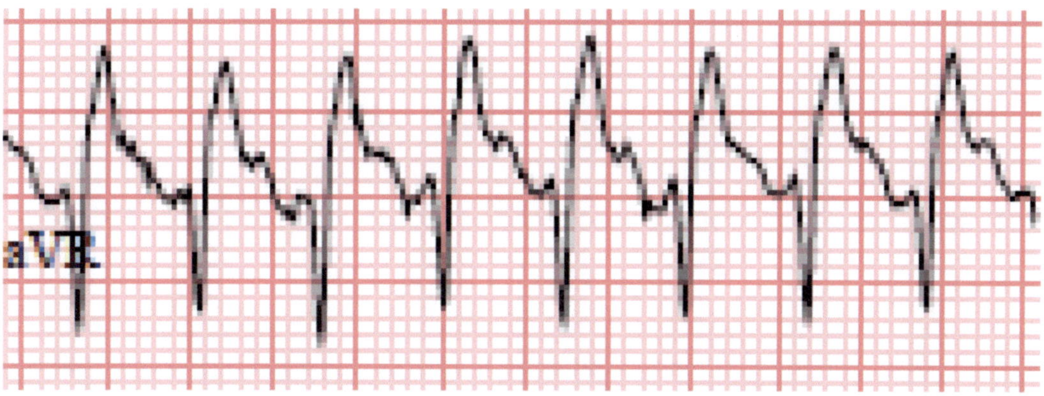

Fig. 7 Lead aVR from the ECG from Fig. 1 showing the absence of a tall initial R wave, argument not in favor of ventricular tachycardia (but not excluding it either)

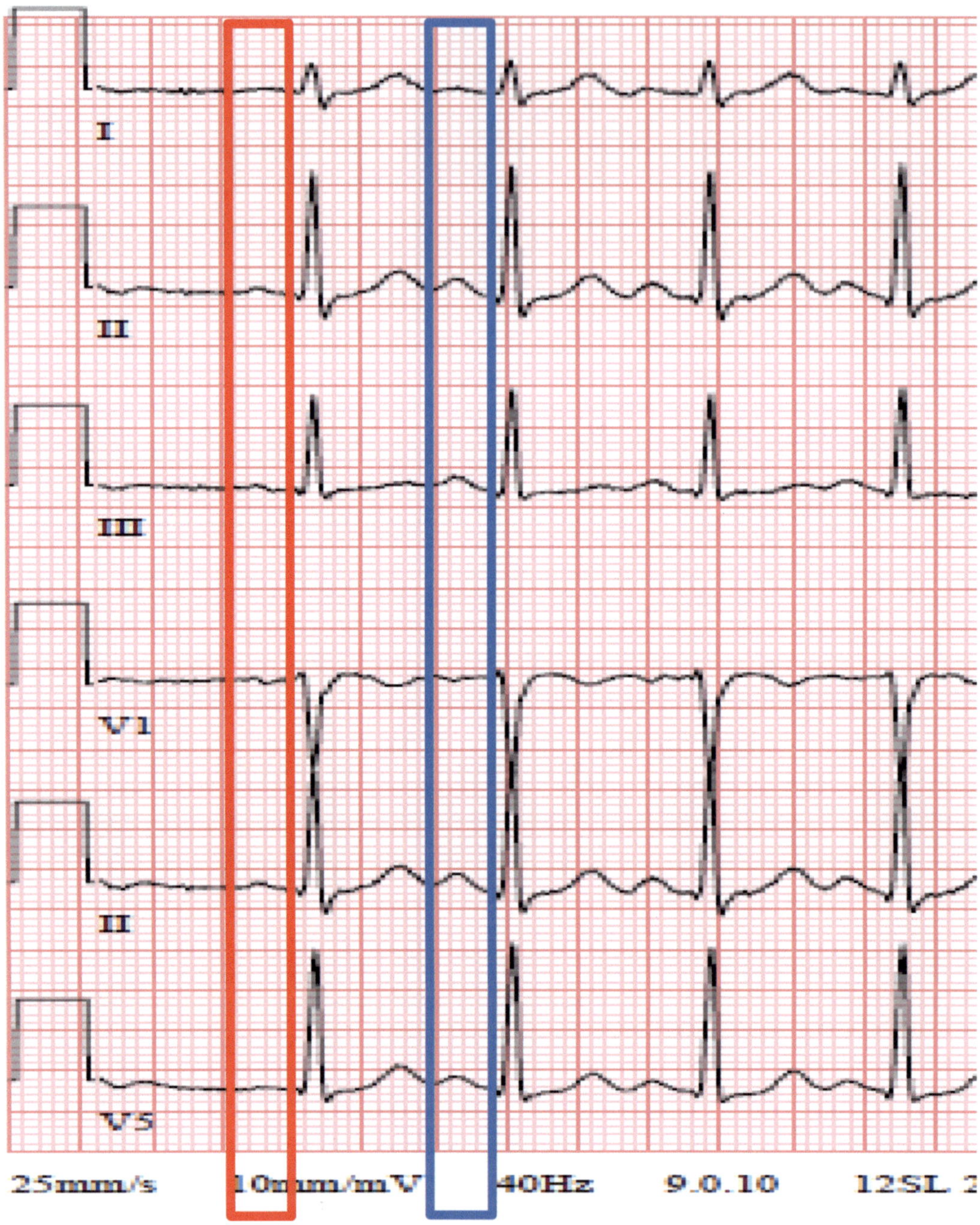

Fig. 8 Leads I, II, III, V1, II, and V5 from the ECG from Fig. 2 showing two different morphologies of the P wave: the first (red rectangle) corresponds to the sinus P wave, and the second (blue rectangle) corresponds to the atrial tachycardia focus (see text for further explanation)

References

1. Brugada P, Brugada J, Mont L, Smeets J, Andries EW. A new approach to the differential diagnosis of a regular tachycardia with a wide QRS complex. Circulation. 1991;83(5):1649–59.
2. Vereckei A, Duray G, Szenasi G, Altemose GT, Miller JM. Application of a new algorithm in the differential diagnosis of wide QRS complex tachycardia. Eur Heart J. 2007;28(5):589–600.

MIX
Papier aus verantwortungsvollen Quellen
Paper from responsible sources
FSC® C105338

If you have any concerns about our products,
you can contact us on
ProductSafety@springernature.com

In case Publisher is established outside the EU,
the EU authorized representative is:
Springer Nature Customer Service Center GmbH
Europaplatz 3, 69115 Heidelberg, Germany

Printed by Libri Plureos GmbH
in Hamburg, Germany